CONTENTS

LIST OF CONTRIBUTORS

R Tubiana   Institut de la Main, Centre Orthopédique Jouvenet, 6 square Jouvenet, Paris 75116, France

J-M Thomine   Clinique Chirurgicale Orthopédique et Traumatologique, Hôpital Charles Nicolle, Rouen Cedex 76031, France

E J Mackin   The Hand Rehabilitation Foundation, 834 Chestnut Street, G1114, Philadelphia, PA 19107, USA

F Brunelli   Institut de la Main, Centre Orthopédique Jouvenet, 6 square Jouvenet, Paris 75116, France

J P Melki   Clinique Bizet, 23 rue Georges Bizet, Paris 75016, France

Ph Saffar   Centre Chirurgical de la Main, 5 rue du Dôme, Paris 75116, France

P Seror   146 Avenue Ledru-Rollin, Paris 75011, France

FOREWORD

One would call Raoul Tubiana the grand old man of world hand surgery were it not for the fact that in spirit and appearance he looks a young man. There is no doubt, however, that he is one of the outstanding world leaders in the field of hand surgery. He has pioneered so many different surgical procedures, has written and edited outstanding and authoritative texts on all aspects of hand surgery, and has created a world-famous institute for hand surgery in the heart of Paris. His affection and dedication to his trainees is legendary, and as important is his nurturing, stimulation and encouragement of hand therapists.

Those of us who have dedicated our lives to rehabilitation of the upper limb owe him a great debt for his example and his encouragement. Successful surgery of the hand depends vitally on a correct diagnosis and an assessment of the functional capacity of the hand and to what use the patient wishes to put it when the surgeon has done his best. It is therefore essential that the budding hand surgeon have a detailed knowledge of anatomy and physiology, both structural and functional. There are few more complicated areas than the hand, and it is a tribute to the brilliance of this text that these most complex areas are beautifully and simply described and illustrated. Indeed, the line drawings are a work of art in themselves. One would mention, among many, the transverse metacarpal tunnel, the transverse fascia and the pulley system of the fingers, the intrinsic musculature, the ligamentous system of the wrist, the anatomy of the triangular fibrocartilage and the spiral organization of the phalanges and joints. These drawings will not only elucidate some of the complexities of hand anatomy but will also reveal aspects of function that have been mysterious and unknown heretofore or not widely recognized.

Throughout the text, clinical conditions illustrate the lessons that anatomy has to teach us. This is particularly true in the case of pathology of Dupuytren's contracture, rheumatoid arthritis, and claw hand and ulnar palsy. It is thrilling to see Fibonacci's series applied to finger movements. The reader throughout will be enchanted by references to art and culture. Raoul Tubiana is in the great tradition of the natural philosophers; for so designated were the scientists of old who explored nature, revealing its mysteries with love and fascination and transmitting them down the generations. Throughout this text Tubiana speculates and thinks with an original mind about the function of the various parts of the hand. The fact that Tubiana applies his critical

v

faculties to the assessment of other writers' work makes this much more than a text of anatomy and examination; it embraces the whole field of previous and contemporary workers so that one has the feeling of a great family of surgeons and anatomists exploring the mysteries and delights of the hand.

In the section on clinical examination the reader will find description of all the tests for different deformities and disorders. One was particularly impressed by the assessment of the tests for carpal instability, and for tendon function, and the various methods for the management of swan neck, mallet finger and the boutonnière finger which can cause such confusion to the tyro. There is an illuminating chapter on imaging techniques which contributes so much to better understanding of wrist pathology in particular. The value of this text is greatly enhanced by the collaboration of an orthopaedic specialist, Professor Thomine, and of the world-famous hand therapist Evelyn Mackin. As the author comments in his Preface, this is far more than a new edition of the original 1984 text; it totally supersedes the earlier work, pioneering and brilliant as that was. There will be other editions to come, for this is a constantly developing area. New discoveries will be made in the field of functional anatomy and in the understanding of the pathophysiology of many clinical hand problems. There will be advances particularly in sensory assessment and sensory rehabilitation as we begin, with the help of the anatomist and the physiologist, to understand more the complexities of peripheral and central neural encoding, and one will see more retraining procedures developed. It is difficult to see how this book can have a rival; impossible to imagine it being exceeded in its comprehensiveness, the beauty of its illustration and the love and dedication of the writing that has gone into it.

C B Wynn Parry

PREFACE

This book is much more than a new edition of *Examination of the Hand and Upper Limb* (WB Saunders, 1984). Anatomy is a cornerstone of examination of the hand and wrist, and therefore an important section of this book is devoted to anatomy – not the static anatomy found in most text books, but functional and surgical anatomy, providing the information needed by surgeons, microsurgeons, physiotherapists, neurologists, in fact anyone with an interest in the normal anatomy and physiology and the pathology of the hand and wrist. The section on clinical examination has been divided into examination of the teguments, skeleton and musculotendinous apparatus. Clinical examination must be augmented by imaging, which has progressed rapidly, and this is discussed in the third section of the book. Electrodiagnosis and the other modalities are described in this edition. Examination of the peripheral nerve function has been described for the whole upper limb as innervation of the hand cannot be dissociated from the rest of the limb. It comprises assessment of motor function and evaluation of sensation and of the clinical features of nerve paralysis.

I wish to thank the authors who have participated in this work, and my friends Adalbert Kapandji and William Littler for their clear and attractive drawings, and also Léon Dorn, whose beautiful work has illustrated my books for more than 20 years. This book contains some text and illustrations taken from the five volumes of *The Hand* published by WB Saunders and Masson.

R Tubiana

ACKNOWLEDGEMENTS

Figure 1.40 appears by courtesy of Professor F Bonnel, Laboratoire d'Anatomie, Montpellier; Figure 3.47 by courtesy of Dr O Judet and Professor L Lacombe, Hôpital A Paré, Paris; Figure 4.24a,b by courtesy of Dr L Mannerfelt.

The following are reproduced with the kind permission of the publishers:

Brand PW, Beach RB, Thomsen DE (1981) Relative tension and potential excursion of muscles in the forearm and hand, *J Hand Surg*, **6**:201–9 (Figures 1.47–50);

Hakstian RW, Tubiana R (1967) Ulnar deviation of the fingers, *J Bone Joint Surg*, **49A**:299 (Figure 1.78);

Kapandji Al (1963) *Physiologie articulaire*, volume 1 (Librarie Maloine: Paris) (Figure 1.10b).

Lundborg G, Myrhage R, Rydevik B (1977) The vascularization of human flexor tendons within the digital synovial region – structural and functional aspects, *J Hand Surg*, **11A**:692–6 (Figure 1.88c);

Ochiai N et al (1979) Vascular anatomy of flexor tendons, *J Hand Surg*, **2**: 417 (Figure 1.88a);

Penfield WG, Rasmussen T (1950) *The Cerebral Cortex of Man* (Macmillan: New York) (Figure 1.181);

Tubiana R, ed (1981) *The Hand*, volume 1 (WB Saunders: Philadelphia): from the chapter by Aubriot (Figure 2.33); Backhouse (Figure 3.30); de la Caffinière (Figure 2.36); Fahrer (Figures 1.137 and 1.138); Kapandji (Figures 1.124 and 2.19); Pallardy et al (Figures 3.8, 3.18a and 3.45a); Pieron (Figure 1.125); Rabischong (Figure 1.152); Thomine (Figures 1.151 and 2.29); Tubiana (Figures 1.37b, 1.69, 1.112, 1.116, 1.119, 1.173); Valentin (Figures 1.103, 1.104, 1.106 and 1.114);

Tubiana R, ed (1985) *The Hand*, volume 2 (WB Saunders: Philadelphia): from the chapter by Curtis (Figure 2.39); Gilbert (Figure 1.29); Kuhlmann et al (Figures 1.34, 1.38b, 1.53, 1.56, 1.58); Tubiana (Figures 1.36b, 1.41a, 1.144, 1.146, 1.167, 2.30);

Tubiana R, ed (1988) *The Hand*, volume 3 (WB Saunders: Philadelphia) from the chapter by Albertoni (Figure 2.51); Jupiter and Kleinert (Figure 2.9b); Melki (Figure

3.36); Tubiana (Figures 1.85, 1.86, 1.115, 1.164, 2.37, 2.40, 2.42, 2.43a, 2.44a, 2.45b and 2.46–49);

Tubiana R, ed (1993) *The Hand*, volume 4 (WB Saunders: Philadelphia): from the chapters by Tubiana (Figures 1.60, 1.62, 1.109, 1.110, 1.121b, 1.131–135, 2.27, 2.28 and 4.20–4.22);

Tubiana R, Malek R (1968) Paralysis of the intrinsic muscles of the fingers, *Surg Clin North Am*, **48**:1140 (Figure 1.111);

Tubiana R, McCullough CJ, Masquelet AC (1990) *An Atlas of Surgical Exposures of the Upper Extremity* (Martin Dunitz and JB Lippincott: London and Philadelphia) (Figures 1.12b, 1.13c, 1.20, 1.21, 1.42b, 1.43, 1.92, 1.159–162, 1.166, 2.7, 2.8, 2.35, 2.38, 3.31–35, 3.45, 3.46, 4.2, 4.15).

Tables 1.2 and 1.3 originally appeared in Brand PW, Beach RB, Thomsen DE (1981) Relative tension and potential excursion of muscles in the forearm and hand, *J Hand Surg*, **6**:201–9.

Table 1.6 originally appeared in Kelleher JC, Robinson JH, Yanik MA (1985) The pattern abdominal pedicle flap. In: Tubiana R, ed, *The Hand*, volume 2 (WB Saunders: Philadelphia).

Portions of Section 4.4 have appeared in Tubiana R, Nerve regeneration and prognosis following peripheral nerve injury. In: Tubiana R, ed, *The Hand*, volume 3 (WB Saunders: Philadelphia).

The following are redrawn with the kind permission of the publishers:

Capener N (1956) The hand in surgery, *J Bone Joint Surg*, **38B**:128 (Figure 1.61b);

Cauna M (1954) Nature and functions of the papillary ridges of the digital skin, *Anat Rec*, **119**:449 (Figure 1.154);

Hagert CG (1992) The distal radioulnar joint in relation to the whole forearm, *Clin Orthopaedics*, **275**:56–64 (Figure 1.52);

Kapandji AI (1963) *Physiologie articulaire*, volume 1 (Librarie Maloine: Paris) (Figures 1.51, 1.55a,b);

Kelleher JC (1982) Large combined axial vessel pattern abdominal pedicle flap, *Am J Anesthesiol*, **11**:33–48 (Figure 1.165);

Kuczynski K (1974) Functional micro-anatomy of the peripheral nerve trunks, *Hand*, **6**:1–10 (Figure 1.124);

Lundborg G, Myrhage R (1977) The vascularization and structure of the human digital tendon sheath, *Scand J Plast Reconstr Surg*, **11**:195–203 (Figure 1.89);

Martineaud JP, Seroussi S (1977) *Physiologie de la circulation cutanée* (Masson: Paris) (Figure 1.145);

Rabischong P (1963) Innervation proprioceptive des muscles lombricaux de la main chez l'homme, *Rev Chir Orthop*, **25**:927 (Figure 1.168);

Stack GH (1962) Muscle function in the fingers, *J Bone Joint Surg*, **44B**:899–909 (Figure 1.120);

Stack GH, Vaughan-Jackson OJ (1971) The zig-zag deformity in the rheumatoid hand, *Hand*, **3**: 62–7 (Figure 1.61a);

Tubiana R, ed (1981) *The Hand*, volume 1 (WB Saunders: Philadelphia): from the chapter by Dubousset (Figures 1.73b, 1.74, 1.79); Fahrer (Figure 1.136);

Tubiana R, ed (1985) *The Hand*, volume 2 (WB Saunders: Philadelphia): from the chapter by Tubiana (Figure 2.18); Weber (Figure 1.57);

Tubiana R, ed (1993) *The Hand*, volume 4 (WB Saunders: Philadelphia): from the chapter by Narakas (Figure 4.1c); Tubiana (Figure 4.24c);

Wynn Parry CB (1981) *Rehabilitation of the Hand*, 4th edn (Butterworth: London) (Figure 4.91);

Zancolli E (1979) *Structural and Dynamic Basis of Hand Surgery*, 3rd edn (JB Lippincott: Philadelphia) (Figure 1.82).

Evelyn Mackin would like to thank Teri Stahller for her excellent photographic assistance, and Kathryn Maynes for her excellent secretarial assistance, in the preparation of Section 4.3.

1 FUNCTIONAL ANATOMY

INTRODUCTION

Recent developments in hand surgery have come about as a result of a better understanding of the dynamic anatomy and function of the hand. This new concept of functional rather than static anatomy is the subject of this section.

The hand is both an organ designed to obtain information and an organ of execution. Its very specialized anatomy expresses these two functions, which are both essential in our dealings with the environment. We will first discuss the architecture and then the functions of the hand.

The hand gives the upper limb its importance and uniqueness. It is located at the extremity of the upper limb, which functions as its vector. The hand functions efficiently only if the proximal joints of the limb are stable and yet mobile; they are oriented so that the hand is almost always under visual control.

The hand moves within a large volume of space, the shoulder being the apex; it can reach any part of the body fairly easily because of the mobility of the shoulder as well as that of the elbow and the wrist, all operating in different planes (Figure 1.1). The shoulder is the most mobile joint in the body and it allows orientation of the upper limb as required. The movements of the clavicle amplify those of the shoulder (von Lanz and Wachsmuth, 1959). The arm assures projection of the limb from the trunk. The elbow, through flexion–extension movements, brings the hand closer to or moves it away from the body.

Distal to the elbow, there is in effect only one physiological unit. The combined movements of the wrist and forearm place the hand in a position for grasping. For gripping, the wrist is usually in flexion when close to the trunk and in extension when placed at a distance. Forearm rotation (pronation–supination) plays an important role too, particularly for bringing food to the mouth.

The hand's blood and nerve supplies are continuous with those of the rest of the limb. Some of its muscles, the extrinsic muscles, arise in the arm and forearm. Thus the hand must be studied as an integral part of the upper extremity.

The open hand, with fingers extended and in contact, forms a balanced graceful oval in its longitudinal axis. Its proximal "carpometacarpal" half is flattened, presenting two faces, each with a unique anatomical and functional significance. The back of the hand

1

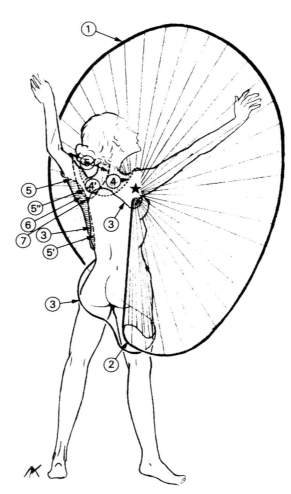

Figure 1.1. The range of movements of the upper extremity, and the body regions accessible to the right hand (by Kapandji). The spherical section of the space centered at the shoulder is contained in the cone of circumduction (1), within which the hand may grasp an object or food and carry it back to the mouth. Its posterior aspect (2) projects slightly backward. Zones of body access (for the right upper extremity): The dorsal zone (3) is reached by the arm carried backward, downward, and inward, with the elbow flexed and the forearm pronated or supinated for the lower half and supinated for the upper half and the perineal region. The cervical–trapezius zone (4) is reached by passing to the right of the head. The contralateral cervical–deltoid zone (5) is reached by passing in front of the left side of the head. The contralateral lateral–dorsal zone (6) is reached by passing in front of the trunk. Certain zones are partially overlapping, especially zones 3, 5, and 6 at the triple point (7) of the opposite scapula, accessible with difficulty by three different routes.

(the dorsum) is the surface that is usually visible and is therefore aesthetically important; the palmar surface, which is usually hidden, is the functional surface. The posterior or dorsal aspect is convex, and the anterior, palmar or volar aspect is concave. The distal half of the hand is separated into five digits, which flex toward the palm. They converge in closing—that is, they flex and adduct—and diverge in opening—that is, they extend and abduct.

The digits are divided into the thumb and four fingers. The thumb has a more proximal and lateral position, allowing movement inward and outward from the palm. The four fingers are the distal extension of the carpometacarpal part of the hand, and they

2

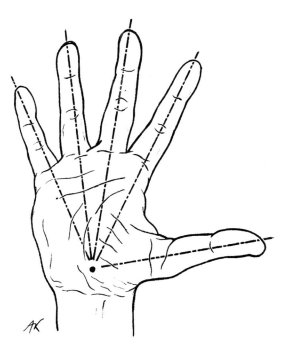

Figure 1.2. The five rays of the hand. Each is a polyarticular chain composed of a metacarpal and three phalanges, except the thumb, which has only two phalanges. When the digits are flexed separately, they converge toward a proximal point situated at the base of the palm. The thumb ray, being the shortest, is clearly separated from the fingers and is implanted proximally.

can be flexed from a distal position to a proximal position on the palm. The hinges of these movements are not at the bases of the digits, but at the thenar crease and at the transverse distal palmar crease.

The digits are of different lengths. When the digits are fully extended and touching each other, the tips almost describe a regular curve, the peripheral digits being the shortest. When the digits are separated, they diverge irregularly, the web space of the thumb being the largest and deepest (Figure 1.2). When the fingers are extended and separated, the tips of the fingers lie on the circumference of a circle whose center is the head of the third metacarpal (Littler, 1977; see Figure 1.8).

The hand is remarkably mobile and malleable. It is capable of conforming to the shape of objects to be grasped or studied, and of emphasizing an idea being expressed. These possibilities and varieties of function are realized through the unique structure of this organ, which consists of 19 bones, 17 articulations, and 19 muscles situated entirely within the hand, and about the same number of tendons activated by the forearm muscles.

We will consider the osseous and fibrous skeleton of the hand, the movements of the hand and the wrist, the functional value of the digits, and the cutaneous covering of the hand.

1.1 SKELETON OF THE HAND

The architecture of the hand enables it to form a strong grip and also to have a wide freedom of movement. This is achieved through a bony skeleton of many small bones associated with a highly developed and supple fibrous skeleton.

The osseous skeleton

The rays of the hand

The skeleton of the hand and wrist consists of 27 bones, of which 19 are long bones. The skeleton is divided into five rays, each ray making up a polyarticulated chain comprising the metacarpals and phalanges. The base of each metacarpal articulates with the distal row of the carpus (Figure 1.3). The carpus articulates with the skeleton of the forearm through its proximal row. The radioulno-carpal articulation has two axes of movement to which is added a third—pronation and supination from the forearm. Therefore, the wrist has three axes of movement, permitting the hand to be positioned in any spatial configuration and allowing it to be placed as needed for grasping.

Since the skeleton of the hand consists of five polyarticulated chains, it is susceptible to deformation. The radial ray or first ray, which is the shortest, is made up of only three bones—a metacarpal and two phalanges; its considerable functional importance and originality stem essentially from its great freedom of movement. The

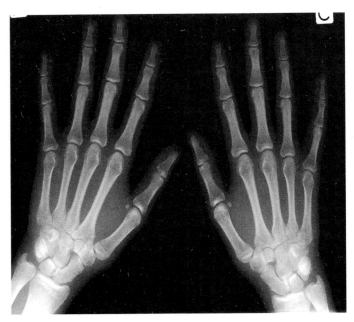

Figure 1.3. Radiographs of the skeleton of both hands. The thumb metacarpal is the shortest and the index metacarpal by far the longest. The proximal and middle phalanges of the long and ring fingers are longer than those of the index finger. Note the interlocking design of the carpometacarpal articulations and the saddle shape in opposing planes of the articular surfaces of the trapezium and the base of the first metacarpal.

first ray continues the external column of the carpus formed by the scaphoid and trapezium. This column is endowed with a relative autonomy, owing to scapholunate mobility. Moreover, the trapezium is clearly angled out in front of the carpal plane so that the first metacarpal makes an angle of about 45 degrees with the second metacarpal in the sagittal plane. This position, along with the shape of the metacarpotrapezial joint, explains the gap between the first ray and the palm, and allows the thumb metacarpal to oppose the other four digital rays (Figure 1.4). These other rays are of unequal length and are formed by four skeletal segments—a metacarpal and three phalanges.

Precise relationships exist among the length, mobility, and position of each ray. The lengths of the metacarpals vary, the thumb metacarpal being the shortest, the index finger the longest, and the others decreasing in length from the third to the fifth digits. However, the proximal and particularly the middle phalanges of the middle and ring fingers are longer than those of the index finger so that the long finger, and usually the ring finger, are longer than the index finger.

Not only does each skeletal segment and each ray have a different absolute length, but the relative lengths also vary with the movements of opening and closing the fist in such a manner that the digital extremes of each ray converge in flexion either toward the pulp of the thumb for thumb pinch or toward the base of the thenar eminence for power grip (digitopalmar grip). This convergence away from the median axis means that the more ulnar the digit, the more obliquely it must deviate as it approaches the

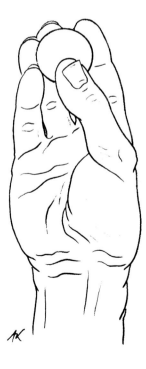

Figure 1.4. The thumb ray—more mobile, shorter, and more proximal than the others—can project in front of the plane of the palm to oppose itself to the other four rays.

palm (Figure 1.5). The two ulnar metacarpals, especially the fifth, have slightly more mobility in flexion–rotation, compensating for their lack of length. The convergence of the palmar digits toward the scaphoid tubercle results from the orientation of their distal segments in flexion, and it is essentially at the level of the metacarpophalangeal and the proximal interphalangeal articulations that these deviations are produced, as demonstrated by Dubousset (1971) and Kuczynski (1975).

Thus, there is a precise relationship between the length and mobility of the thumb and the length and mobility of the rest of the fingers. This architectural relationship could be described as a positioning for grip.

The skeleton of the hand presents a longitudinal and transverse concavity, giving it the shape of a cup with a palmar concavity when the thumb is placed next to the index finger. When the thumb spreads to grasp an object, the cup becomes a gutter whose major oblique axis follows the thumb crease. It is essential for the prehensile role of the hand that these curvatures be respected in both their longitudinal and transverse axes.

The transverse axis of the palm, which corresponds to the metacarpophalangeal articulations, is not perpendicular to the longitudinal axis, represented by the median ray.

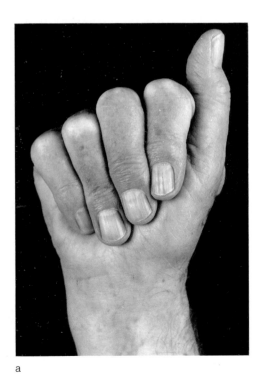

a

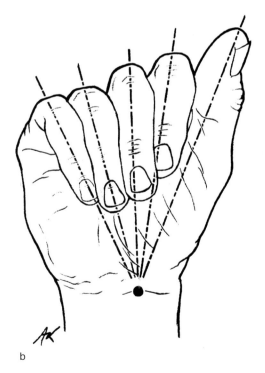

b

Figure 1.5a and b. The oblique flexion of the ulnar three digits. Only the index ray flexes in a sagittal plane. The more ulnar the digit, the more obliquely it flexes toward the median axis. Thus, when the last four digits are flexed separately at the metacarpophalangeal and proximal interphalangeal joints, their axes converge toward the scaphoid tubercle.

Instead, this transverse axis is oblique, more distal at the metacarpophalangeal joint of the index finger and more proximal at the fifth metacarpophalangeal joint. Thus it forms an acute angle of approximately 75 degrees with the longitudinal axis (Figure 1.6). It is necessary to take this obliquity into account when applying plaster casts or splints and also in the positioning of crutch and cane handles.

The epiphyseal plates are located at the proximal ends of the phalanges and the first metacarpal (which can be considered a phalanx), whereas they are located at the distal ends of the other metacarpals (Figure 1.7).

Fixed and mobile elements of the skeleton

One might schematically distinguish two groups in the skeleton of the hand: the fixed and the mobile elements (Littler, 1960; Figure 1.8). The fixed elements include the

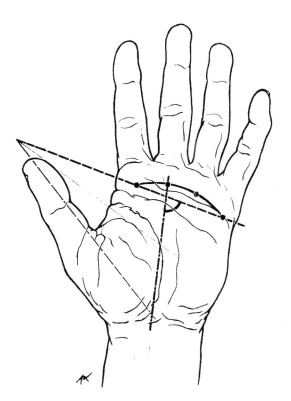

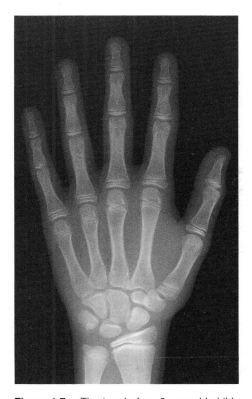

Figure 1.6. The obliquity of the transverse palmar axis. The transverse palmar axis passes along the line from the second to the fifth metacarpal head and forms an angle of 75 degrees with the axis of the third ray. The axis of the palmar groove is more oblique and follows closely the distal part of the oppositional crease of the thumb.

Figure 1.7. The hand of an 8-year-old child. Notice that the epiphyseal plates are located at the proximal ends of the phalanges and the first metacarpal (which could be considered a phalanx) whereas they are located at the distal ends of the other metacarpals.

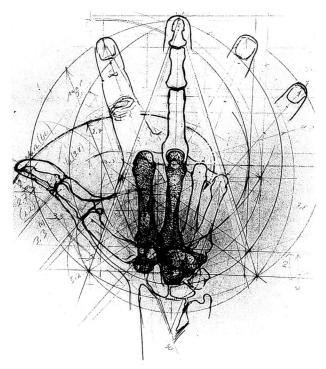

Figure 1.8. Geometric representation of the hand (by Littler). The fixed elements of the skeleton are represented by the stippled areas. In the hand, with the fingers extended and abducted, the finger tips lie on the circumference of a circle whose center is in the third metacarpal head. The circumference of this circle also runs along the articular surface of the distal radius. The carpus lies within a smaller circle whose center is the head of the capitate. The longitudinal axis of the hand passes through the middle finger, the third metacarpal, and the head of the capitate. The movements of the thumb for opposition, i.e. from extension–abduction to flexion–adduction, form a spiral equiangular curve.

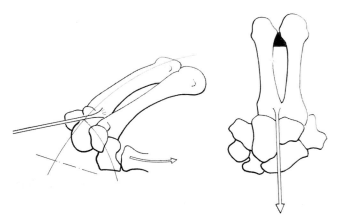

Figure 1.9. The fixed elements of the skeleton of the hand: the distal row of the carpal bones and the second and third metacarpals is extended by the extensor carpi radialis brevis.

distal row of the carpal bones and the second and third metacarpals (Figure 1.9). Between the different skeletal pieces composing the so-called fixed portion, the articulations are allowed some degree of independence, sufficient to insure a discrete suppleness yet permitting stability without rigidity. The mobile elements include two parts:

8

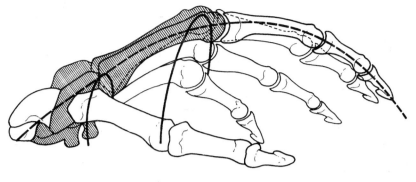

Figure 1.10a. Side view of the longitudinal arches and the transverse arches of the hand. The shaded areas show the fixed part of the skeleton.

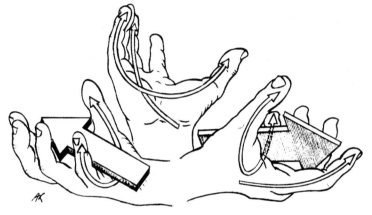

Figure 1.10b. The thumb forms, along with the other digits, four oblique arches of opposition. The most useful and most functionally important arch is between the thumb and the index finger, used for precision grip. The farthermost arch, between the thumb and little finger, insures a locking mechanism on the ulnar side of the hand in power grips.

- the distal elements—the phalanges—which form the skeleton of the digits and make closure of the fingers possible, and
- the peripheral metacarpals, essentially the thumb and the fifth metacarpals.

The arches of the hand

Usually two transverse arches—a carpal and a metacarpal arch—and one longitudinal arch are described (Figure 1.10a). To these one may also add the oblique arches of opposition between the thumb and each of the fingers (Figure 1.10b; Kapandji, 1963).

The transverse arches

The carpal arch
The carpal arch has a deep palmar concavity, which at first sight resembles a rigid osseous mass sometimes incorrectly termed the "carpal block" (Figure 1.11).

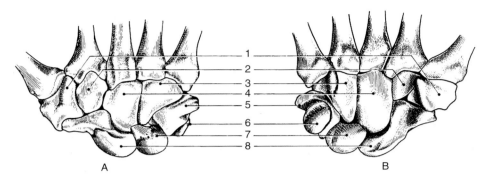

Figure 1.11. The carpal bones. (A) Dorsal view. (1) Trapezium; (2) trapezoid; (3) hamate; (4) capitate; (5) triquetrum; (6) pisiform; (7) lunate; (8) scaphoid. (B) Palmar view.

Two classifications of the carpal bones have been described. Both can help in understanding the mechanisms of stability.

1 The horizontal classification stresses the transverse cohesion of the bones. Two rows of carpal bones—proximal and distal—are considered. The proximal row is intercalated between the radius and the distal row. It relates simultaneously to the articular surfaces of both the radius and the second carpal row and must constantly adapt to these mobile surfaces (see Figure 1.42).
2 The vertical classification emphasizes the longitudinal coherence, essential for the transmission of muscular forces (see Figure 1.53). Only the radial (scaphoid) and central (capitate articulated with the lunate) columns articulate with the radius. In the ulnar column there is a gap between the ulna and the triquetrum.

The proximal row of carpal bones is mobile because of its connections to the radius and the distal row. Moreover, each of the bones that make up this row (scaphoid, lunate, and triquetrum) has its own distinct movements. The scaphoid, as it cradles the capitate, also articulates distally with the trapezium and the trapezoid and so contributes to the stability of the midcarpus.

The transverse arch of the distal carpal row is much more rigid. The keystone of this arch is formed by the capitate, which moves with the fixed metacarpals.

The wrist is more stable in flexion than in extension. This stability is due not so much to the interlocking of different pieces of the skeleton as to the strength of the various capsules and ligaments, structures to which we will return in studying the fibrous skeleton.

The flexor retinaculum

The flexor retinaculum distal to the radial joint forms a roof over the carpal gutter and transforms it into a tunnel (Figure 1.12). Its role in effecting stability of the wrist is questionable. The massive and powerful finger flexor tendons are retained close to the axes of flexion–extension and medial–lateral deviation by the flexor retinaculum. In this

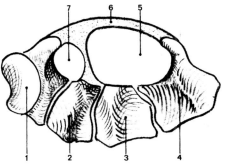

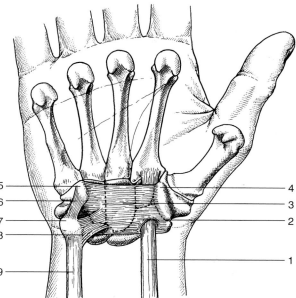

Figure 1.12a. The carpal canal. The carpal groove with an anterior concavity is formed into an osteofibrous tunnel by the flexor retinaculum, which inserts on its two borders. The tunnel is subdivided into two parts by a sagittal septum that separates the carpal canal proper (situated medially and containing the flexor tendons and the median nerve) from the lateral tunnel (containing the tendon of the flexor carpi radialis). (1) Trapezium; (2) trapezoid; (3) capitate; (4) hamate; (5) carpal tunnel; (6) flexor retinaculum; (7) tunnel for flexor carpi radialis.

Figure 1.12b. (1) Flexor carpi radialis; (2) scaphoid tubercle; (3) flexor retinaculum; (4) ridge on trapezium; (5) hook of the hamate; (6) pisohamate ligament; (7) pisiform; (8) volar carpal ligament; (9) flexor carpi ulnaris.

way, the flexors generate almost no torque at the radiocarpal joint while acting on the digits. These tendons, along with the median nerve, are surrounded by their synovial sheaths as they enter the carpal tunnel (Figure 1.13).

The narrowness of this osteofibrous tunnel explains why syndromes of irritation and compression of the median nerve are so common. The nerve, which is more superficial than the tendons, is compressed by them when the wrist is in the flexed position (Phalen's sign; Phalen, 1951).

The metacarpal arch

The metacarpal arch, by contrast, is endowed with a great deal of adaptability because of the mobility of the peripheral metacarpals. These peripheral metacarpals form the sides of the cup or the palmar gutter and can deepen the concavity as they approach each other, both being attached to the fixed element, i.e. the middle metacarpals (Figure 1.14).

The thumb metacarpal is independent and articulates with the trapezium. The middle metacarpals are united to the carpus by the intrinsic interlocking encasement of the bones themselves.

The index metacarpal is the most firmly fixed. The ring metacarpal is a transitional element to the fifth metacarpal and has about 10 degrees of mobility in flexion and extension. The fifth metacarpal is semi-independent; it articulates with the hamate and

11

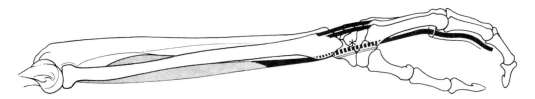

Figure 1.13a. The flexor retinaculum maintains and restrains the tendons of the extrinsic flexors of the digits within the carpal canal. Thus, these palmar tendons and especially the profundus are kept close to the axis of flexion–extension of the wrist. The extensors of the wrist, although less powerful than the flexors digitorum, are more distant from the axis of flexion–extension and therefore have a mechanical advantage that compensates for the difference in power and enables them to act synergistically with the flexors in the power grip.

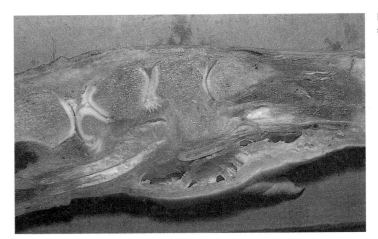

Figure 1.13b. Longitudinal section of the carpal canal.

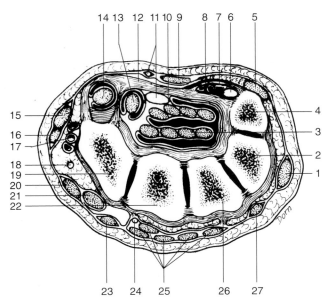

Figure 1.13c. Cross section of the carpal canal (1) extensor carpi ulnaris; (2) triquetrum; (3) flexor digitorum profundus; (4) pisiform; (5) flexor carpi ulnaris; (6) ulnar nerve; (7) volar carpal ligament; (8) ulnar artery and venae comitantes; (9) palmaris longus; (10) flexor digitorum superficialis; (11) median nerve and palmar cutaneous branch; (12) flexor retinaculum; (13) flexor pollicis longus; (14) flexor carpi radialis; (15) abductor pollicis longus; (16) extensor pollicis brevis; (17) radial artery and venae comitantes; (18) superficial branch of radial nerve; (19) scaphoid; (20) extensor carpi radialis longus; (21) extensor carpi radialis brevis; (22) capitate; (23) extensor pollicis longus; (24) posterior interosseous nerve; (25) extensor digitorum communis and extensor indicis propius; (26) hamate; (27) extensor digiti minimi.

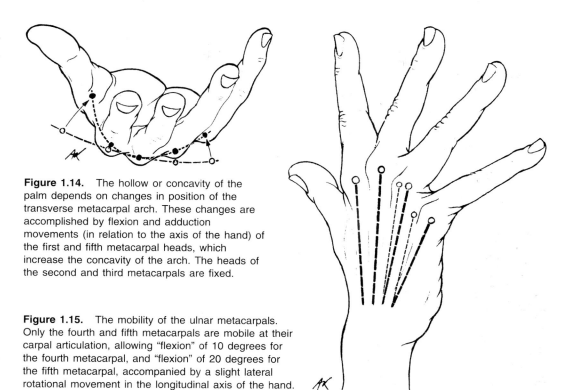

Figure 1.14. The hollow or concavity of the palm depends on changes in position of the transverse metacarpal arch. These changes are accomplished by flexion and adduction movements (in relation to the axis of the hand) of the first and fifth metacarpal heads, which increase the concavity of the arch. The heads of the second and third metacarpals are fixed.

Figure 1.15. The mobility of the ulnar metacarpals. Only the fourth and fifth metacarpals are mobile at their carpal articulation, allowing "flexion" of 10 degrees for the fourth metacarpal, and "flexion" of 20 degrees for the fifth metacarpal, accompanied by a slight lateral rotational movement in the longitudinal axis of the hand.

is restrained on its radial side by its articulation with the base of the fourth metacarpal. It has a range of flexion–extension of approximately 20 degrees (Figure 1.15), which is well utilized and can be increased by phalangization (Tubiana and Roux, 1974).

The second to fifth metacarpals are all bound together by various fibrous structures, the most distal of which is the deep transverse intermetacarpal ligament. This ligament is better named the interglenoid ligament, because it ties together the anterior "glenoid ligaments" of the metacarpophalangeal articulations, known as the "volar plates."

The longitudinal arches

The longitudinal arches are composed of a fixed portion, the carpometacarpal, and a mobile portion, the digits (Figure 1.16). For every ray there is a longitudinal arch. They diverge distally according to their different obliquities when the digits extend, the thumb ray being the most divergent. The keystones of these arches are the metacarpophalangeal articulations, whose thick anterior glenoid capsules, the volar plates, prevent hyperextension (Figure 1.17). We have just mentioned that the volar plates are interconnected by the transverse interglenoid ligament (see Figure 1.30). Thus the stability of the

13

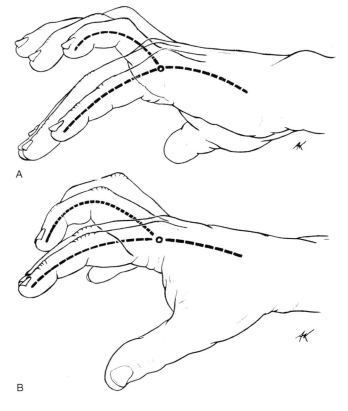

Figure 1.16. The carpometacarpal longitudinal arch. (A) View of the ulnar side. (B) View of the radial arch. Normally its curve is smooth, but an imbalance between the three muscular systems, especially an "intrinsic-minus" situation (loss of the intrinsic muscles), results in a break in the continuity of the curves at the level of the metacarpophalangeal joint, considered to be the keystone of this arch.

A

B

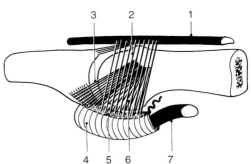

Figure 1.17. Schematic view of the metacarpophalangeal joint, keystone of the longitudinal arch of the hand. This joint is stabilized by the collateral ligaments and by the thick volar articular capsule, the volar plate, on which the lateral accessory ligaments, the sagittal bands of the extensor apparatus, and the first annular segment of the pulley of the flexor tendons insert. (1) Extensor tendon; (2) sagittal band; (3) collateral ligament; (4) flexor tendon sheath; (5) volar plate; (6) accessory collateral ligament; (7) flexor tendon.

metacarpophalangeal joints is essential to the support of the longitudinal arch as well as of the transverse metacarpal arch.

The five rays of the hand differ in mobility and independence. These are considerable for the thumb, much less for the fifth ray, and even less for the others. However, the index ray has a certain degree of independence, not at the metacarpal level (which is fixed) but at the phalangeal level, owing to the arrangement of its flexor and extensor muscles.

Figure 1.18. The three functional zones of the hand. (I) The thumb, master digit of the hand, represents the dominant element, which gives value to all the others. (II) The highly mobile index and middle fingers participate in precision grips separately or together with the thumb. They play a dynamic role. (III) The ring and little finger generally work together with the others in power grips against the palm. They have a more static role and often remain "in reserve".

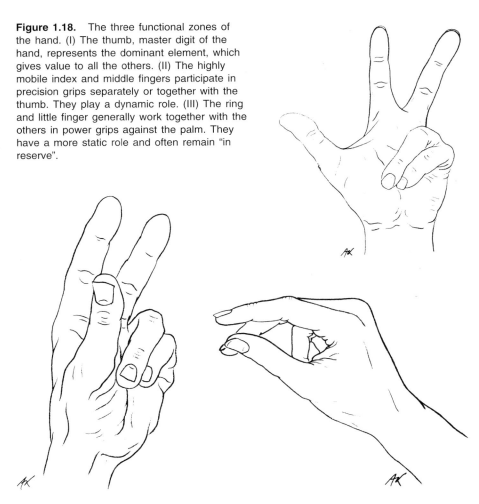

Figure 1.19. The tridactyl configuration. The first three digits work in close synergy for most grips not requiring force. This functional configuration, often utilized, constitutes (according to Capener, 1956) the "dynamic tripod".

Working with the thumb, the index finger manipulates objects with dexterity. However, there is a specialization of the radial and ulnar rays (Figure 1.18). The two ulnar digits customarily act together, especially in a palmar grip, to provide support and static control, the radial digits have a rather dynamic action; the thumb and the index and middle fingers work together to form the elements of the "dynamic tripod" for precision handling (Capener, 1956); this could be better named the "dynamic tridactyl" (Figure 1.19). This specialization of the digits is by no means absolute: the middle finger especially, owing to its position, can be integrated with the index finger for opposition to the thumb in precision grip, or with the ulnar digits in a power grip.

15

The fibrous skeleton

The osseous skeleton is complemented by a fibrous skeleton that reinforces it while allowing considerable adaptability; the fibrous skeleton comprises the aponeuroses, ligamentous structures, and fibrous sheaths attached to the bones and to the dermis.

The superficial palmar aponeurosis

The superficial palmar fasciae stretch between the flexor retinaculum, which forms their proximal boundary, and the root of the fingers, which is their distal limit.

The central zone is anatomically and pathologically the most important. This is the mid-palmar aponeurosis, which roofs the compartment of the hand where the flexor tendons and neurovascular bundles diverge. It forms an aponeurotic triangle with the apex proximally, the ulnar border coinciding with the hypothenar muscles, and the radial border with the lateral thenar muscles.

It is this midpalmar aponeurosis which must be considered when studying Dupuytren's disease. It comprises longitudinal, transverse and sagittal fibers.

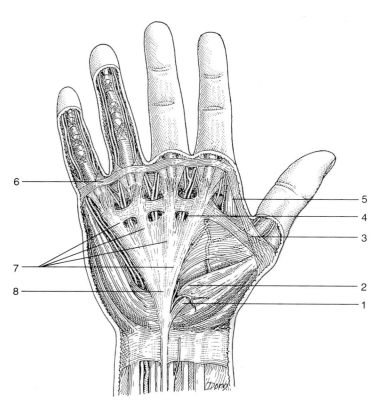

Figure 1.20. Dupuytren's contracture. (1) Radial division of tendon of palmaris longus; (2) palmar cutaneous branch of median nerve; (3) proximal commissural ligament of the first web space; (4) superficial transverse ligament; (5) distal commissural ligament of the first web space; (6) natatory ligament; (7) pretendinous bands; (8) ulnar division of tendon of palmaris longus.

16

1 The longitudinal formations span the palm across its middle third, and become more condensed in front of the flexor tendons of the long fingers, where they form the four pretendinous bands. A fifth band in front of the first ray is less well defined (Figure 1.20).

   These bands are in continuity with the palmaris longus tendon but are anatomically distinct structures. The mid-palmar fascia exists even in the absence of palmaris longus where their fibers blend with the antebrachial fascia, and Dupuytren's disease can still occur in these circumstances. Distally, the pretendinous bands disappear about at the level of the distal palmar crease. Most of the fibers insert into the deep surface of the dermis between the distal transverse palmar crease and the proximal digital flexion crease. A small proportion of these longitudinal fibers penetrate on either side of the metacarpophalangeal (MP) joint and
   • terminate on the deep surface of the web space;
   • blend with the deep palmar fascia;
   • continue into the finger on both sides of the digit.
2 The transverse formations, one proximal and the other distal, enclose the MP joint within the palm (Figure 1.21).

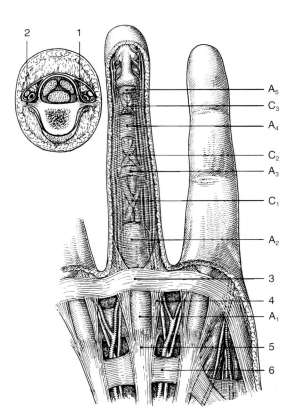

Figure 1.21. (1) Grayson's ligament; (2) Cleland's ligament; (3) natatory ligament; (4) spiral band; (5) pretendinous band; (6) superficial transverse ligament; A_1–A_5, C_1–C_3 pulleys.

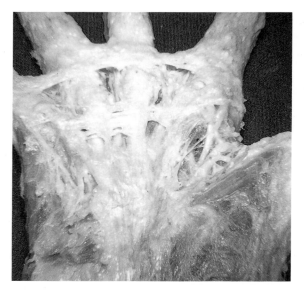

Figure 1.22. Superficial palmar aponeurosis. Note the longitudinal fibers in front of the tendons and the two transverse ligaments; the proximal ligament is called superficial (actually these fibers are deep in comparison to the longitudinal fibers) and the distal transverse ligament is called commissural (or natatory).

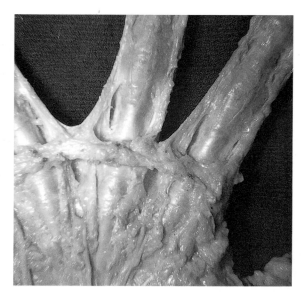

Figure 1.23. The distal transverse formation and the longitudinal fibrous structures on either side of the fingers which extend to the distal phalanx.

The transverse superficial ligament is located on the deep surface of the pretendinous bands. The distal border of this "ligament" is situated at approximately the level of the distal palmar skin crease. The proximal border is just distal to the superficial palmar arterial arch.

Between the proximal border of the superficial transverse ligament and the diverging borders of the pretendinous bands, there are triangular-shaped spaces in the fascia filled with adipose tissue. The lumbrical muscles and the digital neurovascular bundles (which run on the surface of the muscles) lie in these spaces. In the radial part of the palm, the fibers of the superficial transverse ligament continue in the first web space to form the proximal commissural ligament.

The distal transverse formation (see Figure 1.22 and Figure 1.23) crosses the base of the proximal phalanges of the long fingers superficially and forms the fibrous skeleton of the interdigital folds, the interdigital ligament or natatory ligament. Its proximal borders are well defined, and extend from the radial border of the index finger to the ulnar border of the little finger. Its distal border extends into the digital fascia. It covers the palmar neurovascular pedicles of each of the fingers as well as the flexor tendons.

At the base of the little finger, the natatory ligament divides to surround the abductor digiti minimi and the ulnar neurovascular pedicle. At the base of the index finger, the ligament continues to the first webspace where it forms the commissural crest and becomes the distal commissural ligament described by Grapow (1887).

The natatory ligament consists of more than just transverse fibers. It has additional longitudinal fibers on either side of the fingers extending to the distal phalanx. These fibers lie deep to the digital neurovascular bundles which are enclosed at the base of the fingers by the natatory ligament superficially and the retrovascular band (Thomine, 1965).

This fibrous lateral digital formation also receives deep fibers originating from the palmar sagittal septa and from the division of the longitudinal bands. Thus, in each web space a commissural chiasma results which is adherent to the skin of the interdigital folds, but the skin at the lateral part of the web space is usually free of adhesions. It is this mobile zone that is the point of departure for the digital dissection of Dupuytren's disease.

3 The palmar sagittal septa bands run from the deep surface of the mid-palmar fascia towards the deep palmar fascia that covers the musculoskeletal structures. These septa begin at the proximal border of the superficial transverse ligament, and end distally at approximately the same level as the pretendinous bands. They form a series of eight vertical septa described by Legueu and Juvara (1892), situated on either side of the flexor apparatus of the fingers (Figure 1.24). These septa limit the longitudinal compartments which contain the flexor tendons, the lumbrical muscles and the digital neurovascular pedicles. They are formed by longitudinal fibers which reach the depth of the palm, passing between the transverse fibers of the midpalmar fascia (Poirier and Charpy, 1926).

The *digital fascia* consists of a circular fascia which splits on the anterolateral aspects of the fingers to surround the neurovascular bundles. It comprises various elements (see Figure 1.21):

- a fine subcutaneous, circular envelope separated from the palmar skin by cellular adipose tissue, partitioned by fibrous strands that connect with the deep surface of the dermis. These adipose cushions disappear at the level of the digital flexion creases. The circular fascia adheres laterally to the flexor tendon sheaths but does not adhere with its volar surface except in the region of the proximal interphalangeal (PIP) joint.

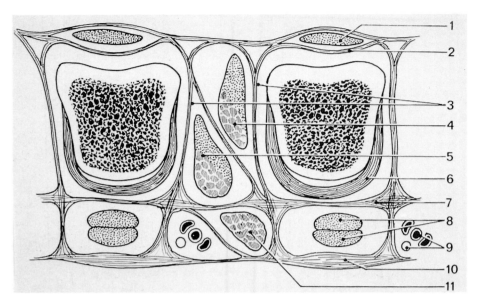

Figure 1.24. The palmar sagittal septa bands (from Legueu and Juvara, 1892).
(1) Extensor tendon; (2) dorsal aponeurosis; (3) perforating fibers; (4) dorsal interosseous muscle; (5) palmar interosseous muscle; (6) proximal part of volar plate; (7) deep palmar aponeurosis; (8) flexor tendons; (9) neurovascular bundles; (10) pretendinous band; (11) lumbrical muscle.

- a fibrous division between the phalanges and the dermis that is dorsal to the palmar collateral neurovascular pedicles, first described by Cleland (1878). These Cleland's ligaments are perforated by numerous orifices for the passage of the neurovascular elements destined for the dorsal surface of the finger. Cleland's ligaments seem to blend partially with the retrovascular band but McFarlane (1974) believes these two formations are distinct.
- a very fine membrane that corresponds to the "ligament" described by Grayson (1941) which lies in front of the palmar neurovascular pedicle. This represents the anterior layer of the fibrous sheath surrounding the pedicles.

The aponeurotic formations of the radial part of the hand
These formations are located in the first webspace, the thenar eminence and the thumb (Figure 1.25).

In the first web space there are two transverse formations as mentioned above: the proximal and distal commissural ligaments. These converge toward a fibrous junction located in front of the MP joint of the thumb (DeFrenne 1977).

The most lateral of the longitudinal fibers of the superficial palmar fascia are directed toward the thumb. The deep fibres attach to either side of the flexor pollicis longus

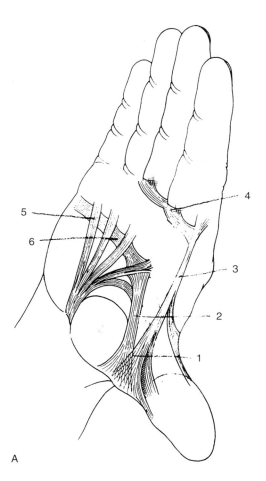

A

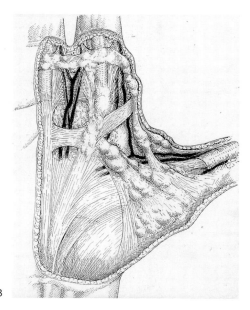

B

Figure 1.25. (A) Aponeurotic formation of the radial part of the hand: (1) fibrous complex in front of the metacarpophalangeal joint of the thumb; (2) proximal commissural ligament of the first web space; (3) distal commissural ligament of the first web space (Grapow); (4) interdigital or natatory ligament; (5) pretendinous bands; (6) transverse superficial ligament. (B) Localization of Dupuytren's disease in the radial part of the hand.

tendon sheath, whereas the superficial fibres attach to the dermis analogous to the other longitudinal formations of the superficial palmar fascia.

In the thumb, part of the dense intersection is located in front of the MP joint. More distally, the fibrous arrangement is similar to that of the fingers with a circular fascia. The prevascular and retrovascular fibers insert into the dermis of each side of the thumb and also into the skeleton, extending to the distal phalanx.

The deep palmar aponeurosis

The deep palmar aponeurosis lines the anterior aspect of the interosseous muscles and metacarpals, to each of which it is connected. Its transverse continuity is broken, however, opposite the third metacarpal by the insertion of the transverse fibers of the adductor pollicis. It is weak and thin proximally, but its distal part merges with the deep transverse intermetacarpal ligament, which is itself anchored to the volar plates of the metacarpophalangeal joints. It is connected to the superficial palmar aponeurosis by the fascial septa that divide the midpalmar space.

The palmar compartments

The palmar compartments (Figure 1.26) are defined in terms of the various fascial septa.

The midpalmar space is bounded superficially by the palmar aponeurosis; posteriorly it corresponds to the deep palmar fascia opposite the last two intermetacarpal spaces, while laterally it corresponds to the adductor muscle, which is lined by the corresponding portion of the thenar fascia. It is bounded medially by the hypothenar aponeurosis and laterally by the thenar aponeurosis. It contains the superficial and deep common flexor tendons and their sheaths, the superficial palmar arch, and the digital vessels and digital nerves.

The lateral palmar space, or thenar compartment, is limited posteriorly by the deep palmar fascia of the two first interspaces and anteriorly by the thenar aponeurosis. It contains the four thenar muscles and the tendon of the flexor pollicis and its sheath.

The medial palmar space, the smallest, lies in front of the fifth metacarpal, which makes up its floor. It is closed anteriorly by the medial (or hypothenar) palmar fascia and contains the three hypothenar muscles.

The interosseous space consists in fact of four compartments separated by the metacarpals, each one having as its posterior wall the deep dorsal fascia. They each contain the interosseous muscle of the corresponding space.

The dorsal aponeuroses

The superficial dorsal fascia is a thin subcutaneous sheet which lines the superficial aspect of the extensor tendons. Proximally it merges with the extensor retinaculum. It stretches across from the first to the fifth metacarpal.

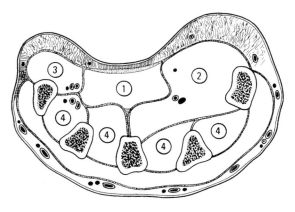

Figure 1.26. Palmar septa. (1) Middle palmar septum; (2) thenar or lateral palmar septum; (3) hypothenar or medial palmar septum; (4) the four interosseous septa.

The deep dorsal fascia, a slender cellular network, lines the dorsal aspect of the metacarpals and interosseous muscles. Between these two sheets there is a cellular gliding space through which the extensor tendons run.

Functions of the fibrous skeleton

The fibrous skeleton of the hand has many important functions:

- stability
- skin fixation
- containment
- partition
- protection and padding
- connection
- co-ordination
- tendon guidance
- restraint.

Stability

The fibrous skeleton plays an essential role of support in uniting bone segments and stabilizing the transverse and longitudinal arches of the hand. Each of the five rays contains three segments, which are mobile within certain limits. To stabilize one of these requires three supports—two collateral ligaments and one volar plate for each joint—which means 45 stays necessary for the five rays (Moberg, 1976).

The *volar plates* reinforce the capsules of the digital joints anteriorly. They are thick and resistant and have a firm distal insertion on the anterior aspect of the base of the phalanges (Figure 1.27). This insertion is thicker in its middle part, where it is adjacent to the bone. The proximal insertion is supple and thin and allows the movement of flexion–extension. The thickness of the volar plates increases the distance between the flexor tendons and the axis of the joint and thus improves the efficiency of the flexors. The main function of this reinforcement of the anterior capsule is to prevent hyper-extension.

The range of extension varies from joint to joint. Owing to the presence of two firm lateral check attachments proximally (Eaton, 1971), the volar plate limits extension in the proximal interphalangeal joint more than in the other digital joints. It is essential that the

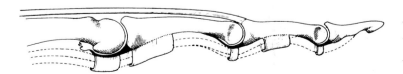

Figure 1.27. The three volar plates of the fingers and the five annular portions (pulleys) of the flexor tendon's fibrous sheath.

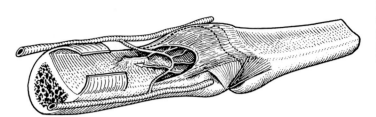

Figure 1.28. The proximal attachments of the PIP volar plate insert into the proximal phalanx each side of the flexor tendons.

middle phalanx never be hyperextended; this position triggers a zig-zag (swan-neck) deformity and severely impairs function. The two proximal attachments of the volar plate of the proximal interphalangeal joint insert into the proximal phalanx on each side of the flexor tendons (Figure 1.28) and blend with their fibrous sheath. By contrast, some hyperextension is possible at the MP and distal interphalangeal joints. This accounts for the fact that resistance to rupture is three times greater at the proximal interphalangeal joints than at the MP joints (between 16 and 21 kg for the proximal interphalangeal joint and between 5 and 8 kg for the MP joint, according to Weeks and Wray, 1978). There is also a significant difference in physiological extension from person to person and from race to race.

The blood supply of the volar plates comes from transverse arcades between the two palmar collateral digital arteries (Figure 1.29). These arcades run deep to the flexor tendons and some branches of the PIP arcade vascularize the flexor tendons through the vinculum longus.

The *deep transverse intermetacarpal or interglenoid ligament* connects the volar plates of the metacarpophalangeal joints (Figure 1.30). This ligament is attached at its extremities to the first dorsal interosseous muscle, which inserts on the radial border of the volar plate of the index finger, and to the abductor digiti minimi, which inserts on the ulnar border of the volar plate of this digit (Figure 1.31).

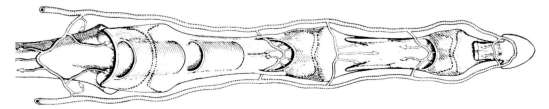

Figure 1.29. Blood supply of the volar plates. Some branches of the arcade run toward the attachment of the flexor tendon vincula.

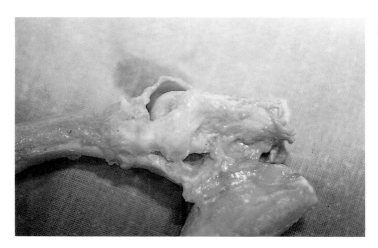

Figure 1.30. The deep transverse intermetacarpal ligament connects the volar plates of the metacarpophalangeal joints.

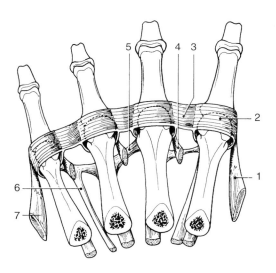

Figure 1.31. The fibrous skeleton of the transverse metacarpophalangeal arch. The metacarpophalangeal arch is supported by the extremely important fibrous skeleton. It is formed in front by the thick anterior capsular reinforcements of the metacarpophalangeal joints (or volar plates) joined together by the deep transverse metacarpal ligament (also called the interglenoid ligament). On the dorsal aspect the extensor communis tendons are joined together by the juncturae tendinum (conexus intertendineus). The common extensor digitorum sends to each side of the joint the sagittal bands that insert on the interglenoid ligament. This fibrous skeleton is tightened by the intrinsic muscles, in particular by the first dorsal interosseous muscle on the radial side and by the abductor digiti minimi on the ulnar side. (1) First dorsal interosseous muscle; (2) volar plate; (3) intermetacarpal ligament; (4) interosseous muscle; (5) conexus intertendineus; (6) extensor digitorum communis tendon; (7) abductor digiti minimum.

The *deep dorsal aponeurosis*, which inserts on the four ulnar metacarpals, forms a true posterior intermetacarpal ligament.

Fixation of the skin
Fixation of the skin is found in the zones of prehension in the palm (dermal insertions of the superficial palmar aponeurosis) and in the digits (Cleland's ligaments, dermal insertions of the fibrous structures in the finger pulp).

Containment

The superficial palmar aponeurosis, digital aponeurosis, and dorsal aponeurosis insure containment of the structures of the hand.

Partition

The deep palmar aponeurosis and septa separate the hand into compartments.

Protection and padding

The fibrous meshwork is found in the subcutaneous tissue of the distal part of the palm in front of the metacarpal heads, in the hypothenar eminence, and in the finger pulp.

Connection

The transverse interglenoid ligament, or deep intermetacarpal ligament, connects the volar plates. The juncturae tendinum, or connexus intertendineus, connect the extensor digitorum communis (EDC) tendons.

Co-ordination

The oblique retinacular (Landsmeer's) ligaments provide co-ordination between the interphalangeal joints of the fingers.

Tendon guidance

The various digital fibrous sheaths of the flexor tendons prevent the tendons from bowstringing as they cross the individual joints. The retinacula of the wrist are palmar and dorsal. The flexor retinaculum, as already stated, inserts on the carpal bones, whereas the extensor retinaculum inserts proximally on the distal end of the radius. This dorsal structure has six compartments for the tendons of the muscles of the posterior compartment of the forearm (see Figure 1.37).

All these features keep the tendons applied against the skeleton and permit their changes of direction at the level of the reflexion pulleys. They also contribute to the stability of the wrist and fingers.

Restraint

Restraint is provided by the sagittal bands of the common extensor and the check rein ligaments of the volar plates. This complex fibrous apparatus allows each segment of the digit to have great freedom of movement, to be stable, to remain within a small volume, and to be highly mobile without the need for bulky muscle bellies.

During active utilization of the hand, the fibrous skeleton has zones of condensation, kept under tension by a balance of forces exerted in different directions. Thus, the fibrous skeleton has not only distinct important anatomical components, but in a functional sense has balance and equilibrium in its dynamics. Zancolli (1979) has especially emphasized that this assemblage of fibrous structures on each side of the palmar surface of the MP joints forms a true fibrous nucleus (force nucleus; Figure

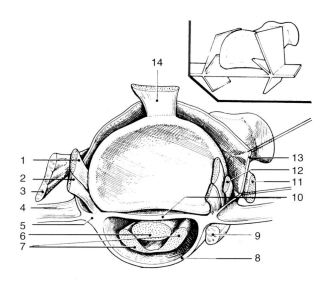

Figure 1.32. The fibrous nucleus (force nucleus of Zancolli) is located on each side of the palmar aspect of the metacarpophalangeal articulation and is formed by the convergence of the transverse interglenoid ligament, the volar plate, the sagittal bands of the extensor communis, the fibrous flexor tendon sheath, and the lateral accessory metacarpoglenoid ligaments. (1) Collateral ligament; (2) accessory collateral ligament; (3) interosseous muscle; (4) intermetacarpal ligament; (5) fibrous nucleus; (6) flexor digitorum profundus; (7) flexor digitorum superficialis; (8) flexor tendon sheath; (9) lubrical muscle; (10) volar plate; (11) interosseous muscle; (12) insertion of interosseous muscle into base of phalanx; (13) sagittal band; (14) central slip of extensor tendon inserting on base of proximal phalanx.

1.32). Indeed, the structures converging toward this nucleus are multiple—the deep transverse intermetacarpal ligament, the anterior articular capsule (the volar plate), the sagittal bands of the extensor, the proximal portion of the proximal flexor annular pulley (A_1), and the accessory collateral ligaments of the MP joints. If this fibrous complex is destroyed or simply displaced (as for example by distention of the MP joint, a condition frequently seen in rheumatoid arthritis) the balance of forces converging at this level will be disturbed, the transverse arch will flatten, the finger will be deformed, and its function will be compromised.

At the level of the proximal interphalangeal joint a similar fibrous arrangement can be seen. In front the fibrous flexor tendon sheath is suspended from the volar plate. Laterally, Cleland's ligaments are attached to the skin, and the oblique retinacular ligaments cross the joint obliquely, while the transverse fibers of the retinacular ligament are the more superficial.

1.2 SKELETON OF THE WRIST

The wrist is of special importance because its mobility and stability are essential for good hand function. Wrist mobility is a sum of all the movements of an articular complex made up of the radiocarpal joint, the mid-carpal joint, the ulnocarpal joint and the radioulnar joint.

Its stability depends on the equilibrium of the bony morphology at each joint and the passive resistance of the fibrous skeleton.

The osseous skeleton

The distal radial articular surface has a double obliquity (12–15 degrees in the lateral view and 15–20 degrees in the anteroposterior (AP) view (Figure 1.33). The posterior lip and the radial styloid thus have a buttressing effect.

The carpal articular surface ("the carpal condyle") has a smaller diameter of curvature than the radius and its precarious stability in the medial and palmar aspects depends upon ligamentous and capsular resistance.

The carpus, because of its anterior concavity, is more stable in flexion than extension. It does not form a single rigid bony block, because the eight small bones of the carpus all have different degrees of movement: the distal row is quite rigid, but the three proximal row bones are relatively mobile.

The stability of the carpal bones does not rely upon tendon insertions (with the obvious exception of the pisiform which is a sesamoid in flexor carpi ulnaris tendon). Rather, carpal stability is largely due to interosseous ligaments and bony configuration of these carpal bones.

The triquetrum is not in contact with the ulna head; a fibro-cartilage disc, the triangular ligament, separates the two bones. The scaphoid and lunate articulate with the radius; the scaphoid presents a long axis inclined by 45 degrees to the long axis of the radius. Its distal pole has a tubercle which lies palmarly. The lunate also has a palmar tubercle. The lunate sits on the capitate and has anterior and posterior horns. A line

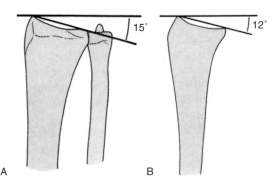

Figure 1.33. The biconcave articular surface of the distal end of the radius. (A) Anteroposterior view. A line joining the end of the radial styloid and the ulnar border of the distal end of the radius forms an angle with the horizontal of approximately 15 degrees that opens medially. (B) Side view. The posterior margin of the distal end of the radius forms with the anterior rim a 12 degree angle that opens forward.

drawn between the anterior and posterior horns lies perpendicular to the long axis of the wrist in neutral position.

The distance between the distal articular surface of the radius and the base of the metacarpals is constant (McMurty R et al, 1978). During movements of the wrist the relationship between the carpal bones changes. For example, rotation of the scaphoid and lunate as the wrist moves from extension to flexion has a double "cam" effect. Rotation in a sagittal plane allows the persistent adaptation of the carpal articular surface in order to present the correct diameter of curvature to the distal radius. Thus the carpus is a "condyle of variable geometric form" (Kuhlmann, 1977). Kinematics of the carpal bones are described in section 1.3.

The ulnar head sits proximal to the distal radius and has only an indirect effect on stability of the wrist. The triangular ligament extends the distal radial articular surface to the ulnar styloid and forms the principal link between the two bones.

The fibrous skeleton

The fibrous skeleton is composed of intra-articular ligaments, the fibrous joint capsule and extrinsic capsular ligaments and two extra-articular ligaments or retinacula.

The intra-articular ligaments

These comprise the carpal interosseous ligaments, the radioscapholunate ligament and the triangular radio-ulnar ligament or triangular fibro-cartilage. The triangular fibro-cartilage is described with the distal radio-ulnar joint.

The interosseous ligaments

The interosseous or "intrinsic" ligaments connect the carpal bones (Figure 1.34).

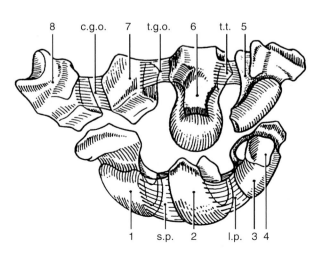

Figure 1.34. Horizontal classification of the carpus. Proximal row: (1) scaphoid; (2) lunate; (3) triquetrum, which articulates with the pisiform (4) anteriorly. These bones are held together by interosseous ligaments (sp, scapholunate; lp, lunotriquetral). Distal row: (5) hamate; (6) capitate; (7) trapezoid; (8) trapezium. These bones are linked by three interosseous ligaments (tt, trapezio-trapezoid; tgo, trapezoid–capitate; cgo, capitate–hamate).

29

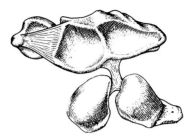

Figure 1.35. The radioscapholunate ligament inserts on the volar aspect of the articular surface of the radius. It transmits blood vessels to the two carpal bones (Testut and Kuenz, 1928). The radioscaphoid fibers, longer than the radiolunate ones, allow for the differences in the range of movement of these bones.

The three proximal row carpal bones are connected by particularly strong interosseous ligaments, which are made up of fibers of different lengths inserted around the proximal part of each bone. These ligaments are able to transmit sagittal displacement from one bone to the next.

The four distal row carpal bones form a rigid block, owing to their intrinsic ligaments. Between the proximal and distal row, the intrinsic ligaments should not impede mid-carpal joint movement. There are no intrinsic ligaments centrally connecting the capitate to lunate but they are present in the medial and lateral columns of the carpus. Therefore, the distal scaphoid is attached palmarly to the distal row by a lateral ligament to the trapezium and a medial ligament to the trapezoid and capitate. This distal fibrous complex of the scaphoid acts to oppose forces which tend to pull the scaphoid horizontally.

At the ulnar side of the mid-carpal joint, the triquetrum is attached to the capitate by a volar oblique ligament which allows sliding of the triquetrum on the inclined surface of the hamate. The pisiform is fixed to neighbouring bones by a series of ligaments which allow little displacement.

The radioscapholunate ligament

The radioscapholunate ligament of Testut and Kuenz (1928) brings only a small contribution to wrist stability, but it contains numerous blood and lymph vessels and can be involved in diseases such as rheumatoid arthritis (Mannerfelt and Raven, 1978) (Figure 1.35).

The fibrous joint capsule and extrinsic capsular ligaments

There are anterior, posterior and ulnar condensations of the capsule which form the extrinsic ligaments. The strongest part lies anteriorly so as to resist the tendency to anterior subluxation due to the inclination of the distal radial articular surface. The palmar capsule is thickened to form a strap joining the anterior border of the radial articular surface to the ulnar styloid with attachment to the anterior horn of the lunate and proximal pole of the triquetrum. The capsule is reinforced by powerful ligaments (Figure 1.36).

The description of the anterior ligaments varies with different authors. Most often it has been described as a "V"-shaped ligament with symmetrical limbs from the radial and ulnar sides converging on the capitate for their insertion. Others have described a

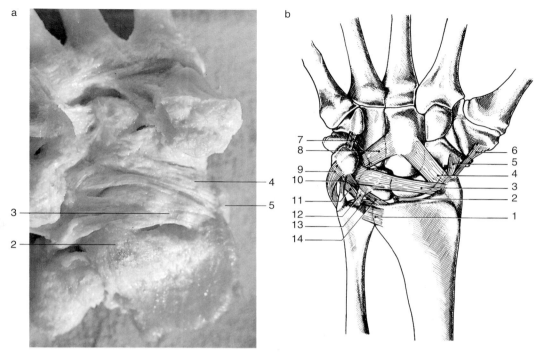

Figure 1.36 a and b. Volar extrinsic ligaments of the wrist. (1) Palmar ligament of distal radioulnar joint; (2) radioscapholunate ligament; (3) stylolunate–triquetral bundle of the volar radiocarpal ligament—there are weak points in the anterior capsule between these bundles; (4) stylocapitate bundle of volar radiocarpal ligament—this thick ligament, which crosses the waist of the scaphoid, is the only ligamentous structure linking the radius to the distal carpal row; (5) styloscaphoid bundle of volar radiocarpal ligament; (6) radial collateral ligament; (7) palmar triquetrocapitate ligament—medial branch of volar ligamentous V, the other branch being formed by the volar radiocapitate ligament; (8) pisohamate ligament; (9) extensor retinaculum; (10) ulnar collateral ligament; (11) radiotriquetral meniscus; (12) radioulnar triangular fibrocartilage; (13) ulnotriquetral band of palmar ulnocarpal ligament; (14) palmar radiotriquetral ligament.

double "V" inserting on the capitate, one "V" distally and one "V" proximally, the ulnar limb of this being the capitotriquetral ligament. Also some have emphasized the importance of the radiolunotriquetral band.

The ligaments from the radius are much stronger than those from the ulnar. This is particularly true of the volar radiocarpal ligament; arising from the radial styloid it fans out into a number of bands. It is possible to recognize a proximal radiolunotriquetral band and a stronger, more distal band passing anterior to the scaphoid neck, acting as a pivot for the rotation of the scaphoid, before inserting on to the capitate. As Verdan (1954) has pointed out, in pronation to supination movements, this ligament presses on the scaphoid; for this reason he recommends that the elbow be immobilized in cases of fracture of the scaphoid. This band is the only ligament between the radius and the distal carpal row and has a restraining function.

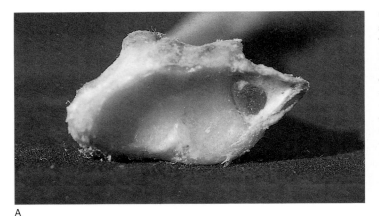

A

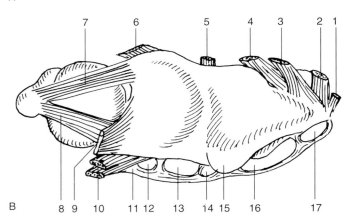

B

Figure 1.37. (A) The articular surfaces of the distal radius and the triangular fibrocartilage. (B) Schematic distal view of the radius and ulna. (1) Radial collateral ligament; (2) radio-scaphoid band of the palmar radiocarpal ligament; (3) radio-capitate band of the same ligament; (4) radiotriquetral band of the palmar radiocarpal ligament; (5) the radio-scapholunate ligament; (6) palmar radiotriquetral ligament; (7) anterior pillar of the triangular fibrocartilage; (8) posterior pillar of the triangular fibrocartilage; (9) radiotriquetral meniscus; (10) radiotriquetral band of the dorsal radiocarpal ligament; (11) extensor retinaculum; (12) the compartments for the tendons of the extensor digiti minimi; (13) the extensor digitorum and extensor indicis; (14) the extensor pollicis longus; (15) the dorsal tubercle of the radius or Lister's tubercle; (16) the extensores carpi radiales; (17) the extensor pollicis brevis and abductor pollicis longus.

Between these two bands, Poirier and Charpy (1926) noted an interval which corresponds to the lunocapitate joint line. This represents a weak point in the volar capsule which is particularly vulnerable because there is no lunocapitate ligament (Figures 1.36 and 1.37).

The dorsal capsule

The dorsal capsule is much weaker but is reinforced by a "V"-shaped transverse ligament with its apex on the triquetrum (Figure 1.38). The posterior radio-triquetral ligament inserts on the posteromedial aspect of the distal radius. It forms the posterior band of the triquetral sling.

The general direction of these anterior and posterior ligaments originating from the radius is oblique distally and medially. In this way they counteract the tendency for ulnar subluxation. The proximal portion of these ligaments converges to the triquetrum, a true osteofibrous knot acting as the "stone in a sling" (Kuhlmann, 1977) surrounding the

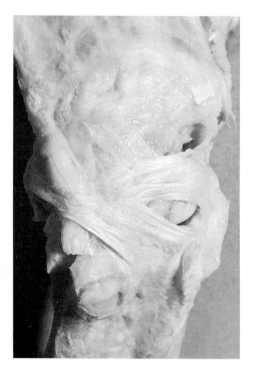

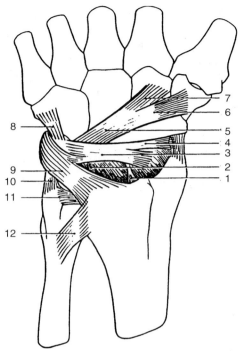

Figure 1.38a. The dorsal ligament is reinforced by a "V" shaped transverse ligament with its apex on the triquetrum.

Figure 1.38b. The dorsal ligaments: the posterior radioscapholunate ligament (1), the posterior radiotriquetral ligament (2), the horizontal band (3) of the triquetral sling, which gives off an expansion (4) toward the radial collateral ligament, the oblique band (5), which inserts into the trapezium (6) and the trapezoid (7), the posterior triquetrohamate ligament (8), the posterior band (9), the ulnar collateral ligament (10), the triangular ligament (11), and the posterior radioulnar ligament (12).

ulnar aspect of the wrist. The ulnar sling and the palmar strap are interdependent and their permanent adaptation is the key to auto-locking of the wrist in all positions.

Few ligaments have a longitudinal axis in the wrist: the radioscapholunate ligament and the so called collateral ligaments are the exceptions.

Collateral supporting structures

These have been described as radial and ulnar collateral ligaments but they only have a little influence on stability because the wrist needs to have freedom of lateral movements and cannot be fixed by rigid lateral structures. The majority of lateral support is provided by the tendons of the extrinsic muscles which cross the wrist to the hand and allow active stabilization to reinforce the skeletal stability.

The ulnar fibrous structures

These structures play an important role in resisting the tendency for ulnar subluxation of the wrist caused by the obliquity of the distal radial articular surface. They include the dorsal and palmar radioulnar ligaments, the triangular fibrocartilate, the ulnar collateral ligament, the anterior and posterior radio-triquetral ligaments and the ECU fibrous sheath. Taleisnik (1976) describes in addition a "meniscus" between the radius and triquetrum, which has a common origin with the triangular fibrocartilage ligament from the dorso-ulnar corner of the radius. From here the meniscus swings around the ulnar border of the wrist to insert onto the triquetrum (see Figure 1.39). In summary, the carpus is essentially suspended from the radius, with the help of two oblique ligamentary systems whose insertions are diagonally opposed (see Figure 1.37b): the anterolateral fibrous complex, which inserts on the styloid process of the radius and is distributed in a fan shape—this reinforces the palmar capsular strap which contains the pressure toward the front; the posteromedial fibrous complex, which inserts on the posteromedial distal angle of the radius and opposes ulnar displacement.

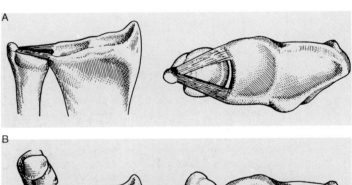

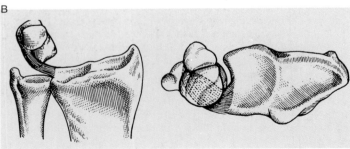

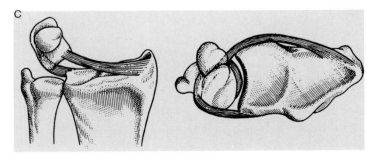

Figure 1.39. The ulnar fibrous structures. (A) Triangular fibrocartilage ligament. (B) Taleisnik's meniscus. (C) Anterior and posterior radio-triquetral ligaments forming the "Kuhlmann sling".

Distal radioulnar joint and triangular fibrocartilage complex

For many years the interest of surgeons has been focused on the radial part of the wrist. Only recently has attention moved to the ulnar side, particularly the distal radioulnar joint (DRUJ) and the triangular fibrocartilage complex (TFCC). The most important functional movement of the wrist (pronosupination) occurs at the DRUJ and the TFCC is the most important stabilizer of the ulnar carpus. The DRUJ involves the sigmoid notch of the radius and the ulnar head, three-quarters of which is covered by articular cartilage. The head of the ulna has two articular surfaces: one in the sagittal plane articulated with the radius and another in the horizontal plane in the form of a crescent articulated with the fibrocartilage ligament. In the frontal plane, the articular surface of the radius, in front of the ulnar surface has an angle of divergence of 15–20 degrees with the axis of the ulna (Bonnel, 1994). The curves of the two surfaces are not symmetrical. The radius of the circle of the radial surface is 1.8 times superior to the ulnar head radius (Ekenstam, 1985). The head of the ulna does not simply rotate but makes a combined sliding-rotation movement. In neutral position the articulating surface of the sigmoid notch is optimally covering the articulating surface of the ulnar head. This contact area is gradually diminished during pronation-supination until only a marginal contact remains at the end of each movement. In extreme movements this incongruence, a factor in instability, necessitates

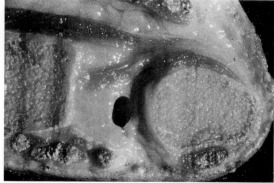

B

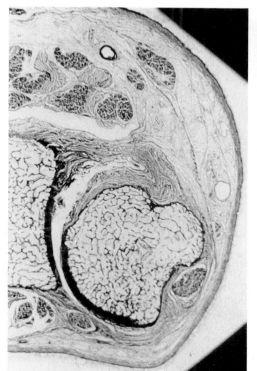

A

Figure 1.40. (A) Transverse section of the DRUJ showing the difference of radius of circle between the articular surfaces of the two bones. Note also the position of ECU tendon which stabilizes the ulna head in supination. (B) Transverse section of the DRUJ showing the superior articular surface of the triangular ligament and the two heads (deep and superficial) of the pronator quadratus.

the addition of the distal radioulnar ligaments and of the ulno-triquetral ligaments, the action of muscular support: the tendons of extensor carpi ulnaris in supination (Figure 1.40a) and to a lesser degree of the flexor carpi ulnaris. The deep head of the pronator quadratus brings the ulna nearer to the radius and the superficial head limits the dorsal displacement of the ulna during pronation (Figure 1.40b). The interosseous membrane, which inserts distally at 3 cm of the ulnar styloid process, may play a role in its stability.

In addition to all the extrinsic structures, the *triangular fibrocartilage* provides intrinsic stability and is the principal stabilizer of the distal radioulnar joint. Several fibrous structures are associated with the articular disc, forming the TFCC. In spite of some confusion in anatomical terminologies, for most authors the TFCC also includes the articular triangular ligament, the volar ulno-triquetral ligament, the dorsal radio-triquetral ligament, the Taleisnik meniscus and the extensor carpi ulnaris sheath (Figures 1.41 and 1.42).

The articular disc is triangular, the base of the triangle is inserted on the radius and its ulnar extremity is inserted at the base of the radial side of the ulnar styloid process. It extends the radial articular surface to the ulnar styloid. The volar and dorsal margins of the disc are thick and called ligaments, the center is thin and is perforated in half of patients over 50 years of age (Mikic, 1989). The articular disc is 2 mm thick at its radial origin and 5 mm thick at its ulnar insertion.

Besides stability, the triangular ligament has a function in the transmission of forces. The center of the disc assures the transmission of forces and the palmar and dorsal ligaments have a dynamic stabilization function. Stability of the DRUJ is accomplished by joint congruity combined with tightening of the volar ligament fibers of the articular disc in pronation and dorsal fibers in supination (Ekenstam and Hagert, 1984). For these authors, intact dorsal and volar parts of the triangular ligament are the main stabilizing factors of the DRUJ joint.

The extra-articular ligaments of the wrist

Two strong extra-articular ligaments or retinacula provide further support. The *transverse carpal ligament* or flexor retinaculum has been already described (see Figures 1.12 and 1.13).

The *posterior retinaculum* is composed of two parts (Figure 1.43):

1 a transverse portion, which has a series of proximal insertions into the distal radius forming six osteofibrous tunnels or compartments. These compartments serve as pulleys for the extensor tendons of the wrist, fingers and thumb; and

2 an oblique portion, which turns around the ulnar part of the carpus and extensor carpi ulnaris tendon and finishes by insertion on the pisiform and triquetrium. In this way it forms an extra-articular sling. It is important to note that though the distal fibers are the strongest, these lie distal to the ulna head and so are unable to contribute to its stability (Figure 1.44). In Figure 1.44 the extensor retinaculum distal fibers continue proximally to the pisiform with the proximal fibers of the flexor retinaculum. This connection occurs deeply with respect to the flexor carpi ulnaris tendon at the floor of the Guyon space (Zancolli and Cozzi; 1992).

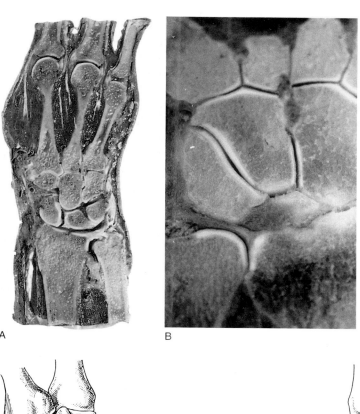

Figure 1.41a and b. The triangular fibrocartilage complex, frontal section.

A

B

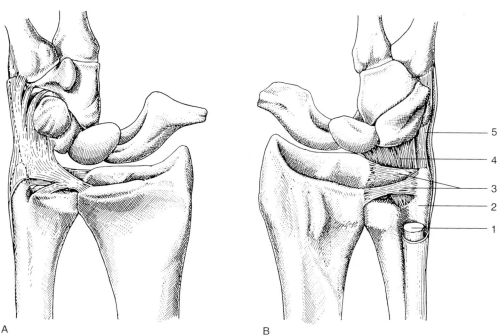

A

B

Figure 1.42. Triangular fibrocartilage complex. (A) Volar view. (B) Dorsal view: (1) ECU tendon; (2) fibrous sheath of ECU tendon; (3) dorsal and volar ligaments of the triangular fibrocartilage; (4) ulnar-luno-triquetral ligament; (5) ulnar collateral ligament.

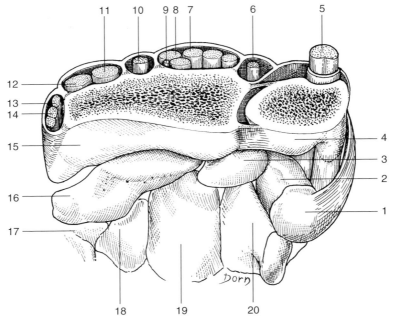

Figure 1.43. The posterior retinaculum: (1) pisiform; (2) triquetrum; (3) lunate; (4) ulna; (5) extensor carpi ulnaris; (6) extensor digiti minimi; (7) extensor digitorum communis; (8) extensor indicis prorius; (9) posterior interosseous nerve; (10) extensor pollicis longus; (11) extensor carpi radialis brevis; (12) extensor carpi radialis longus; (13) extensor pollicis brevis; (14) abductor pollicis longus; (15) radius; (16) scaphoid; (17) trapezium; (18) trapezoid; (19) capitate; (20) hamate.

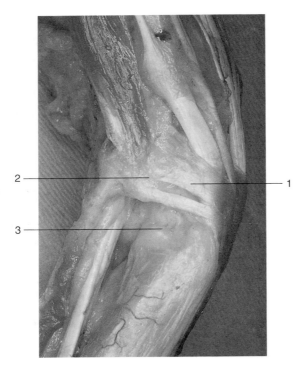

Figure 1.44. The extensor retinaculum distal fibers continue proximally to the pisiform with the proximal fibers of the flexor retinaculum. (1) Oblique portion of the dorsal retinaculum; (2) pisiform; (3) ulna head.

A knowledge of the different elements of the fibrous skeleton of the wrist is indispensable for understanding the physiology of this articular complex and the secondary deformities of traumatic or rheumatic origin which can affect it, and for treating in a rational way fractures, instabilities or deformities of the wrist.

Vascularization of the wrist bones

Blood supply of the wrist bones is provided by the dorsal and palmar transverse vascular arches.

The scaphoid

The scaphoid receives its blood supply mainly from branches of the radial artery. These branches can be grouped into three systems (Taleisnik and Kelly, 1966; Mestdagh et al, 1979):

- the dorsal group, which penetrates the dorsum of the scaphoid along the spiral waist;
- the laterovolar vessels, which approach the scaphoid immediately distal and lateral to the radial articular surface; and
- the distal vessels which enter it on the volar aspect of the tubercle of the scaphoid. Gelberman and Menon (1980) in a more recent study describe two vascular systems instead of three: a dorsal and a volar system limited to the scaphoid tubercle.

The important point in all these descriptions is that there are no intraosseous anastomoses between the arteries to the tuberosity and the remainder of the intraosseous vessels. In the case of a fracture, the proximal part of the bone is therefore exposed to avascular necrosis if it is not supplied by a direct arterial branch.

The lunate

The lunate is supplied by volar and dorsal vessels. In Lee's study of the intraosseous arterial pattern of the lunate (1963), numerous dorsal and volar vessels were present in 66 per cent of cases, and these vessels anastomosed within the bone; in 26 per cent there was a single volar or a single dorsal vessel, and in 7.5 per cent supply was via volar or dorsal arteries that did not connect with each other.

Post-traumatic avascular necrosis is a danger in the absence of any anastomosis between the anterior and posterior vessels or in case of a unilateral blood supply.

1.3 MOVEMENTS OF THE HAND AND WRIST

The hand is essentially a mobile organ. It can coordinate an infinite variety of movements in relation to each of its elements. This blending of movements of the wrist and digits allows the hand to mold itself to the shape of the object for palpation or grasp. We will consider the factors involved in the mobility of the hand and the movements of each functional unit of the hand.

Factors involved in mobility

The great freedom of movement of the hand is due to:

- gliding mechanisms;
- the articular systems;
- the muscles; and
- the tendons.

Gliding mechanisms

Most of the structures in the hand glide in relation to the neighboring structures.

The dorsal integument must be supple, elastic, and malleable. The skin of the back of the hand slides distally to allow metacarpophalangeal joint flexion. Interphalangeal flexion is accomplished by means of a special arrangement of skin folds on the dorsum of each articulation.

The vessels and nerves adapt themselves to differences in length and are surrounded by loose fibroadipose connective tissue.

The extrinsic muscles continue into the tendons, which, in order to perform their function, must glide in relation to the other elements of the hand. The gliding mechanism, which has an essential role, depends on two main factors: the nature of the anatomic area through which it moves, and the direction and amplitude of tendon movement. In the unrestricted areas, where the tendon has a straight trajectory, it is surrounded by the paratenon, areolar connective tissue arranged in layers. This is the pattern for most of the extensor tendons except on the dorsal aspect of the wrist.

In narrow crowded areas, the gliding mechanism is assured by the synovial sheath, which allows a considerable amplitude of movement. The synovial sheaths at specific sites are surrounded by fibrous sheaths that keep the tendon close to the skeleton, in particular when the pulling tendons cross the sinus of an articular angle, as on the anterior and posterior aspects of the wrist or on the palmar aspect of the digital joints. The fibrous sheath assumes the role of a pulley when the tendon changes direction.

The gliding mechanism represented by the synovial sheaths is much more developed on the palmar aspect. There are three synovial sheaths for the flexor tendons of the index finger, long finger, and ring finger extending from the neck of the metacarpals to the DIP joint (Figure 1.45). The superficial and deep flexor tendons of the digits also glide over each other. In the little finger the sheath is continued proximally, joining

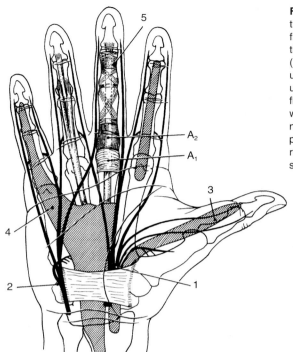

Figure 1.45. Diagram showing the different relations of the flexor tendons of the fingers at the wrist and in the hand: (1) the median nerve; (2) the ulnar nerve; the radial (3) and ulnar (4) synovial sheaths of the flexors extend proximally to the wrist. In the fibrous sheaths, note the important mechanical pulleys. (For additional details relating to the pulley system, see Figure 1.72.)

the common flexor tendon sheath which surrounds all the finger flexor tendons in the distal forearm and proximal palm. The flexor pollicis longus tendon also runs within a sheath commencing proximal to the carpal tunnel and extending distally to the thumb interphalangeal joint level.

On the dorsal aspect, the extensor synovial tendon sheaths are present only at the level of the wrist, which is the only joint in the hand capable of active dorsal flexion. Each synovial sheath has a visceral and parietal component separated by a potential synovial cavity containing a very thin layer of synovial fluid, which constitutes the basic gliding and nutritional mechanism. Any alteration of these gliding mechanisms has important functional repercussions.

The articular system

The skeleton of the hand has many articulations. No single articulation is an isolated mechanical entity in itself. The articulations of the hand form functional groups arranged in kinetic chains (Figure 1.46).

A certain interdependence exists between the various articulations and the architectural structure of the wrist and hand. The position of each articulation depends on the equilibrium of forces acting at that level. The equilibrium and the interdependence between the elements in the same osteoarticular chain are the result of

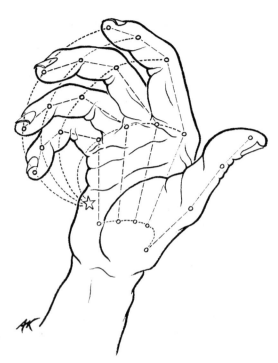

Figure 1.46. The architectural and functional harmony of the hand. In a normal hand the kinetic chains that make up the digits are not arranged at random. The phalanges and joints of the fingers are organized in regular curves—for the most part spirals (see Figure 1.70)—that give a spatial value to the functional equilibrium.

several factors, both active and passive. The active factor is the dynamic balance between antagonist muscles (Duchenne, 1867), while the passive factors include the restraining action of ligaments (Landsmeer, 1955; Milford, 1968) and muscular "viscoelasticity," to use the term coined by Long and Brown (1964), which facilitates the coordination of motion. Single articular movements around a fixed perpendicular axis simply do not exist in the hand. Almost all the movements are around oblique and variable axes, resulting in combined movements permitting optimal orientation of the phalanges at the time of prehension.

Muscles

When considering the 17 mobile articulations of the digits and those of the wrist, the actions of the numerous muscles that act upon them must be kept in mind.

Muscles move joints by creating tension and excursion in an intermediary structure, the tendon, which then translates them into joint motion. All skeletal muscles are striated muscles that are made up of muscles fibers. The sarcomere is the basic unit of muscle tissue in the muscle fiber. Sarcomeres are composed of interacting molecules of myosin and actin. With sarcolemmal contraction, there is overlap and interdigitation of these molecules and physical shortening of the sarcomere. With maximum interdigitation, there is a maximal force of contraction. The force of active contracture is diminished if

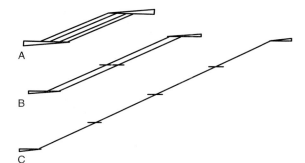

Figure 1.47. (A) Four muscle fibers in parallel. (B) Two muscle fibers in parallel, each twice the length of fibers in A. (C) One muscle fiber, four times as long as fibers in A. System A can exert four times the tension of C. System C has four times the excursion of A. Systems A, B, and C are each capable of the same amount of work. (Work = tension × excursion.)

the molecules are pulled apart or pushed too close together, thus losing the interdigitations by "bunching up" the molecules.

The sarcomeres are arranged in two ways in muscle (Figure 1.47):

• they are lined up in a series one after another and in this way determine the length of a muscle fiber—this directly affects the distance through which a muscle can contract (its excursion); and

• they are positioned next to one another in parallel, thus establishing the cross-sectional area of a muscle—this determines the overall force or tension that the muscle can generate.

Muscle tension is created not only by active contracture of its sarcomeres, but also by passive recoil. When a muscle is stretched, it stores potential energy, much like an elastic band. When released, the muscle contracts. This is an elastic, completely passive contracture, not an active one. It is therefore not under nervous system control but nevertheless plays an important role in the total muscle tension. Figure 1.48 shows the relationship between length and tension in a muscle fiber during passive stretch alone and active contraction alone. Figure 1.49 shows the Blix curve, which combines the

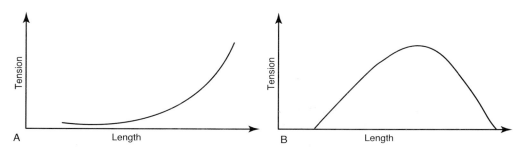

Figure 1.48. (A) General shape of the length–tension curve of a muscle when it is passively stretched. The muscle may require only a little tension to result in lengthening when it is close to the resting length of the muscle. It will require more tension to produce less lengthening as it gets near its elastic limit. (B) General shape of active contraction of a muscle fiber. Muscle fiber produces its highest tension at its resting length and less active tension when it gets shorter or longer.

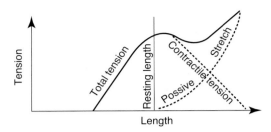

Figure 1.49. Basic concept of the Blix curve.

two. Note the high tensions created with increasing length; most of this is a result of the passive components and is therefore not under voluntary control.

The muscles of the hand are customarily divided into two groups: the intrinsic and the extrinsic muscles. One may add a third group, namely, the muscles of the wrist. Both the origins and the insertions of the intrinsic muscles are in the hand, whereas the origins of the extrinsic muscles are in the arm and forearm and the insertions are in the hand. This topographic distinction has only limited value functionally, however, because each movement is the result of many muscular actions.

Numerous muscles power the movements of the hand and wrist—20 extrinsic muscles (five muscles for the movements of pronation-supination, six for the movements of the wrist, and nine for flexion or extension of the digits) and 19 intrinsic muscles that permit the independent action of each phalanx. (The physical examination of each of these muscles is described in Section 2.3.) Over and above the details of their anatomical insertions, the examiner needs to know the movement generated by each muscle, its stabilizing role in controlling an articulation, its force, and the excursion of its tendon. Knowledge of these motions is particularly valuable when one is planning to re-establish the action of a muscle or a group of muscles through a transfer.

The actions of the individual muscles of the hand were hard to interpret when we were limited to clinical or anatomical information. The development of electrical stimulation (Duchenne, 1867) and electromyography has brought a great degree of precision to the study of normal function. The muscles involved in free movement of the digits, power grip, and precision movements are not the same.

Muscle power

The power of a healthy muscle depends on the number of the muscle fibers and on their angle of insertion into the tendon. Muscular contraction becomes stronger as the number of fibers is increased and as the angle with its tendon diminishes (Zachary, 1946).

Evaluation of muscular force lacks precision. Since each movement involves several muscles, dynamic methods that used to be at our disposal were not sufficiently selective; electric methods should allow a more precise evaluation.

The method usually used to calculate muscular force has been that developed by Fick (1911) and Steindler (1940) in their anatomical studies. According to these authors:

$$\text{Force of a muscle} \quad = \quad \frac{\text{cross-sectional area of the muscle in square centimetres}}{} \quad \times \quad \text{coefficient}$$

The coefficient is 10 kg.cm^{-2} with the Fick method and 3.65 kg.cm^{-2} with the Steindler method. The figures most often cited for the strengths of the extrinsic muscles of the hand are those of von Lanz and Wachsmuth (1959), who themselves cite Fick (1911). Their values in kilogram.meters are given in Table 1.1 (Boyes, 1962).

The following figures have been calculated by Fahrer (1981b) for the thenar muscles: abductor pollicis brevis, 0.50; opponens pollicis, 0.40; flexor pollicis brevis, 0.50; and adductor pollicis, 1.50. These figures are open to the following criticisms:

1 The value for the force of a muscle is obtained by multiplying the physiological surface area by a coefficient. The physiological surface is difficult to measure with precision because the muscle fibers are seldom parallel. As for the coefficient, its value is quite arbitrary.

2 The values are given in terms of working power, i.e. kg.m. In mechanical terms, working power is defined as the force of a muscle, expressed in kilograms, multiplied

Muscle	Strength (kg.m)
Brachioradialis	1.9
Pronator teres	1.2
Extensor carpi radialis brevis	1.1
Extensor carpi radialis longus	0.9
Extensor carpi ulnaris	1.1
Flexor carpi radialis	0.8
Flexor carpi ulnaris	2.0
Palmaris longus	0.1
Flexor pollicis longus	1.2
Extensor pollicis longus	0.1
Abductor pollicis longus	
as a wrist flexor	0.1
as a wrist abductor	0.4
Extensor pollicis brevis	0.1
Flexor digitorum superficialis	4.8
Flexor digitorum profundus communis	4.5
Extensor digitorum communis	1.7
Extensor indicis proprius	0.5

Table 1.1. Strength values of the extrinsic muscles of the hand

by the distance of displacement of its insertion, expressed in meters. The displacement of the insertion is represented by the tendon excursion. Thus, a muscle developing a force of 50 kg whose tendon moves 5 cm will do the same work as a muscle developing a force of 100 kg whose tendon moves only 2.5 cm. It would be more useful to have these evaluations in kilogram.force units or in newtons and not in kg.m (Fahrer and Pineau, 1976).

The values of the cross-section as calculated by Fick are not absolute. Fahrer and Pineau (1976), for example, reported a mean value of 12 cm^2 on one cadaver, compared to 21 cm^2 given by Fick for the flexor digitorum superficialis. When the limb is at rest, the muscles are balanced, and the muscles fibers (and therefore the sarcomeres) assume what is defined as their resting lengths. This is also the length at which the greatest tension can be produced by active contraction.

Muscle excursion
Resting length is approximately equal to the distance between maximal stretch and maximal contracture of a fiber. This is called the potential excursion. At the two extremes of its potential excursion, the ability of a muscle to form an active contraction will be close to zero. This is a useful parameter because it can be measured with ease, and the relative potential excursions allow comparison of muscles. However, this excursion is theoretical and does not reflect *in vivo* conditions (e.g. soft tissue constraints in normal and unhealthy tissues), nor does it reflect the range of excursion in which there is useful muscle contraction.

Two other terms are therefore useful when considering muscle excursion:

• The required excursion (Brand, 1985), or that necessary to move all the joints that a muscle–tendon unit crosses through the full range of motion; and
• The available excursion (Freehafer et al, 1979), which is a measure of the maximum excursion of a muscle that has been freed from its insertion.

Required and available excursion are usually approximately equal for a muscle. Available excursion is dependent on the soft tissue restraints of paratenon. Connective tissue and collagen can be increased by stretching exercises or decreased by post-traumatic or postoperative adhesions.

Muscle fiber length
Muscle fiber length must not be confused with muscle length. Certain muscles have fibers almost equal to the length of the muscle and therefore have the maximum potential for excursion. The lumbricals are an example. When additional strength is necessary, this arrangement becomes unsatisfactory, as many fibers would be necessary to generate the required strength and would give unwieldy bulk to the muscle, especially with contraction. Therefore, most extrinsic muscles of the hand have long tendons with shorter muscle fibers inserting along a certain portion of the length of insertion in the forearm. In this way a strong muscle is created, and the diminished bulk is exchanged for the decreased excursion that results with shorter fibers.

Relative strength

The absolute strength of muscles varies considerably between individuals and can change with exercise in the same person. However, the relative strength of the forearm muscles does not change very much between individuals.

Observations made by Brand et al (1981) in cadaver arms are reproduced in Tables 1.2 and 1.3. These compare three parameters:

- the mass fraction, which is related to the relative amount of work performed by each muscle (recall that work is the force generated by a muscle multiplied by the distance through which it moves);
- the tension fraction, which is a reflection of the cross-sectional area; and
- the resting fiber length, which is related to the potential muscle excursion.

This information is helpful for choosing muscles for transfer.

Tendons

Muscles generate the tension and create excursion, but tendons are responsible for transmitting the muscle work to the part of the skeleton that is to be moved. To facilitate discussion of the properties of tendons, certain commonly used terms must be defined.

Axis of a joint

When bones move around each other at a joint there is a line, usually through one of the bones, that remains stationary (i.e. that does not change its relationship to either bone throughout the arc of motion). This is the axis of the joint. There is an axis for each plane of joint motion, and that axis is perpendicular to the plane of motion. A joint that has more than one plane of motion will have more than one axis. Joints may have axes for flexion–extension, abduction–adduction, and rotation.

Forces and vectors

Forces must be thought of as having magnitude and direction. Vectors, used as diagrammatic expressions of these properties of forces, are practical tools, as they can be geometrically combined to determine resultant forces or broken down into component vectors, which are useful for determining the effect a force will have on a particular joint. The aspect of a force perpendicular to the bone in a given plane of motion will be that part of the force responsible for movement through the joint in that plane.

Moment and torque

The effect that a force has on the movement of a bone is called the moment of the force. In general, because we are referring to circular movement around the joint axis, the term becomes equivalent to torque.

Moment is different from force because it takes into account the point of application of the force. The distance between the joint axis and the point of application of the force on the bone (which is the lever arm in the musculoskeletal system) is called the moment

Muscle	Resting fiber length (cm) Mean*	Mass fraction (%) Mean*	SD*	Tension fraction (%) Mean*
Abductor digiti quinti	4.0	1.1	0.23	1.4
Adductor pollicis	3.6	2.1	0.40	3.0
Abductor pollicis brevis	3.7	0.8	0.18	1.1
Abductor pollicis longus	4.6	2.8	0.34	3.1
Brachioradialis	16.1	7.7	2.00	2.4
shortest fibers	10.9			
longest fibers	21.3			
First dorsal interosseous				
first metacarpal origin	3.1	0.8	0.25	1.3
second metacarpal origin	1.6	0.6	0.11	1.9
total first dorsal interosseous	2.5	1.4	0.29	3.2
Second dorsal interosseous	1.4	0.7	0.17	2.5
Third dorsal interosseous	1.5	0.6	0.19	2.0
Fourth dorsal interosseous	1.5	0.5	0.13	1.7
Extensor carpi radialis brevis	6.1	5.1	1.30	4.2
Extensor carpi radialis longus	9.3	6.5	0.77	3.5
shortest fibers	6.3			
longest fibers	12.3			
Extensor carpi ulnaris	4.5	4.0	0.52	4.5
Extensor digitorum communis				
index finger	5.5	1.1	0.20	1.0
middle finger	6.0	2.2	0.51	1.9
ring finger	5.8	2.0	0.35	1.7
little finger	5.9	1.0	0.41	0.9
Extensor digiti quinti	5.9	1.2	0.35	1.0
Extensor indicis proprius	5.5	1.1	0.36	1.0
Extensor pollicis brevis	4.3	0.7	0.32	0.8
Extensor pollicis longus	5.7	1.5	0.48	1.3
Flexor carpi radialis	5.2	4.2	0.87	4.1
Flexor carpi ulnaris	5.2	5.6	0.66	6.7
Flexor digitorum profundus				
index finger	6.6	3.5	0.76	2.7
middle finger	6.6	4.4	0.94	3.4
ring finger	6.8	4.1	1.10	3.0
little finger	6.2	3.4	0.93	2.8

Muscle	Resting fiber length (cm) Mean*	Mass fraction (%) Mean*	Mass fraction (%) SD*	Tension fraction (%) Mean*
Flexor digitorum superficialis				
index finger	7.2	2.9	0.64	2.0
middle finger	7.0	4.7	1.10	3.4
ring finger	7.3	3.0	0.84	2.0
little finger	7.0	1.3	0.81	0.9
Flexor digiti quinti	3.4	0.3	0.10	0.4
Flexor pollicis brevis	3.6	0.9	0.22	1.3
Flexor pollicis longus	5.9	3.2	0.42	2.7
Lumbrical				
index finger	5.5	0.2	0.08	0.2
middle finger	6.6	0.2	0.06	0.2
ring finger	6.0	0.1	0.06	0.1
little finger	4.9	0.1	0.05	0.1
Opponens digiti quinti	1.5†	0.6	0.20	2.0
Opponens pollicis	2.4†	0.9	0.26	1.9
Palmar interosseous				
first	1.5	0.4	0.12	1.3
second	1.7	0.4	0.11	1.2
third	1.5	0.3	0.08	1.0
Pollicis longus	5.0	1.2	0.34	1.2
Pronator quadratus	3.0†	1.8	0.32	3.0
Pronator teres	5.1	5.6	1.24	5.5
superficial fibers	6.5			
deep fibers	3.7			
Supinator	2.7†	3.8	0.95	7.1

*Data from 15 hands determined the mean and standard deviation of the mass fraction for each muscle. Mass and fiber length measurements from the last five of these hands were used to calculate tension fractions.
†The fibers of these four muscles cross the joint axis with wide variation in fiber length. The figures quoted here for the mean fiber length of these four muscles are more visual estimates than mathematical averages. The mass fraction is accurate, but the tension fraction for these four muscles is only as true as the fiber length. Mean fiber lengths are included for the shortest and longest fibers of BR, ECRL, and PT because of the large range of fiber lengths. Values are included for the two segments of the first DI, as well as total values. The data were not normalized for skeletal size differences.

Table 1.2. Alphabetical reference list of normal expected values for fiber length, mass fraction, and tension fraction in adult males and females (Brand et al, 1981)

Muscle	Mean resting fiber length (cm)	Muscle	Mass fraction (%)	Muscle	Tension fraction (%)
Brachioradialis	16.1	Brachioradialis	7.7	Supinator*	7.1
Extensor carpi radialis longus	9.3	Extensor carpi radialis longus	6.5	Flexor carpi ulnaris	6.7
Flexor digitorum superficialis (ring finger)	7.3	Flexor carpi ulnaris	5.6	Pronator teres*	5.5
Flexor digitorum superficialis (index finger)	7.2	Pronator teres	5.6	Extensor carpi ulnaris	4.5
Flexor digitorum superficialis (little finger)	7.0	Extensor carpi radialis brevis	5.1	Extensor carpi radialis brevis	4.2
Flexor digitorum superficialis (middle finger)	7.0	Flexor digitorum superficialis (middle finger)	4.7	Flexor carpi radialis	4.1
Flexor digitorum profundus (ring finger)	6.8	Flexor digitorum profundus (middle finger)	4.4	Extensor carpi radialis longus	3.5
Flexor digitorum profundus (index finger)	6.6	Flexor carpi radialis	4.2	Flexor digitorum profundus (middle finger)	3.4
Flexor digitorum profundus (middle finger)	6.6	Flexor digitorum profundus (ring finger)	4.1	Flexor digitorum superficialis (middle finger)	3.4
Lumbrical (middle finger)	6.6	Extensor carpi ulnaris	4.0	First dorsal interosseous	3.2
Flexor digitorum profundus (little finger)	6.2	Supinator	3.8	Abductor pollicis longus	3.1
Extensor carpi radialis brevis	6.1	Extensor digitorum profundus (index finger)	3.5	Adductor pollicis	3.0
Extensor digitorum communis (middle finger)	6.0	Flexor digitorum profundus (little finger)	3.4	Flexor digitorum profundus (ring finger)	3.0
Lumbrical (ring finger)	6.0	Flexor pollicis longus	3.2	Pronator quadratus*	3.0
Extensor digitorum communis (little finger)	5.9	Flexor digitorum superficialis (ring finger)	3.0	Flexor digitorum profundus (little finger)	2.8
Extensor digiti quinti	5.9	Flexor digitorum superficialis (index finger)	2.9	Flexor digitorum profundus (index finger)	2.7
Flexor pollicis longus	5.9	Abductor pollicis longus	2.8	Flexor pollicis longus	2.7
Extensor digitorum communis (ring finger)	5.8	Extensor digitorum communis (middle finger)	2.2	Second dorsal interosseous	2.5
Extensor pollicis longus	5.7	Adductor pollicis	2.1	Brachioradialis	2.4
Extensor digitorum communis (index finger)	5.5	Extensor digitorum communis (ring finger)	2.0	Third dorsal interosseous	2.0
Extensor indicis proprius	5.5	Pronator quadratus	1.8	Flexor digitorum superficialis (index finger)	2.0
Lumbrical (index finger)	5.5	Extensor pollicis longus	1.5	Flexor digitorum superficialis (ring finger)	2.0
Flexor carpi radialis	5.2	First dorsal interosseous	1.4	Opponens digiti quinti*	2.0
Pronator teres	5.1	Flexor digitorum superficialis (little finger)	1.3	Extensor digitorum communis (middle finger)	1.9
Pollicis longus	5.0	Extensor digiti quinti	1.2	Opponens pollicis*	1.9
Lumbrical (little finger)	4.9	Pollicis longus	1.2	Fourth dorsal interosseous	1.7

Muscle	Value	Muscle	Value	Muscle	Value
Abductor pollicis longus	4.6	Abductor digiti quinti	1.1	Extensor digitorum communis (ring finger)	1.7
Extensor carpi ulnaris	4.5	Extensor digitorum communis (index finger)	1.1	Abductor digiti quinti	1.4
Extensor pollicis brevis	4.3	Extensor indicis proprius	1.1	Extensor pollicis longus	1.3
Flexor carpi ulnaris	4.2	Extensor digitorum communis (little finger)	1.0	Flexor pollicis brevis	1.3
Abductor digiti quinti	4.0	Opponens pollicis	0.9	First palmar interosseous	1.3
Abductor pollicis brevis	3.7	Flexor pollicis brevis	0.9	Second palmar interosseous	1.2
Adductor pollicis	3.6	Abductor pollicis brevis	0.9	Pollicis longus	1.2
Flexor pollicis brevis	3.6	Second dorsal interosseous	0.7	Abductor pollicis brevis	1.1
Flexor digiti quinti	3.4	Extensor pollicis brevis	0.7	Extensor digitorum communis (index finger)	1.0
Pronator quadratus	3.0	Third dorsal interosseous	0.6	Extensor digiti quinti	1.0
Supinator	2.7	Opponens digiti quinti	0.6	Extensor indicis proprius	1.0
First dorsal interosseous	2.5	Fourth dorsal interosseous	0.5	Third palmar interosseous	1.0
Opponens pollicis	2.4	First palmar interosseous	0.4	Extensor digitorum communis (little finger)	0.9
Second palmar interosseous	1.7	Second palmar interosseous	0.4	Flexor digitorum superficialis (little finger)	0.9
Third dorsal interosseous	1.5	Flexor digiti quinti	0.3	Extensor pollicis brevis	0.8
Fourth dorsal interosseous	1.5	Third palmar interosseous	0.3	Flexor digiti quinti	0.4
Opponens digiti quinti	1.5	Lumbrical (index finger)	0.2	Lumbrical (index finger)	0.2
First palmar interosseous	1.5	Lumbrical (middle finger)	0.2	Lumbrical (middle finger)	0.2
Third palmar interosseous	1.5	Lumbrical (ring finger)	0.1	Lumbrical (ring finger)	0.1
Second dorsal interosseous	1.4	Lumbrical (little finger)	0.1	Lumbrical (little finger)	0.1

*See † footnote for Table 1.

Table 1.3. Normal values listed in order of magnitude for mean fiber length, mass fraction, and tension fraction for adults (Brand et al, 1981)

arm of that force if the force is perpendicular to the lever. However, in general, forces that move the bones (e.g. forces created by muscles) are not perpendicular to the bone. In these cases, the perpendicular component of the force must be used to calculate the moment. One can use the perpendicular distance between the joint axis and the force as the moment arm. This is geometrically equivalent and easier to conceptualize (Figure 1.50). Thus:

moment = force × perpendicular moment arm

Hereafter, the term moment arm is used to refer to the perpendicular moment arm.

Mechanical advantage

To maintain a state of equilibrium around a joint, the sum of the moments (torque) acting around it must be equal. If two forces act at different distances from a joint (i.e. that have different moment arms), one of them will have a mechanical advantage. This is defined as the moment arm of one force acting at a joint divided by the moment arm of a second force acting in the same plane around that joint.

Amplitude of tendon excursion

The amplitude of gliding of a tendon depends especially on muscular contraction. The amplitude of contraction of a muscle reflects the muscle's ability to shorten as its fibers retract, and is about one third the length of the muscle's resting fleshy belly. It also is a function of the direction of its fibers. The amplitude increases if the fibers are longer and if the angle they make with the tendon is acute (Zachary, 1946).

The amplitude of tendon excursion is also controlled by other factors, such as the adherence of muscle to its aponeurosis, the freedom of gliding of the tendon with its paratenon, the changes in the direction around a pulley, and the crossing of one or more articulations. Also the amplitude of gliding of the tendons of the extrinsic muscles

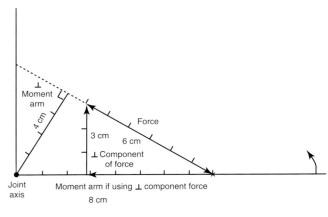

Figure 1.50. Force is divided into two components. The vertical one is perpendicular to the lever arm to be moved. The point of application of force is marked with an X. Either of the two methods indicated can be used to determine the moment of force around the joint axis.

of the hand varies in the same tendon, depending on its physical and metabolic integrity and on the level at which it is measured. Thus, the extensor digitorum has an amplitude of approximately 4 mm at the distal interphalangeal joint, 8 mm at the proximal interphalangeal joint, 15 mm at the metacarpophalangeal joint, and 45 mm at the wrist. The flexor tendons of the fingers have a much larger excursion. According to Verdan (1976), the amplitude of gliding is 5 mm for the profundus at the distal interphalangeal joint and, for the superficialis and profundus, respectively, 16 mm and 17 mm at the proximal interphalangeal joint, 26 mm and 23 mm for the profundus at the metacarpophalangeal joint, 46 mm and 38 mm at the carpal canal, and 88 mm and 85 mm in the distal forearm. These values are slightly greater than those noted by Boyes (1970). Large variations certainly exist from person to person.

The maximal excursion for each tendon in the adult is as shown in Table 1.4 (Boyes, 1970). Note that the motor muscles of the wrist have a tendinous excursion of approximately 3.5 cm. The common extensor of the fingers and the long flexor of the thumb have an excursion of approximately 4–5 cm, and the tendons of the long flexors of the fingers have the greatest excursion of all the muscles in the hand.

All the notions of topographical relationships of the muscles, their relative strengths, and their tendinous excursions are insufficient for appreciation of the movements. The muscles are not controlled individually: "Movements, not muscles, are represented in the cerebral cortex" (Wood-Jones, 1942). No muscle works alone, and the simplest action always requires the participation of antagonists. Movements are determined by the modulation of their respective forces. This is the important concept of "synergistic antagonism," which states that all movements are merely the result of a "displacement of dynamic equilibrium" between two or more muscles or groups of muscles (Kapandji, 1963).

Tendon	Maximal excursion (cm)
Pronator teres	5.0
Extensor carpi radialis brevis	3.7
Extensor carpi radialis longus	3.7
Flexor carpi radialis	4.0
Flexor carpi ulnaris	3.3
Flexor pollicis longus	5.0
Extensor pollicis brevis	2.8
Extensor pollicis longus	5.0
Abductor pollicis longus	2.8
Flexor digitorum profundus	7.0
Flexor digitorum superficialis	6.4
Extensor digitorum	4.5

Table 1.4. Maximal excursion of the tendons in the adult hand according to Bunnell (1956)

Movements of the functional units

The movements of the hand may be schematically divided into movements of the wrist, movements of the fingers, and movements of the thumb.

Movements of the wrist

"The wrist is the key joint of the hand" (Bunnell). The study of the wrist and forearm is inseparable from that of the hand. From the elbow distally, there is only one physiological unit. For example, in pronation–supination the movement of the radius in relation to the ulna is in fact the movement of the hand around its longitudinal axis.

Wrist movements occur around three principal functional axes: longitudinal, transverse, and anteroposterior. Yet all these movements are complex and are not restricted to a fixed geometric axis.

Pronation–supination: the movement of longitudinal rotation

Schematically, the radius forms an arched bone which moves around the ulna in pronation. The distal radioulnar joint cannot be dissociated mechanically from the proximal radio-ulnar joint. Their stability and function depend on the length of the two bones, on a constant distance between radius and ulna to maintain ligaments and muscle tension, and the respect of the pronation curvature of the radius (Bonnel and Allieu, 1984). A diminution of the length of the ulna of 2 mm or a lengthening of 2.5 mm entails a corresponding variation in the transmission of forces of 5% to 40% (Palmer, 1987). For Hagert (1992) the proximal and distal radio-ulnar joints together form a bicondylar joint "the forearm joint". The proximal condyle, the radial head, rotates axially whereas the distal condyle, the ulnar head, is fixed with respect to rotation. The mobile radius is distally attached to the stable ulnar head, and the ulnar head serves as a keystone, carrying the load of the radius. Resection of the ulnar head deprives the wrist of its keystone. In fact, the radius does not revolve around a fixed axis of the distal ulna in this movement. The distal ulna itself moves in a small circle, within the arch of the radius, opposite in direction and situated in a more posterior plane (Capener, 1956; Vallois, 1926). In effect, the real axis of the hand and forearm for this motion may be situated anywhere between the radial and ulnar styloid according to each respective arc (Figure 1.51). Thus there is not one but many pronation–supinations (Kapandji, 1963).

The results of the preceding studies (see pages 33–36) are important for the management of the fractures of the forearm:

1 The equality of length of the two bones must be preserved.
2 Following a fracture of the distal radius (Figure 1.52), the ulnar head will no longer be congruent to the sigmoid notch of the radius due to the displacement of the radius into dorsal and radial angulation. The TFCC will also be ruptured to some extent at least involving disruption of the dorsal portion of the TFCC, the part that stabilizes the joint in supination. Thus the reduction of the displacement must be perfect.

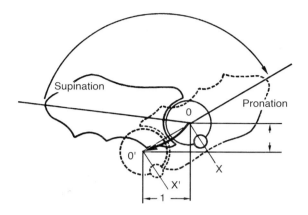

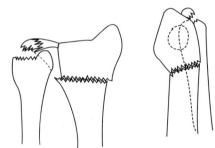

Figure 1.51. Pronation–supination at the wrist level. Pronation–supination is a complex movement that mobilizes the lower end of the radius and ulna. The radius undergoes a rotation of almost 180 degrees, and the ulna undergoes a movement on the arc of a circle. The center of these two movements has no fixed location. It is located somewhere in the distal end of the ulna, but the axis of pronation–supination is variable, not only from movement to movement but also during the course of the same movement.

Figure 1.52. Feature of the distal extremity of the forearm with displacement. The ulnar head is no longer congruent to the sigmoid notch of the radius.

3 The stability on a well reduced extra-articular fracture is optimal with the forearm immobilized in pronation.

4 A fracture with displacement of the ulnar styoid process must be reduced and stabilized.

5 Resection of the ulnar head should be avoided.

6 After a malunited fracture of the distal radius, or of any site of the radius or ulna, the DRUJ function should be restored if necessary by corrective osteotomy wherever possible.

Movement of the hand on the forearm

This brings into play the two series of articulations of the wrist—the radiocarpal and the midcarpal. These articulations allow motion into two axes: anteroposterior in flexion–extension and transverse in lateral deviation. These movements are complicated by the morphology of the wrist, which is a zone of architectural transition between the two bones of the forearm and the five metacarpals forming the palmar concavity necessary to facilitate opposition of the thumb. The anterior concavity of the wrist also plays an important role in balancing the forces of the long tendons in the synergistic action of the finger flexors and the extensors of the wrist (see Figure 1.13a).

Proximal row and distal row

The eight bones of the carpus are schematically arranged into a proximal row and a distal row, although the scaphoid straddles the lunate–capitate interspace, articulating with both the trapezoid and the trapezium (see Figure 1.11). Destot (1923) likened the distal aspect of the two bones of the forearm with the triangular ligament to a third carpal row. He described the scapholunate as a "mobile and supple meniscus," since the articulations of its component bones are united by the interosseous ligaments. These permit the bones to arrange themselves according to wrist movements.

Extensive carpal mobility would be impossible without scapholunate action, as was first described by Henke (1859). Later Fick (1901, 1911) described the mutual displacement of the ossicles as indispensable in allowing the proximal row to articulate with the distal row. He offered the hypothesis that the scaphoid always maintains contact with the trapezium by flexing and pivoting. According to Destot, "the scapholunate joint appears essential" not only for the physiology of the wrist, but also because "all the traumatic pathology of the wrist concentrates in the lesions of these ossicles." This is now accepted as being only partially true.

The bones of the proximal row do not form a simple articular surface opposed to the articular surface of the forearm bones and moving around two well defined axes. The motion of each of its ossicles should be studied individually. Navarro (1937), Landsmeer (1968, 1976), and Kauer (1964), among others, have compared the mechanism of the carpus to that of longitudinal parallel chains (Figure 1.53):

1 An external chain is composed of the radius, scaphoid, and trapezium prolonged by the column of the thumb.
2 A middle chain is formed by the radius, lunate, capitate, and the third metacarpal. The lunate tilts slightly toward the ulnar side so that a small part of its proximal articular surface lies in contact with the triangular ligament. These two chains are connected by the scapholunate ligament whose fibers of unequal length allow the mutual displacement of the two ossicles, and by the capitate, which articulates with

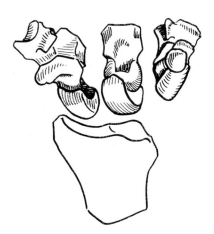

Figure 1.53. The carpus can be considered as three longitudinal columns: the radial column comprises the scaphoid, trapezium, and trapezoid; the intermediate column comprises the lunate and capitate; and the ulnar column is formed by the triquetrum and the hamate. Only the radial and intermediate columns articulate with the articular surface of the radius.

the scaphoid and the lunate through two distinct articular facets. In a sense, then, the scaphoid and the lunate are "intercalary" bones.

3 Finally, the medial chain formed by the triquetrum and the hamate constitutes the axis of pronosupination. It has been called the column of rotation (Taleisnik, 1976).

Taleisnik points out that the distal row of the carpus can be regarded as a single anatomical and functional unit that, with the lunate, makes up the central column of flexion–extension. This leaves the scaphoid as the only mobile part of the lateral column and the triquetrum as the only part of the medial column (Figure 1.54).

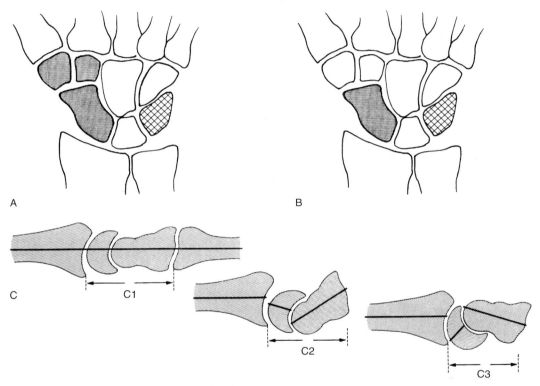

Figure 1.54. The columnar or vertical carpus. The carpal bones are grouped into three vertical columns. (A) According to Navarro (1937), the lateral or mobile column is composed of the scaphoid, trapezium, and trapezoid; the central or flexion–extension column is formed by the lunate, capitate, and hamate; and the medial or rotation column is composed of the triquetrum. (B) A modification of this concept (Taleisnik, 1976). The central column is expanded to include the lunate and the four distal bones, reducing the lateral column to the scaphoid. The central column forms, with the radius, a longitudinal three-segment link. Each column is a functional unit. This concept helps in understanding the physiology and pathology of the wrist. It has practical applications in the treatment of instability of the wrist and avascular necrosis of the carpolunate joint. (C) The lunate and capitate are intercalary bones between the radius and the third metacarpal. In pathological situations these bones are displaced in flexion or extension, according to the location of ligamentous changes. Schematically, in the course of rheumatoid arthritis, the lunate rocks into flexion (VISI: volar intercalated segment instability), whereas in traumatic ligamentous conditions, it levers into extension (dorsal: DISI) (Linscheid and Dobyns, 1971). The tilt of the carpus is accompanied by a shortening of the distance between the radius and the metacarpals. C1, normal; C2, VISI; C3, DISI.

The assimilation of the carpal bones into chains of longitudinal bones permits an explanation of opposite displacements after certain traumatic lesions or in rheumatoid arthritis.

Lateral movements

It must be noted that there is a physiological ulnar deviation at rest, easily demonstrated clinically and radiologically. The collateral movements of the wrist have an ulnar amplitude of approximately 40 degrees and a radial amplitude not greater than 15 degrees (Figure 1.55). The muscle with the best momentum for ulnar deviation of the wrist in pronation is the extensor carpi ulnaris; the abductor pollicis longus and extensor pollicis brevis have the best momentum for abduction of the wrist. This motion occurs at the radiocarpal articulation as well as at the mid-carpal level, but in different proportions: 55 to 60 per cent

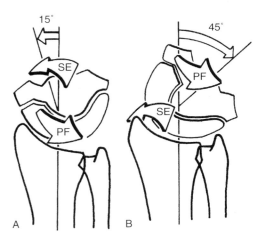

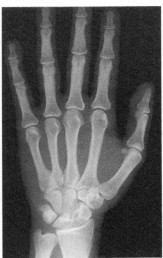

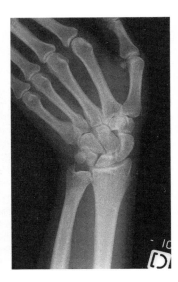

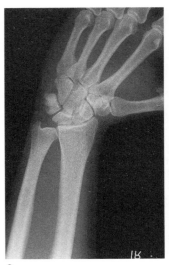

Figure 1.55. Lateral movements of the wrist. Abduction (radial inclination) and adduction (ulnar inclination) of the wrist consist of movements occurring at the radiocarpal joint and midcarpal joints. (A) During abduction, the proximal row also executes a pronation–flexion (PF) and the distal row a supination–extension movement (SE). (B) During adduction, the movements are in reverse: supination–extension (SE) for the proximal row and pronation–flexion (PF) for the distal row. In both instances these accessory movements cancel each other out. Note that the ulnar inclination is three times the radial inclination. (C) Radiograph views showing complete radial and ulnar inclination.

occurs at the radiocarpal joint in ulnar deviation and 60 to 65 per cent occurs at the midcarpal joint in radial deviation (Kaplan, 1975), but individual variations are considerable. The axis of these movements runs through the capitate (Santos-Gutierez, 1964). However, these movements are not simple inclinations in abduction and adduction. Extension of the wrist facilitates radial deviation, and flexion of the wrist facilitates ulnar deviation (Figure 1.56).

Anteroposterior movements

The anteroposterior movements of flexion and extension of the wrist have a range of approximately 80 degrees in each direction, distributed among the radiocarpal articulation and the mediocarpal articulation in proportions that vary among different studies (Fick, 1911; MacConaill, 1941). These are not simple displacements in flexion or in extension; rotation and a rocking motion are present simultaneously.

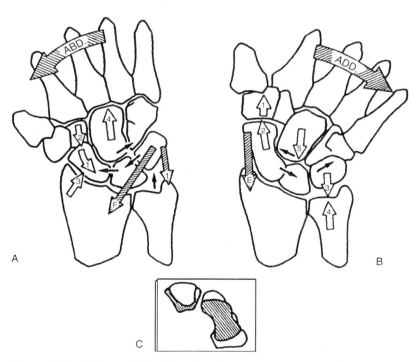

Figure 1.56. (A) In radial deviation, the ulnar displacement of the proximal carpal row is checked by band F of the ulnar collateral ligament such that the distal row continues to turn; the scaphoid (1) is compressed between the distal radius (3) and the trapezium (2), and the lunate is blocked by the triquetrum. Simultaneously, the capitate (4) is pulled distally, allowing greater space for the lunate. (B) In ulnar deviation the trapezium (1) moves distally, checked by the radial collateral ligament (E), allowing the scaphoid (2) to assume a more vertical position. The triquetrum is limited by the ulnar head (4) and triangular ligament, and the capitate (5) compresses the lunate, which tilts in a volar direction. (C) The variations in functional distance of the two bones are clearly seen when superimposed (hatched) between radial (gray) and ulnar (clear) deviation.

Wrist kinematics

Valuable contributions to our understanding of wrist mechanics have been made by Dobyns and Linscheid, Kapandji, Kuhlmann, Landsmeer and Kauer, Lichtman, Taleisnik, Weber, Youm and Flatt.

Radial deviation (Figure 1.56a)

As the wrist moves from ulnar to radial deviation, the triquetrum translocates radially and dorsally on the slope of the hamate (Figure 1.57). As this occurs, the lunate is brought coaxially with the capitate as the triquetrum enters the mid-zone on the hamate articulation. Simultaneously the axis of the scaphoid flexes to its neutral position. As radial deviation is continued from the neutral position, the triquetrum continues to translate up the slope of the hamate. As the last 10 degrees of radial deviation is achieved, the triquetrum enters the radial dorsal facet of the hamate articulation. As this occurs, the lunate, by virtue of its ligamentous attachments with the triquetrum, is brought dorsal to the axis of the capitate, and compressive forces transmitted through the capitate cause the lunate to go into slight palmar flexion.

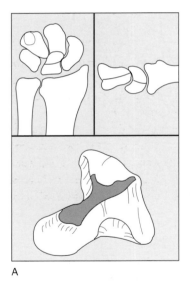 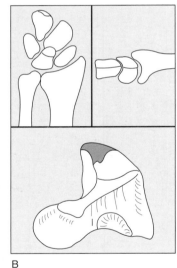

A   B

Figure 1.57. Wrist kinematics.

(A) Ulnar deviation. (*Top*) Line drawings of the wrist deviated towards the ulna with the axis of the capitate and the lunate added. As the axis of the lunate drops below the axis of the capitate, the lunate goes into dorsiflexion. (*Lower*) Position of the triquetrum on the hamate with the wrist in ulnar deviation. View from ulnar side with volar to the left and distal at the bottom of the photograph. Line drawing of the hamate in the same orientation as above. The shaded area is the volar radial facet that is occupied by the triquetrum in ulnar deviation.

(B) Radial deviation. (*Top*) Line tracings of biplanar x-ray views in radial deviation, demonstrating the change in the relationship between the triquetrum and the hamate and the flexed position of the scaphoid which appears shorter. (*Lower*) The position of the triquetrum on the hamate when the wrist is in full radial deviation. Note that the triquetrum has moved dorsally as well as radially. The shaded area is the radial facet occupied by the triquetrum in radial deviation.

Ulnar deviation (Figure 1.56b)

As the hand moves from neutral position to ulnar deviation, the triquetrum is translated ulnarly on the slope of the hamate (Figure 1.57). Because of the relative volar position of the hamate's ulnar facet, the triquetrum is also forced in a palmar direction. This palmar translocation of the triquetrum on the hamate brings the lunate axis palmar to the axis of the capitate. Compressive forces transmitted by the capitate act on the lunate to rotate it into the dorsal facing attitude. This extension of the lunate is transmitted through the scaphoid–lunate articulation by the interosseous ligament and results in elevation of the distal pole of the scaphoid. The extension of the scaphoid is accommodated at the distal scaphoid–trapezium–trapezoid joint.

Extension

When the wrist is extended, the palmar ligaments, radiolunotriquetral and radiocapitate, are stretched, and the radiocapitate ligament which crosses the neck of the scaphoid brings about simultaneous extension of the scaphoid and capitate. This effect is transmitted through the scapholunate ligament and brings the lunate into extension so that the capitate and lunate are co-axial in extension. In contrast, the extension of the scaphoid stops before the lunate stops, which continues to turn by 30 degrees.

Flexion

During the opposite movement of flexion the dorsal ligaments are stretched and the triquetrum is moved towards the radial articular surface of the hamate. The flexion of the mid-carpal joint is more important than the radiocarpal joint, and the capitate is flexed more than the lunate (Figure 1.58). (From Kuhlmann JN et al, 1985.)

Taleisnik (1976) has pointed out that during extension and ulnar deviation the scaphoid becomes longitudinal, the carpus behaves as a single unit, and the wrist motion is predominantly radiocarpal. Conversely, in volar flexion and radial deviation, when the scaphoid position is perpendicular to the long axis of the radius, the mid-carpal joint is "unlocked." Volar flexion and radial deviation are mainly mid-carpal joint motions.

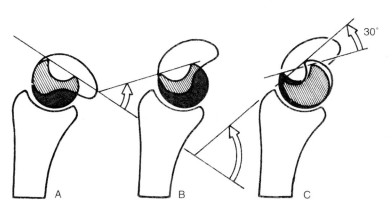

Figure 1.58. The relationship between the scaphoid and lunate in flexion (A) and extreme extension (C). The rotation of the two bones is not equal. The scaphoid extension is maximal in (B), but the lunate dorsiflexes a further 30 degrees (C).

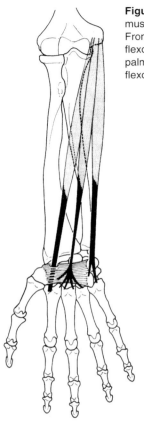

Figure 1.59. The flexor muscles of the wrist. From radial to ulnar: flexor carpi radialis, palmaris longus, and flexor carpi ulnaris.

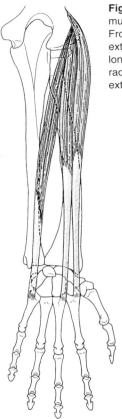

Figure 1.60. Extensor muscles of the wrist. From radial to ulnar: extensor carpi radialis longus, extensor carpi radialis brevis, and extensor carpi ulnaris.

The motion of wrist extension is accompanied by a slight radial deviation and pronation of the forearm. Inversely, the movement of flexion is accompanied by a slight ulnar deviation and supination of the forearm and a synergistic contraction of the biceps, which in effect at the same time limits extension of the elbow (Capener, 1956). Moreover, the position of the wrist in flexion or extension influences the tension of the long or "extrinsic" muscles of the digits, which are "polyarticular" and cross the wrist and finger joints.

The wrist is stabilized by its extrinsic muscles, incorrectly termed "mono-articular." In reality, all the "proper" muscles of the wrist insert beyond the carpus, which constitutes an intercalary system, including the slender and inconstant palmaris longus, whose lateral tendon continues to the base of the proximal phalanx of the thumb (Fahrer and Tubiana, 1976), and the powerful flexor carpi ulnaris, which inserts beyond the pisiform into the fibers continuing with the abductor digiti quinti, thus forming a digastric system (Fahrer, 1975). These "proper" muscles are divided into two groups: three flexor muscles (Figure 1.59) and three antagonistic extensor muscles (Figure 1.60).

Extension of the wrist

Extension of the wrist is functionally more important than its flexion. It reinforces or facilitates the action of the flexor tendons of the fingers. Nothing can replace the extension deficit.

Muscles of wrist extension

Extension of the wrist is dependent on three muscles (Figure 1.60):

- extensor carpi radialis longus (ECRL);
- extensor carpi radialis brevis (ECRB); and
- extensor carpi ulnaris (ECU).

The ECRL, which inserts on the base of the second metacarpal, extends the wrist and draws it into radial deviation.

The ECRB inserts on the radial part of the base of the third metacarpal; this more medial location makes it the primary wrist extensor, but it has also a slight action of radial deviation.

The ECU inserts on the base of the fifth metacarpal and crosses the wrist at the level of the ulna, in contrast to the ECRB and ECRL tendons, which cross at the level of the radius. Furthermore, the ECU tendon rotates around the ulnar head. When the forearm is in pronation, its tendon is situated on the ulnar side of the styloid process, whereas in supination it is on the radial side in a dorsal position closer to the radius (Figure 1.61). Thus the ECU is an extensor of the wrist in supination and primarily causes ulnar deviation of the wrist in pronation. It then works in synergy with the flexor carpi ulnaris and prevents radial deviation during pronation.

ECRB and the ECRL are commonly considered to be similar muscles, but in fact they differ in many respects (Brand, 1985). The ECRL takes its origin at the supracondylar ridge of the humerus about 4–5 cm proximal to the epicondyle, and the thickest part of the muscle is proximal to the elbow joint. It plays a role in elbow flexion and loses a part of its wrist action when the elbow is flexed. In contrast, the ECRB has its origin on the epicondyle and is not affected by the position of the elbow. All of its action is on the wrist. These two tendons are congruent along most of their length in the forearm and often have tendinous connections. However, they diverge distal to the retinaculum so that at their insertions, the center of the ECRL tendon is about 1.5 cm lateral to the center of the ECRB (Figure 1.62).

According to Ketchum and Thomson (1985), the two ECR tendons comprise about 10 per cent of the muscle mass of the forearm and 76 per cent of the muscle mass of the extensors of the wrist. The muscle mass of the ECRB is only 88 per cent when compared with that of the ECRL, but its sole action is on the wrist. The moment arms for extension of the wrist are 16.30 mm for the ECRB and only 12.50 mm for the ECRL (Ketchum et al, 1978). The ECRL has longer muscular fibers, mostly at the level of the elbow.

In the ECRL, the moment arm for elbow flexion and radial deviation is more important than that for wrist extension. The ECRL only becomes a wrist extensor after radial deviation is balanced against the ulnar forces of the ECU. The ECU has the weakest

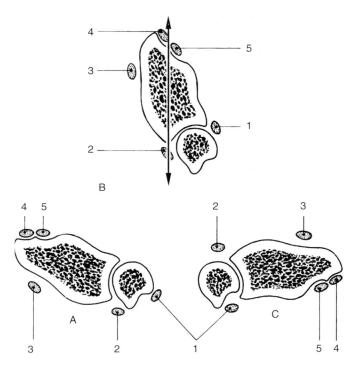

Figure 1.61. Position of the tendons of the flexors and extensors of the wrist during pronation and supination: (1) extensor carpi ulnaris (ECU); (2) flexor carpi ulnaris (FCU); (3) flexor carpi radialis (FCR); (4) extensor carpi radialis longus (ECRL); (5) extensor carpi radialis brevis (ECRB). (A) In pronation, ECRL and RB are extensors of the wrist, and the FCU is a flexor of the wrist. The FCR and ECU are lateral stabilizers. (B) In the neutral position, the axis of movements of the wrist is oblique. This axis is between ECR and FCU. (C) In supination, both the ECR muscles and the ECU act as extensors of the wrist. The FCR and FCU are flexors. The changes in position of the ulna, which are less important than those of the radius, are not shown in these diagrams for the sake of clarity.

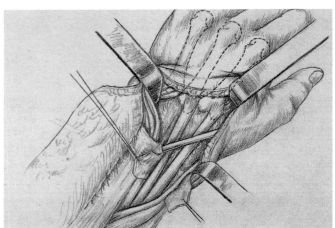

Figure 1.62. Insertion of extensor carpi radialis longus (ECRL) and extensor carpi radialis brevis (ECRB). Distal to the retinaculum, the two tendons diverge. The ECRL inserts on the second metacarpal base, and the ECRB inserts on the third metacarpal base.

moment of extension (6.3 mm in supination), which becomes zero when the wrist is in complete pronation.

Thus the three wrist extensors have very different moment arms of extension. The ECRB is the most effective extensor of the wrist, because it has the greatest tension and the most favorable moment arm. Remember that the most frequently used wrist

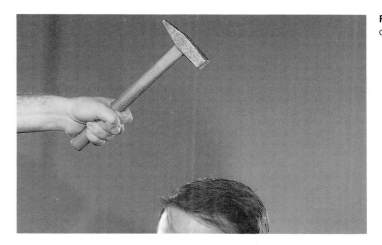

Figure 1.63. Grip power occurs in ulnar deviation.

movements are not those in the axis of flexion–extension, but those in semipronation. The axis of the movements is oblique between the ECRL and ECRB, which produce extension and radial deviation of the wrist, and the flexor carpi ulnaris (FCU), which produces flexion and ulnar deviation of the wrist, explaining the essential importance of this muscle (Figure 1.63). The ECU is the antagonist of extensor pollicis longus (EPL), with the contraction being synergistic; the tension of the ECU is felt when the thumb is abducted.

Effects of loss of wrist extension
Loss of active extension in the wrist constitutes a considerable cosmetic and functional handicap, including the following:

1 A permanent wrist drop (Figure 1.64) that makes gripping with the hand very difficult. Although radial palsy involves only a very small sensory deficit on the dorsal aspect of the hand and palmar surface sensibility is uninvolved, the loss of active extension of the wrist robs this normal palmar sensibility of its functional capacity.
2 Loss of active movement in the wrist, which has serious repercussion on the action of the extrinsic muscles in the hand (Figure 1.65). Flexor action in the thumb and fingers is normally reinforced by extension of the wrist, and therefore palsy of the extensors in the wrist involves a great loss of grip strength. In certain cases this can be the most serious sequela of these palsies.

Wrist movements and the digits
Neither the flexors nor the extensors of the fingers are long enough to allow maximal movements at the wrist and the fingers simultaneously. The restraining action of the long antagonistic muscles explains why complete flexion of the fingers is possible only if the wrist is in slight extension of about 20 degrees (see Figure 1.65). This is the

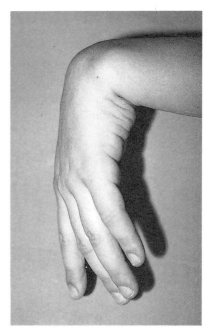

Figure 1.64. Wrist drop (radial palsy).

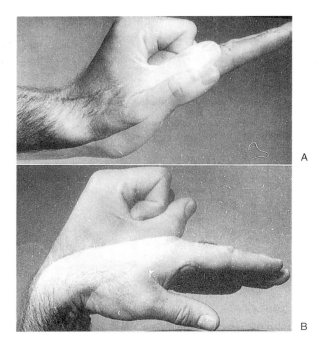

A

B

Figure 1.65. Role of the wrist in positioning of the digits. (A) Extension of the wrist permits full flexion of the digits. The synergistic action of the extensors and flexors of the wrist is made possible by the shape of the transverse carpal arch, which allows the flexor tendons to be kept close to the axis of flexion–extension of the wrist (see Figures 1.13a,b, page 12). If the flexor tendons were displaced volarly, for example by synovitis of the wrist, extension would be reduced and full finger flexion would be impossible. (B) Conversely, wrist flexion places the long extensors under tension and automatically extends the digits.

optimal position for hand function. Conversely, flexion of the wrist puts some tension on the long extensors, resulting in an automatic opening of the fingers.

When the wrist is flexed, the pulp of the thumb reaches the level of the proximal interphalangeal joint of the index finger; when it is in extension, the pulps of the thumb and index finger are passively in contact (Figure 1.66). Thus the position of the wrist has important repercussions on the position of the thumb and fingers. This explains why the movements of the wrist, usually in reverse of the movements of the fingers, reinforce the action of the extrinsic muscles of the fingers. Tenodesis of the motor tendons of the digits, activated by wrist extension, is used in severe paralysis to restore gripping.

Thus the wrist extensors are synergistic with the more powerful digital flexors. The combined movements are facilitated by the architecture of the wrist. The digital flexor tendons cross the wrist within the depths of the carpal arch and are held close to the

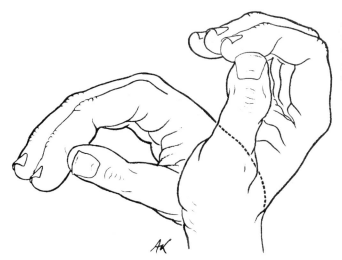

Figure 1.66. When the wrist is flexed, the tip of the thumb is level with the distal interphalangeal joint of the index finger. In wrist extension the pulps of the index finger and thumb come passively into contact.

axis of flexion–extension of the wrist. Therefore, the moment arm in the direction of wrist flexion is minimized, and this allows the wrist extension necessary for full digital flexion (see Figure 1.13). As the wrist position changes, the functional lengths of the digital flexor tendons change and the resultant forces in finger flexion vary. In order for grip to be effective and have maximal force, the wrist must be stable (paralysis of the "proper" wrist muscles, the flexors or extensors, considerably diminishes the force of the digits) and in slight extension and ulnar deviation. In full flexion of the wrist, the grip strength of the hand is 25 per cent of its maximum in extension (Napier, 1966).

Studies with the digital dynamometer and Beckman dynograph recorder have evaluated the effect of wrist position on the force generated at the middle and distal phalanges (Hazelton et al, 1975). The greatest force is exerted is ulnar deviation and then extension; the least force is generated in volar flexion.

The digits in wrist pathology
So far, the influence of wrist position on the more distal joints in the normal hand has been considered. In disease, the wrist position also affects these joints. Thus, lateral deviation of the wrist can involve an opposite deviation of the metacarpophalangeal joint when the stabilizing elements of these joints (lateral ligament and volar plate) are weakened. For example, destruction or distention of the ligaments of the wrist result in ulnar translation of the carpus (Figure 1.67) and radial deviation of the carpometacarpal block: the carpus slides medially on the curve of the distal end of the radius.

The proliferation of rheumatoid synovitis displaces the tendon of the extensor carpi ulnaris forward, and the predominant action of the radial tendons (i.e. the flexor carpi radialis and the extensors carpi radialis longus and brevis) deviates the carpometacarpal

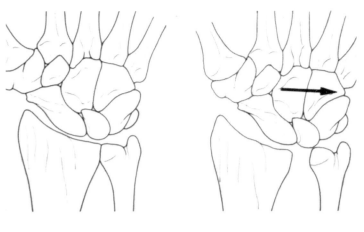

Figure 1.67. Distention of the capsulo-ligamentous structures of the wrist results in ulnar translation of the carpus.

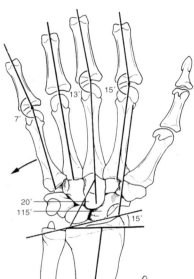

A

Figure 1.68a. The physiological angles between the different skeletal structures of the hand. The articular surface of the distal end of the radius is directed towards the ulna at an angle of approximately 15 degrees. The axis of the lunate forms an angle of approximately 20 degrees with a straight line passing through the capitate and third metacarpal. The axis of the second metacarpal is in line with the longitudinal axis of the radius. The longitudinal axis of the proximal phalanges is inclined towards the ulnar at an angle to the metacarpal axis of approximately 15 degrees for the index finger, 13 degrees for the middle finger, and 7 degrees for the fifth finger. Only the first phalanx of the ring finger is in line with the axis of its metacarpal. The angle between the radial border of the second metacarpal and the lower border of the distal end of the radius is 115 degrees (Shapiro, 1970).

Figure 1.68b and c. Skeletal deformity in rheumatoid arthritis. The carpometacarpal block inclines radially (outward). Shapiro's angle is more than 115 degrees. The proximal phalanges may incline towards the ulnar, thus greatly increasing the digital deformity.

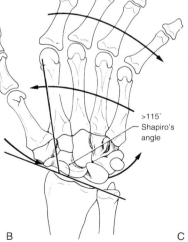

B

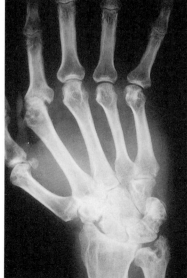

C

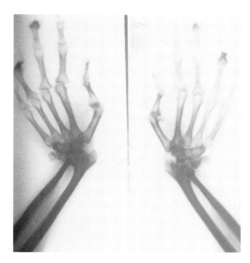

Figure 1.69. Ulnar deviation of the carpometacarpal block in juvenile rheumatoid arthritis. The index and middle fingers of each hand are in radial deviation.

block radially (Figure 1.68b). This inclination increases the angle between the radial border of the second metacarpal and the lower border of the distal radius, which is normally 115 degrees (Shapiro, 1970; Figure 1.68). This radial inclination of the hand causes an important loss of muscular power in the flexors (Hazelton et al, 1975).

The radial deviation of the carpometacarpal block may produce ulnar deviation of the metacarpophalangeal joints because of the interdependence of various articulations in the longitudinal chains (Pahle and Raunio, 1969; Stack and Vaughan-Jackson, 1971). The opposite deviation of the carpometacarpal block, which is seen in juvenile rheumatoid arthritis, may be associated with radial deviation of the digits (Figure 1.69).

Clinically, however, ulnar drift of the metacarpophalangeal articulations often precedes the wrist deformities. This simply means that factors other than deviation of the wrist may be influencing the deviation of the digits.

These concepts of the position of the joints in regard to muscle equilibrium are particularly complex at the digital level (Tubiana and Hakstian, 1969).

All these displacements—carpal ulnar translation and radial deviation, carpal bone shifting, ulnar deviation of the fingers—can be accurately measured whether of traumatic or rheumatoid origin (see Figures 4.7 and 4.8).

Movements of the fingers

Articulations of the fingers

The articulations of the fingers form a triarticular chain that flexes toward the thumb and the palm to allow grasp. This disposition of the fingers in a polyarticular chain permits all varieties of grip, from simple pinch to wrapping around an object. The encompassing movement of the phalanges in going from extension to full flexion

69

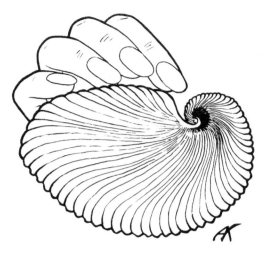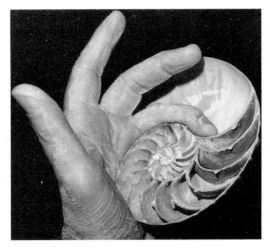

Figure 1.70a and b. The series of Fibonacci and the biological spirals. Fibonacci in 1202 studied the properties of the numerical series 0, 1, 1, 2, 3, 5, 8, 13, 21, . . . (each number is equal to the sum of the two preceding numbers), which corresponds to an "equiangular spiral." Since then biologists have recognized that this typical progressive spiral corresponds to all the spirals seen in flowers and seashells. Littler (1973) has noted that the length of the metacarpal and the phalanges of the same finger resembles the series of Fibonacci; as a matter of fact, in complex flexion a finger describes an equiangular spiral.

becomes an "equiangular spiral," as has been noted by Littler (1973), corresponding to the numerical sequence 0, 1, 1, 2, 3, 5, 8, 13, 21 . . . discovered by Fibonacci in 1202. In this sequence, each number is the sum of the two preceding numbers. It is the natural biological spiral in, amongst others, snails, shells, and flowers (Figure 1.70).

The articulations of the digits have one common, essential feature: they function in the direction of flexion and have two firm collateral ligaments and a thick reinforced anterior capsule, the anterior fibrocartilage, also known as the volar plate. By contrast, the fibrous dorsal capsule is thin and lax (Figure 1.71).

There are notable differences between the interphalangeal and metacarpophalangeal articulations of the digits and even between the articulations at the same level for each digit (Hakstian and Tubiana, 1967; Kuczynski, 1968; Landsmeer 1955; Smith and Kaplan, 1967). These differences are produced by:

- the shape of the articulations,
- the orientation of the articular surface,
- the synovial insertion,
- the disposition of the collateral ligaments,
- the degree of play in the volar plate, and
- the more superficial tissues that encircle these articulations, although these tissues play an uncertain role in their stability.

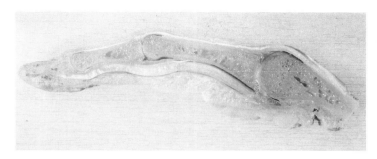

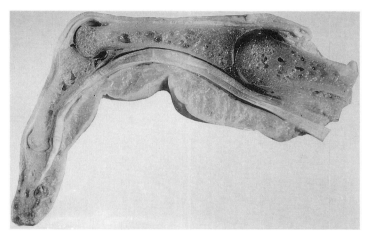

Figure 1.71. Sagittal section of a finger in flexion and extension, demonstrating the osseous chain and the planes of articular and tendinous movements. The volar tendinous apparatus, consisting of the two flexor tendons, is considerably stronger than the dorsal extensor apparatus. Also the capsular structures and the fibro-fatty cushions are much stronger, and even the skin is thicker on the flexor side. The finger is designed to function in flexion.

These elements condition the mobility and stability of these articulations and the orientation of the distal segments. As the thumb pulp pronates in opposition, the pulps of the fingers supinate in external rotation when the metacarpophalangeal joints flex or when the index finger moves radially. These variations in orientation allow for optimal use of the finger pulps (Figure 1.72).

The range of movements of the individual joints of the fingers varies. Flexion of the metacarpophalangeal joint is about 85 degrees, the proximal interphalangeal joint about 115 degrees, and the distal interphalangeal joint 80 degrees. There is also a difference in the range of movements between the thick fingers of the manual worker and the fingers of the non-manual worker. Each finger also has a slightly different range of movements. For example, the index finger is capable of less flexion than the others because it opposes the thumb.

Interphalangeal articulations

The interphalangeal articulations of the digits function uniquely in flexion–extension and their trochlear-shaped articulations are closely congruent throughout excursion of

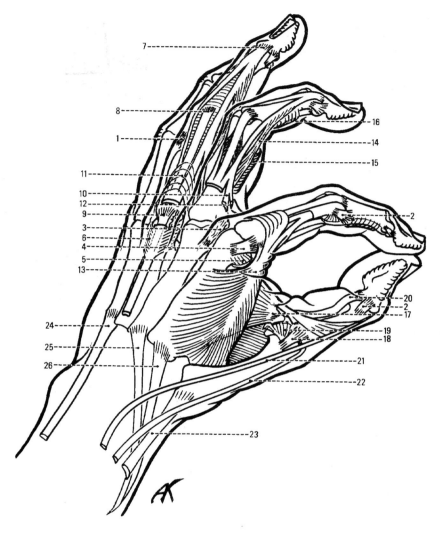

Figure 1.72. The hand with the skin removed (by Kapandji): (1) collateral ligament of the proximal interphalangeal joint slightly relaxed in complete extension and (2) tightened in intermediate flexion; (3) collateral ligament of the metacarpophalangeal joint relaxed in extension and (4) tightened in flexion; (5) accessory fibers of the collateral ligament of the metacarpophalangeal joint inserting on the volar plate; (6) sagittal band of the common extensor inserted on the interglenoid (deep intermetacarpal) ligament; (7) distal insertion of the extensor digitorum on the distal phalanx; (8) insertion of the middle extensor tendon on the middle phalanx; (9) deep insertion on the proximal phalanx; (10) insertion of the interosseous to the lateral band of the extensor digitorum; (11) interosseous hood; (12) lumbrical tendon; (13) first dorsal interosseous with its complete system of insertion and the tendon of the first lumbrical; (14) retinacular ligament; (15) flexor pulley on the first phalanx; (16) distal pulley on the second phalanx; (17) adductor pollicis with its insertions on the internal sesamoid, the base of the proximal phalanx, and the dorsal aponeurosis; (18) medial collateral ligament of the metacarpophalangeal joint of the thumb; (19) accessory collateral ligaments inserted into the volar plate and the sesamoid; (20) flexor pollicis longus; (21) extensor pollicis longus; (22) extensor pollicis brevis; (23) abductor pollicis longus; (24) extensor carpi ulnaris; (25) extensor carpi radialis brevis; (26) extensor carpi radialis longus.

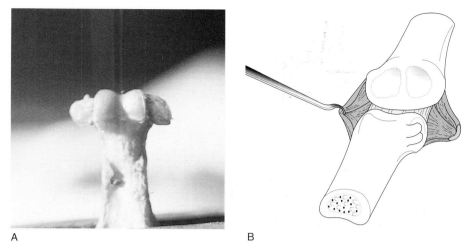

A

B

Figure 1.73. (A) The interphalangeal joint is a stable uniaxial hinge joint. This is the proximal articular surface of the middle phalanx with the two strong collateral ligaments. (B) Proximal interphalangeal joint open to show base of middle phalanx, the two glenoid cavities of which have corresponding condyles on the head of the proximal phalanx. The volar plate is extended laterally by the lateral ligaments.

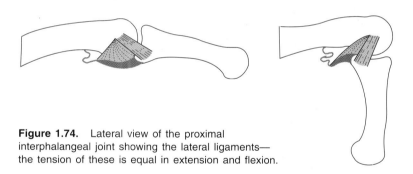

Figure 1.74. Lateral view of the proximal interphalangeal joint showing the lateral ligaments— the tension of these is equal in extension and flexion.

the joint (Figure 1.73). These interphalangeal articulations must have good lateral stability in all positions, achieved by two strong symmetrical collateral ligaments inserting on the axis of rotation of the two epiphyseal regions of the phalanges.

Proximal interphalangeal joint

The proximal interphalangeal joint must be stable in all positions. This is achieved by three main structures.

1 Two strong symmetrical collateral ligaments that arise on the proximal phalanx near the axis of rotation of the joint and insert obliquely into the base of the distal phalanx. These are supported by collateral accessory ligaments whose origin is similar, but they insert volarly into the volar plate (Figure 1.74).

2 The volar plate, which prevents hyperextension, and has a thick distal insertion and two check ligaments proximally inserted on the middle phalanx. It is interesting that traumatic ruptures of the volar plate usually occur in the thicker distal insertion rather than in the thinner proximal insertion. In the case of PIP joint stiffness, resection of the two proximal attachments of the volar plate gives the possibility of freeing the volar plate without opening the joint (Figure 1.75).

3 The fibrous flexor sheath, which is inserted on the volar plate and on the base of the phalanx immediately proximally and distally. This differs from the insertion at the MP joint, where the fibrous flexor sheath inserts on the volar plate and on the base of the proximal phalanx but not on the metacarpal (Figure 1.76).

This arrangement, involving the collateral ligaments, volar plate, and flexor sheath forms a three-dimensional junction, is the key to interphalangeal stability. If the corners of this junction remain intact, significant interphalangeal joint displacement is impossible (Eaton, 1971).

Distal interphalangeal joint
The distal interphalangeal joint has similar structures but less stability and allows some hyperextension, giving a larger pulp contact.

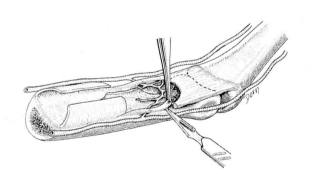

Figure 1.75. Resection of the proximal attachments of the volar plate preserving the transverse arteries for the flexor tendon vincula.

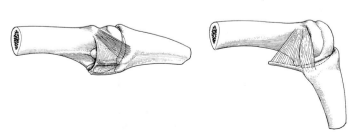

Figure 1.76. The MP volar plate does not insert on the metacarpal, and consequently the fibrous flexor sheath also does not insert there. (A) Extension, (B) flexion.

A   B

Metacarpophalangeal joints

The metacarpophalangeal (MP) joints allow flexion–extension and medial–lateral deviation associated with a slight degree of axial rotation; hence, their capsules are much looser than those of the interphalangeal articulations. The metacarpal condyle, which has a larger anteroposterior axis, articulates with the base of the proximal phalanx, which is smaller and concave and has a larger transverse axis. The surface of the glenoid cavity is amplified by the volar plate and can thus accommodate the metacarpal head. This arrangement allows great amplitude of movement, at the expense of stability, which is provided by the capsuloligamentous apparatus (Flatt and Fischer, 1969).

The lax capsule is considerably reinforced by the radial and ulnar MP ligaments. These are relaxed in extension and tensed in flexion because of their eccentric insertions and the shape of the metacarpal head (narrower posteriorly and more prominent anteriorly; Figure 1.77). This explains why abduction–adduction movements of the MP joints are restricted in flexion and free in extension.

In contrast to the interphalangeal articulations, which are stable throughout most of their range of movements, the MP joints are stable only in flexion. Their configuration also explains why the MP joints should never, under any circumstances, be immobilized in extension or hyperextension, which would result in their locking by retraction of the collateral ligaments.

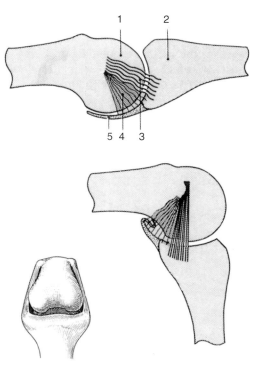

Figure 1.77. Because the metacarpal head is narrow dorsally and because of the projection of the condyle anteriorly, the collateral ligaments are tight in flexion and relaxed in extension. The most proximal fibers of the accessory collateral ligament, which is a proximal prolongation of the collateral ligament and is inserted onto the volar plate, are slack in full flexion. (1) Metacarpal head; (2) proximal phalanx; (3) collateral ligament; (4) accessory collateral ligament; (5) volar plate.

Right hand   Abduction

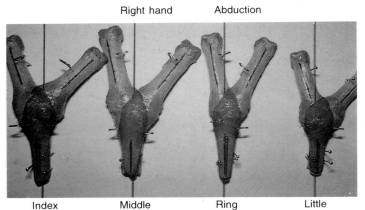

Index   Middle   Ring   Little

Figure 1.78. Anatomical preparation showing that at the level of all the metacarpo-phalangeal joints of the fingers, the ulnar deviation of the first phalanx is much more important than the radial deviation. The radial deviation is approximately 13 degrees for the index finger, 8 degrees for the middle finger, 14 degrees for the ring finger, and 19 degrees for the little finger. Ulnar deviations are 43, 34.5, 20, and 33 degrees respectively.

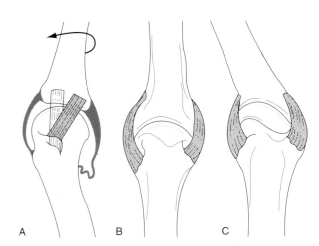

A   B   C

Figure 1.79. The asymmetry in length and direction of the internal and external lateral ligaments of the metacarpo-phalangeal joints explains the necessary movement of rotation of the phalanx during flexion-extension. (A) Profile view. (B) Dorsal view in extension. (C) Dorsal view in flexion.

The lateral accessory metacarpoglenoid ligaments suspend the volar plate, to which is attached the first pulley of the fibrous sheath of the flexor tendons. Any malalignment at the entrance of the fibrous sheath will have important repercussions on the deviation of the digit.

The asymmetry of the metacarpal heads as well as the difference in length and direction of the collateral ligaments also explains the rotational movement of the proximal phalanx during flexion-extension (Figure 1.78), and why the ulnar deviation of the digits normally is greater than the radial deviation.

Normal ulnar inclination of the fingers
The normal ulnar inclination of the fingers occurs at the metacarpophalangeal joints. The inclination is most marked in the index finger, less in the middle and little fingers, and almost non-existent in the ring finger (Figure 1.79). It is due to a number of

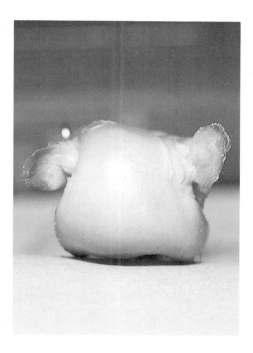

Figure 1.80. Asymmetry of the metacarpal head of the index finger. The ulnar portion of the articular condyle (on the left) is more prominent, while the radial portion is sloping.

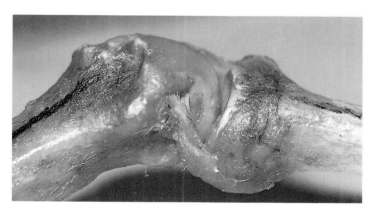

Figure 1.81. Asymmetry of the collateral ligaments of the MP joint of the index finger. The origin of the radial collateral ligament is more distal, closer to the center of the joint space, than is the origin of the ulnar ligament. The radial ligament is longer—thus more ulnar deviation is permitted than radial deviation.

anatomical factors, which have been the subject of numerous studies in recent years as a result of the development of hand surgery for rheumatoid arthritis (Flatt, 1971). These factors have different consequences in different fingers.

1 Articular effects, caused by the asymmetry of the metacarpal heads and the collateral ligaments (Hakstian and Tubiana, 1967) (Figures 1.80 and 1.81).
2 Tendon factors: the extrinsic tendons, extensors and flexors, cross into the hand on the ulnar side of its longitudinal axis (Smith et al, 1964).

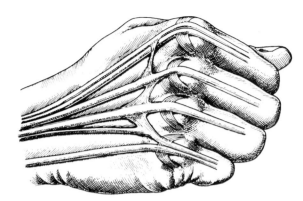

Figure 1.82. The extensor communis tendons of the fingers are joined together at the distal part of the back of the hand by the connexus intertendineus. The tendon of the extensor digitorum for the little finger in the majority of cases leaves the common extensor of the ring finger distally, as shown in the diagram. During closure of the fingers, the fourth and fifth metacarpals flex forward, drawing the extensor tendons down and inward.

3 Muscle factors: the intrinsic muscles with a predominantly ulnar inclination predominate over those with a radial inclination, because their insertions are more distal and especially because of the force of the hypothenar muscles.

4 Zancolli (1979) has emphasized the role of the forward displacement of the two ulnar metacarpals (the "metacarpal descent"), which pull ulnarward the extensor tendons united by their intertendinous connections (juncturae tendinum; Figure 1.82).

To these anatomical factors we must add the physiological action of the thumb, which in lateral grip pushes the fingers ulnarward.

The ulnar inclination is normally limited by the capsuloligamentous resistance at the MP joints and by the action of the interosseous muscles, which act in a radial direction. The weakness of these stabilizing elements, particularly in rheumatoid arthritis, allows the ulnar inclination to be accentuated, resulting in pathological ulnar deviation.

Muscular equilibrium at the level of the digits

Two forearm muscular "extrinsic" systems power the movements of opening and closing the digits (Figure 1.83). The dominance of the flexor system, composed of two strong muscles inserting on the distal phalanges, accounts for the considerable force of the encircling polyarticular chain that ensures grip.The muscular mass of the flexor digitorum profundus for the middle, ring and little fingers is not differentiated. The flexor digitorum profundus for the index finger has a separate muscular head. The flexor digitorum superficialis has independent muscular heads and tendons for the four fingers.

The flexor apparatus

The flexor tendons of the fingers cross five well-defined regions, which are, from proximal to distal:

- the wrist,
- the carpal tunnel,

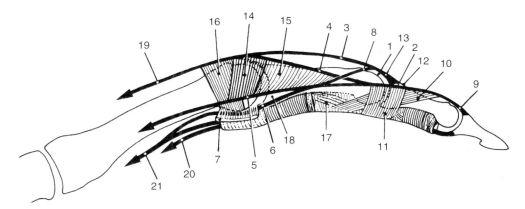

Figure 1.83. Diagrammatic view of the profile of a finger showing the insertions of the intrinsic and extrinsic muscles and the retinacular ligaments. There is a symmetry between the fibrous formations at the level of the metacarpophalangeal joint and the proximal interphalangeal joint. (1) Central or middle extensor tendon; (2) lateral extensor tendon; (3) central band of the extensor communis; (4) lateral band of the extensor; (5) interosseous tendon; (6) lumbrical tendon; (7) deep transverse intermetacarpal (or interglenoid) ligament; (8) central band of the interosseous muscle; (9) terminal extensor tendon; (10) oblique retinacular ligament; (11) transverse retinacular ligament; (12) triangular ligament; (13) insertion of the extensor digitorum into the second phalanx; (14) transverse fibers of the interosseous hoods; (15) oblique fibers of the interosseous hoods; (16) sagittal bands; (17) fibrous sheath of the flexor tendons; (18) insertion of the interosseous muscle on the base of the proximal phalanx; (19) tendon of the extensor digitorum; (20) superficial flexor tendon; (21) deep flexor tendon.

- the part of the palm extending from the exit of the carpal tunnel to the entrance of the fibrous flexor sheath suspended from the volar plate of the MP joint,
- the portion of the osteofibrous canal of the fingers (digital canal) that is common to the deep and superficial flexor tendons and reaches halfway down the middle phalanx, and
- the distal segment of the same tunnel, which transmits only the flexor profundus tendon.

The tendon of the flexor pollicis longus also crosses five regions:

- the wrist,
- the carpal tunnel,
- the palmar region (or more accurately the thenar eminence),
- the digital canal, which extends from the opening of the proximal pulley at the volar plate of the MP joint down to the exit of the "oblique pulley" halfway down the proximal phalanx (Doyle and Blythe, 1975), and
- the distal segment, which reaches the insertion of the tendon on the base of the distal phalanx.

The anatomical relations in these various zones are depicted in Figure 1.84. These diagrams show only too clearly that the danger of adhesions with the fixed structures is greater where the tendon runs within a fibrous sheath, and also that multiple tendon injuries tend to occur in regions where the tendons are bundled together (i.e. the wrist and the carpal tunnel).

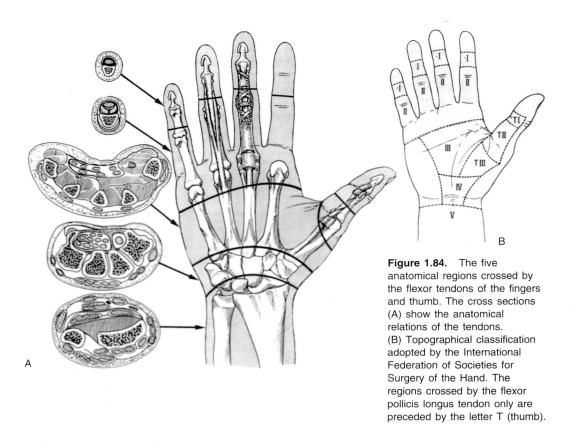

Figure 1.84. The five anatomical regions crossed by the flexor tendons of the fingers and thumb. The cross sections (A) show the anatomical relations of the tendons. (B) Topographical classification adopted by the International Federation of Societies for Surgery of the Hand. The regions crossed by the flexor pollicis longus tendon only are preceded by the letter T (thumb).

The digital flexor tendons pass through the carpal tunnel before they fan out in the palm toward their respective digits. The flexor digitorum profundus tendon passes through the flexor digitorum superficialis tendon. The flexor superficialis tendon is divided into two terminal slips at the level of the proximal phalanx which insert on the middle phalanx and the flexor profundus tendon inserts on the distal phalanx. In each digit the superficial and deep flexor tendons, surrounded by their synovial sheaths for gliding, are kept against the phalanges by their fibrous sheaths. Such a fibrous sheath plays an essential mechanical role in preventing divergence of the tendons from the axis of the digit in both the anteroposterior and lateral directions. This sheath does not have a homogeneous structure because it must adapt to the movement of the phalanges. One can distinguish several segments, some made up of dense annular fibers forming the pulleys and others made up of loose cruciform fibers (Figure 1.85), whose actions have been precisely described by Caffinière (1971), Brand et al (1975), Hunter et al (1980), and Doyle and Blythe (1975). The mechanical role of the pulleys is shown in Figure 1.86. In addition the nutritional action of the sheath is now better understood (Lundborg et al 1977, Manske 1982). This explains why modern techniques of flexor tendon repair favor conservation or reconstruction of the sheaths (Kleinert et al, 1973 and Hunter et al, 1990).

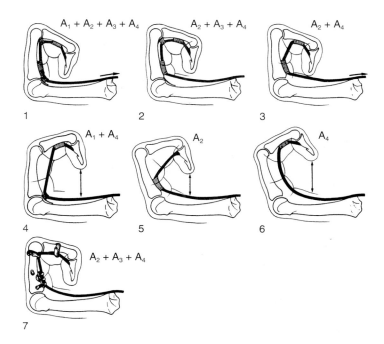

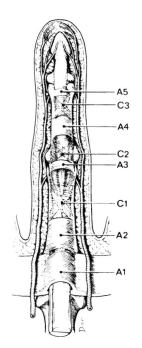

Figure 1.85. The digital flexor tendon sheath is formed by five annular pulleys and three cruciform bands. The second and fourth annular pulleys are the most important for function.

Figure 1.86. Role of the different pulleys in flexion of the fingers. (1) The four normal pulleys ensure complete flexion of the phalanges. (2) Elimination of A_1 does not prevent complete flexion of the fingers. (3) Despite the elimination of A_1 and A_3, complete flexion of the finger remains possible by the presence of A_2 and A_4 only, but the force which the tendon must exert is greater. (4) Persistence of the two pulleys A_1 and A_4 does not permit flexion of the finger. (5) Persistence of pulley A_2 only; flexion is incomplete. (6) Persistence of pulley A_4 only; the deficit is even greater. (7) The three most useful pulleys which must be preserved are A_2, A_4, and A_3 (or a pulley just proximal to the proximal interphalangeal joint).

At the level of the digital sheaths, the flexor tendons have a precarious blood supply through a vinculum longum at the chiasma level, common for both tendons superficial and profundus (Figure 1.87), and vincula brevis for the profundus. Lundborg (1977) has demonstrated the presence of several deprived zones—an "avascular segment" of the flexor superficialis just proximal to the chiasma, and two "avascular segments" of the flexor profundus proximal and distal to the vinculum longum (Figure 1.88). In addition, at the level of the proximal interphalangeal joint, the flexor profundus tendon is vascularized only in its dorsal part—the anterior 1 mm of the tendon, on which considerable pressure force is exerted (Figure 1.89). This segmental supply system, clearly inadequate in some areas, explains the difficulties of surgical repair while emphasizing the importance of the nutritional role of the synovial fluid.

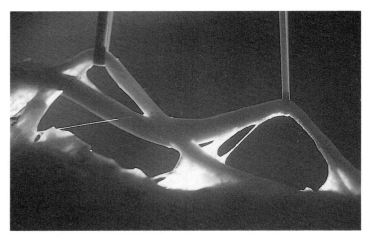

Figure 1.87. Blood supply to superficial and profundus tendons.

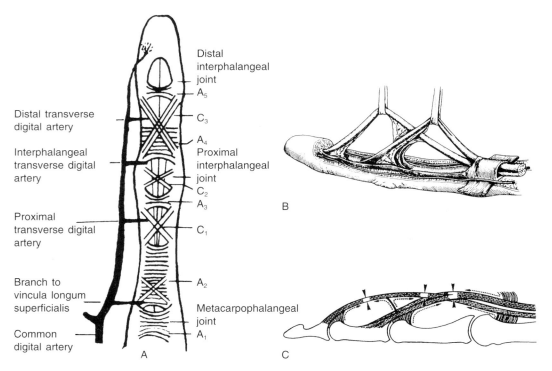

Distal interphalangeal joint

A₅

Distal transverse digital artery

C₃

A₄

Interphalangeal transverse digital artery

Proximal interphalangeal joint

C₂

A₃

Proximal transverse digital artery

C₁

Branch to vincula longum superficialis

A₂

Metacarpophalangeal joint

Common digital artery

A₁

A

B

C

Figure 1.88. Blood supply of the flexor tendons in the digital tunnel. (A) Four transverse tributaries enter the flexor retinaculum at the cruciate areas and feed the fine vincular system. (B) The vincula of the flexor tendons in the digital sheath. One can see that complete removal of the flexor superficialis tendon may devascularize the flexor profundus tendon. (C) The three "avascular" segments of the flexor tendons of the fingers.

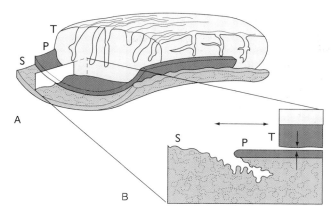

Figure 1.89. Schematic representation of the relationship between the flexor tendon (T), the pulley (P), and the synovial tendon sheath (S). (A) This drawing is based upon observations in the area at the distal border of the second annular ligament (AII). Close to the sharp edge of the pulley there is a deep pocket in the synovial sheath (see below). (B) The "critical zone" around the sharp edge of the pulley. The shaded areas indicate the *avascular parts* of the tendon and the pulley, respectively, where cellular differentiation into chondrocyte-like cells can be observed. The thick arrows indicate the traction and compression forces involved in active finger flexion. The vascular network of the synovial sheath is in continuity with the "outside" of the pulley.

Force of finger flexion

We have already noted that the force of the flexor tendons is influenced by wrist position, but as shown by Hazelton et al (1975), the percentage of total force allocated to each finger is constant, and the difference between the force exerted at the middle and distal phalanges is approximately 32 per cent (in favor of the middle phalanx) regardless of wrist position. The force of flexion of the middle finger is the greatest and accounts for 33.5 per cent of the total force of flexion of the four fingers. The index and ring fingers account for 25 per cent each and the little finger for 16.5 per cent. Thus, the total force exerted by the two ulnar fingers at either the middle or the distal phalanx is only 70 per cent of the total force of the radial fingers. The total force generated in power grip comes not only from the four fingers, but also from the force provided by the thumb and the thenar and hypothenar muscles. The long flexors of the digits essentially flex the distal articulations; it is only at the end of their excursion that they can act on the metacarpophalangeal joints, and eventually on the wrist if the fingers are stabilized in extension.

The extensor apparatus

The extensor apparatus of the fingers is formed by the extrinsic extensor muscles, the intrinsic muscles, and fibrous structures. The extensor apparatus is more complicated than the flexor apparatus.

The extrinsic extensor muscles

The extrinsic extensor apparatus of the fingers is formed by extensor communis and extensor proprius of the index and little fingers. These two extensor proprii, whose tendons are situated medially to the corresponding communis tendons, joint to the communis at the metacarpophalangeal joint. Their function is to give more autonomous movement to the peripheral fingers.

Extensor tendons have the advantage of running an almost entirely extrasynovial course, which facilitates repair. However, they are also thin superficial structures, and when damaged they tend rapidly to become adherent to the underlying bones and joints. The excursion of the extensor tendons of the hand is considerably less than that of the flexors, and thus it is more difficult to compensate for a loss of length.

The nomenclature adopted at the Congress of the International Federation of Societies for Surgery of the Hand established in Rotterdam in 1979 is used to describe the zones of injury (Figure 1.90).

The extensor communis and the two extensor proprius tendons pass under the dorsal retinaculum on the back of the wrist before diverging toward the fingers. On the dorsum of the hand, the extensor communis tendons are interconnected by the juncturae tendinum. These bands assist extension of adjacent connected fingers. Interruption of an extensor tendon proximally may be masked by the effect of these bands. The extensor communis tendon to the little finger may be absent or may be replaced by an oblique junctura from the ring finger (Figure 1.91 and 1.92). This inter-tendinous connection may make the diagnosis of a proximal rupture of the extensor

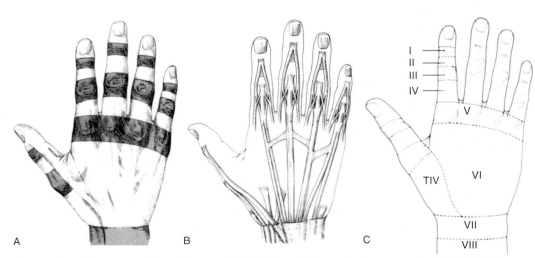

Figure 1.90. Extensor tendons of the hand. (A) Division into topographic zones. (B) Anatomy of the extrinsic extensor tendons. (C) The extensor tendons of the fingers cross eight zones. The extensor tendons of the thumb cross six zones, four specific to the thumb, which are preceded by the letter T (thumb): TI, TII, TIII, and TIV. Two zones are shared with the extensor of the fingers: zones VII (wrist) and VIII (forearm).

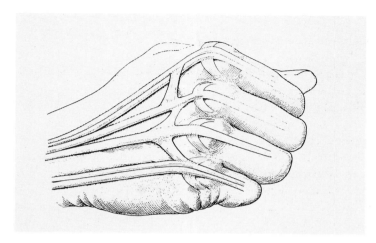

Figure 1.91. The extensor communis tendon to the little finger may be absent and replaced by an oblique junctura from the ring finger.

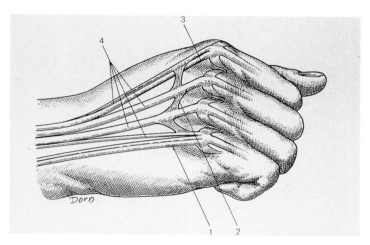

Figure 1.92. (1) Extensor proprius to little finger, (2) extensor digitorum communis, (3) extensor indicis proprius, (4) junctura tendinum or connexus intertendineus.

digiti minimi more difficult. The form of the extensor tendons changes at the level of the MP joints; they become thin and flat. Halfway down the proximal phalanx of each finger the broad flat extensor tendon splits into three parts: an extensor central band and two extensor lateral bands (Figure 1.93).

The extrinsic extensor system has four sites of insertion (Figure 1.94), the most proximal at the level of the interglenoid ligament provided on each side of the metacarpophalangeal articulation by the sagittal bands (Figure 1.95), and the most distal at the level of the base of the distal phalanx. The most important insertion is that of the central tendon into the base of the middle phalanx (Figure 1.96), the insertion at the base of the proximal phalanx being inconstant (Figure 1.97).

These multiple insertions at all the levels of the digital osseous chain distribute the action of the extrinsic extensor tendons to the three phalanges. However, they cannot insure complete extension of the finger. Under normal physiological conditions, isolated

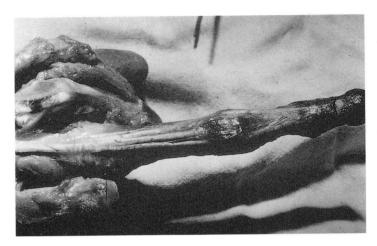

Figure 1.93. The extensor tendon splits into three parts halfway down the proximal phalanx of each finger.

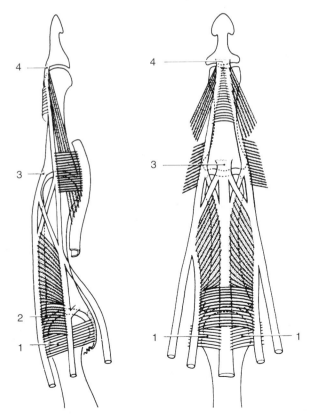

Figure 1.94. The main insertions of the extensor apparatus. The common aponeurosis of the extensor apparatus of the fingers is tensed by the extensor digitorum, by interosseous and lumbrical muscles, and by the retinacular ligaments. The four sites of insertion of the extensor digitorum tendon of the fingers are indicated in these diagrams: (1) the sagittal bands are the most proximal insertion of the extensor tendon. They run into the interglenoid ligament on each side of the metacarpophalangeal joint and contribute to the maintenance of the tendon in the dorsal axis of the finger. (2) Inconstant insertion of the extensor tendon into the base of the proximal phalanx. (3) The insertion of the middle (central) extensor tendon into the base of the middle phalanx is by far the most important. This middle (central) tendon is formed by the junction of the middle bands originating from both the intrinsic muscles and the extensor digitorum. (4) Insertion of the terminal extensor tendon into the distal phalanx. This tendon is formed by the two lateral extensor tendons. In turn, the lateral extensor tendons are formed by the junction of the lateral bands originating from the extensor digitorum tendon as well as from the intrinsic muscles.

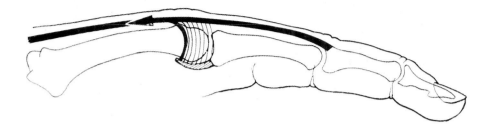

Figure 1.95. The sagittal bands inserted on the MP volar plate are the proximal insertions of the extensor tendon.

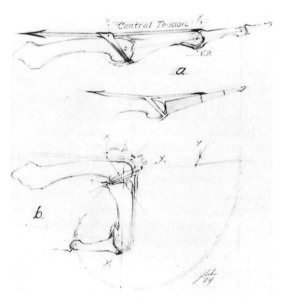

Figure 1.96. The middle or central extensor tendon, which inserts into the base of the second phalanx, has an extremely important action in the extension of all three phalanges: (1) It extends the middle phalanx on which it inserts, except when the metacarpophalangeal joint is in hyperextension (because the action of the extensor is then exhausted on its proximal insertions; shown in the middle diagram). (2) It contributes to extension of the proximal phalanx by pushing back its head when the proximal interphalangeal joint is flexed. (3) It helps extend the distal phalanx owing to the passive coordinating action of the oblique retinacular ligament. Note that in flexion the sagittal bands advance distally (x to x_1). This applies also to the interosseous hood.

contraction of the long extensors extends only the proximal phalanx. The two distal phalanges remain flexed in a clawlike position that is accentuated in paralysis of the lower ulnar nerve. Indeed, the long extensors, whose range of movement is inferior to the range of the flexors, exhaust their action at the level of their proximal insertions, acting solely upon the first phalanx. To act upon the distal phalanges, the long extensors must lose their anchorage to the proximal phalanx, or the antagonist action of the

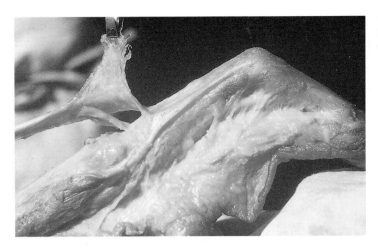

Figure 1.97. The inconstant insertion of the EDC at the base of the proximal phalanx.

long flexors must be suppressed. These are abnormal, pathological conditions. Nature has provided supplementary muscles—the intrinsic muscles—to relay the action of the long extensors and ensure the autonomy in extension of the distal phalanges.

The intrinsic apparatus

Flexion or extension at the level of the three articulations of the digits is not the result of a simple action of the long flexors or the long extensors. These two extrinsic systems, antagonistic to the movement of the distal phalanges but in effect collaborating in the extension of the proximal phalanx (Tubiana and Valentin, 1963), combine with the intrinsic muscular system, consisting of the interosseous and lumbrical muscles.

Anatomy of the intrinsic muscles

Galen, as far back as the second century AD, discovered the anatomy of the interosseous muscles, but the famous anatomist from Pergamum thought that their only action was flexion of the proximal phalanges of the digits. It was only in 1543 that two pupils of Vesalius from Padova, Columbus and Fallope, gave a better anatomical description of these muscles. Columbus described the distal insertion of the lumbricals on the extensor digitorum communis, and Fallope established the action of the interosseous muscles as extensors of the distal phalanges. Winslow (1752) was more precise, for he found that the interosseous and lumbrical muscles act as flexors of the proximal phalanges and extensors of the two distal ones. However, all these investigators considered these muscles to be weak auxiliaries of the long flexors and extensors of the digits.

Duchenne (1867) studied the mechanism of the movements of the digits and demonstrated that the intrinsic muscles were indispensable to ensure the freedom of movement of each phalanx. It is interesting to read the description provided by Duchenne, as translated by Kaplan (Duchenne, 1949):

It would be impossible to imagine a more ingenious mechanism favorable to simultaneous flexion of the proximal phalanx and extension of the two distal phalanges than presented in the anatomic arrangement of the terminal tendons of the [interosseous muscles] and lumbricals.

In the first part of their course from the head and anterolateral aspect of the metacarpal to the dorsal aspect of the head of the proximal phalanx, the tendons of the [interosseous muscles] and lumbricals have an oblique dorsal and distal direction so that during contraction of these muscles, motion occurs in the metacarpophalangeal joint, while the fixed point is at the distal end of the proximal phalanx. This arrangement produces flexion of the proximal phalanx in proportion to the force acting on the distal end of the lever represented by this phalanx.

In the second part of their course from the distal end of the proximal phalanx to the base of the distal phalanx, the same tendons pass over the dorsal aspect of the two distal phalanges, parallel to their longitudinal axis. As a result of this the contraction of the [interosseous muscles] produces only extension of the distal and then the middle phalanges. But the contraction of the [interosseous muscles] and lumbricals acts equally throughout the whole course of these tendons and thus produces simultaneously the two opposite movements of flexion of the proximal phalanx and extension of the two distal phalanges.

To understand well the marvelous ingenuity of the means used by nature to produce the movements and their mechanisms which I explained, it is necessary to obtain the same results by other mechanical combinations. This is exactly what I attempted.

I must confess that it appeared to me that the same movements could be produced by simpler means. Thus, I figured that if nature designed the common extensor of the fingers to extend the proximal phalanx only, why was it not sufficient to limit the insertion of the tendon to the dorsum of this phalanx? . . .

But why should there be a connection of the tendon of the [interosseous muscles] and lumbricals with the middle band of the common extensor? Would it not be simpler to have the tendon of these small muscles glide in an independent synovial sheath acting in the natural direction of the muscles? . . . However, that is where I noticed great difficulties in this mechanical arrangement; extension of the two distal phalanges, instead of being normal, as in the little finger (J) of which my finger (K) pulls the artificial [interosseous muscles] (11), [was] limited, and these phalanges hyperextended to such an extent that they formed an angle at the proximal interphalangeal joint. This is similar to the middle finger (1) in which my finger (K) pulls strongly the artificial dorsal [interosseous muscles] (10) [Figure 1.98].

This mechanical experiment was of great value to me. It showed that the [interosseous muscles] and lumbricals must be limited or regulated in their action on the two distal phalanges without which they reproduce reverse action. . . .

This experiment finally taught me that the middle band of the tendon is continued to its insertion at the proximal and dorsal end of the middle phalanx with the only purpose to limit the action of the [interosseous muscles] and lumbricals.

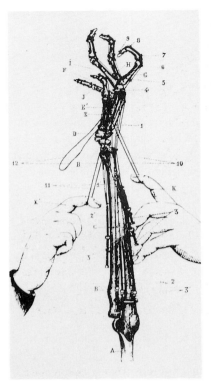

Figure 1.98. Duchenne experiment. The skeleton of a hand and forearm, with the help of artificial muscles (catgut, springs, and screws, which represent tendons attached and directed according to precise anatomical structure), can be made to reproduce natural motions of the phalanges, or to imitate deformities following paralysis of various muscles. (A) Distal end of humerus; (B) and (B′) radius; (C) ulna; (D) wrist; (E) first metacarpal; (E′) second metacarpal; (F) thumb; (G) index finger; (H) fourth finger; (I) middle finger; (J) fifth finger; (K) finger of the operator's left hand; (K′) finger of the operator's right hand. (1) Artificial catgut tendons of the common extensors of the finger. (1′) Cords representing flexors of the fingers; (2) and (2′) springs attached to the cords that represent the extensors and flexors of the fingers and that produce gradual tension or relaxation with the help of screws; (3), (3′), (3″), (4), (5), (6), (7), (8), and (9) small rings fixed at different points of the metacarpals and phalanges in accordance with the anatomical orientation of the interosseous and lumbrical muscles and through which pass the cords representing these small muscles; (10) cords representing the interosseous muscles of the middle finger (I), which is pulled by the operator's left index finger (K); (11) cords representing the interosseous muscles of the fifth finger (J), which are pulled by the operator's right index finger; (12) cords representing the interosseous muscles of the index finger in complete relaxation, imitating paralysis. By reason of this artificial paralysis the index finger (G) whose extensors and flexors are pulled by their corresponding springs assumes the attitude of a claw finger, as observed in individuals whose interosseous muscles are paralyzed and who attempt to extend their fingers.

Mechanisms of finger flexion and extension

Landsmeer (1955) showed that to control two joints of a multiarticular chain in all positions at least three muscles are necessary; all three may cross two joints, or two may be biarticular and one monoarticular. In a polyarticular chain of bones such as the fingers, equilibrium of each intercalated bone is insured by the balanced tensions of the three muscles. The proximal phalanx, which is a typical intercalated bone, is controlled by three muscular systems: two extrinsic muscles (anterior and posterior) and one diagonal intrinsic muscle (lumbrical and interosseous muscles; Figure 1.99). For the middle phalanx, the third diagonal component is not a muscle but the oblique retinacular ligament, which inserts proximally into the flexor pulley and the neck of the proximal phalanx and distally into the lateral extensor tendons (Figure 1.100).

Thus, two oblique structures cross the lateral aspects of the proximal and middle joints of the digital chain. Proximally, they run palmar to the axes of flexion of each joint, and distally they run dorsal to the axes. They can be tightened passively by two mechanisms: the extension of the joint they cross or the flexion of the distal joint. Their tension by the contraction of the long muscles, the tendons of which cross the anterior and posterior aspects of these joints, will trigger the flexion of the corresponding joint. These oblique structures will stabilize the digital chains and will also determine the sequence of the movements of flexion and extension of the phalanges.

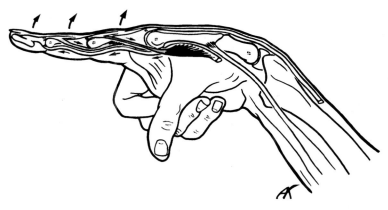

Figure 1.99. The two diagonal systems of digital extension. The first diagonal system is active: it is the lumbrical muscle (hatched) that reduces the tension on the deep flexor and increases the tension on the extensor apparatus leading to and completing the extension of the second and third phalanges. The second diagonal system is passive: it is the retinacular ligament (stippled) that passively contributes to the extension of the second phalanx on the third. The wrist is stabilized in flexion by the flexor carpi radialis, which augments the efficiency of the common extensor in its action of extending the first phalanx. (Diagram by Kapandji, modified from the hand of St. John the Baptist in the altar piece of Isenheim by Mathias Grunewald.)

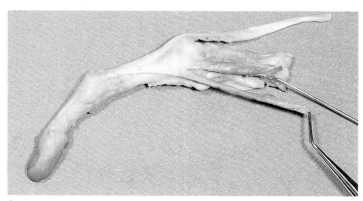

A

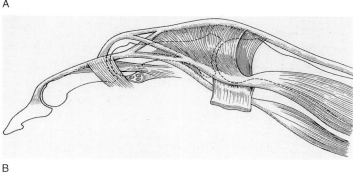

B

Figure 1.100. View from the radial side of a finger showing the elements of the extensor apparatus. At the base of the finger the three muscles acting on the aponeurosis are seen from top to bottom: the extensor digitorum tendon, the interosseous muscle, and the lumbrical muscle.

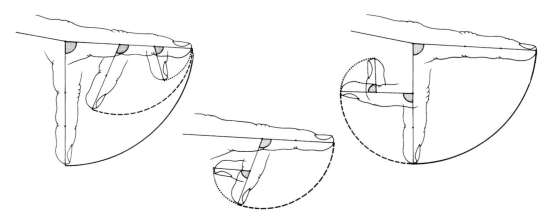

Figure 1.101. The ranges of flexion and extension of the different joints of the fingers. The large arc of flexion of the metacarpophalangeal joint, which represents 77 per cent of flexion of the finger, is under the influence of the intrinsic musculature (reinforced by the long flexors). The arcs of flexion of the interphalangeal joints are totally dependent on the strong extrinsic musculature. They represent only 23 per cent of the flexion, but their function is essential because they are responsible for the completion and strength of grasp. The whole movement describes an equiangular curve (Littler, 1977).

Each phalanx has a wide range of movement in flexion and extension (Figure 1.101). Because flexion is insured by the exceptionally large excursion of the long flexors, that of the long extensors is much less important. Their action has to be relayed by the intrinsic muscles—the interosseous and lumbrical muscles.

The structure of the interosseous muscles is particularly complex. Each interosseous muscle is composed of a number of muscular bundles of different lengths, taking their origins on the lateral or palmar surfaces of the metacarpal shafts. The muscular bundles have a relatively independent nerve supply, arising from the deep branch of the ulnar nerve (Figure 1.102). They continue into tendinous slips, entering the finger posterior to the interglenoid (deep transverse metacarpal) ligament. The tendinous slips insert distally at different levels in the fingers. These anatomical peculiarities allow for several classifications. Albinus (1724) classified the interosseous muscles according to their origins into three palmar adductors and four dorsal abductors of the fingers; this classification was accepted for almost 200 years (Figures 1.103 and 1.104). They can also be classified according to their insertions into deep and superficial, proximal or distal (Salisbury, 1936; Stack, 1962).

The deep insertions are into the lateral tubercles on the base of the proximal phalanx and into the capsule of the MP joint (Figure 1.105). They allow lateral movements of the fingers and prevent posterior dislocation of the muscle (Figure 1.106).

The superficial insertions occur at three separate levels in the finger:

1 One group of muscle bundles runs into the transverse fibers surrounding the posterior aspect of the MP joint and into the base of the proximal phalanx and forms the

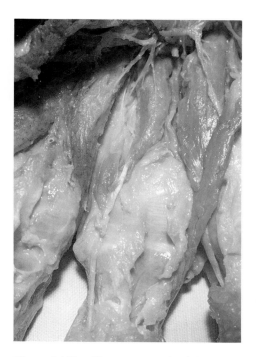
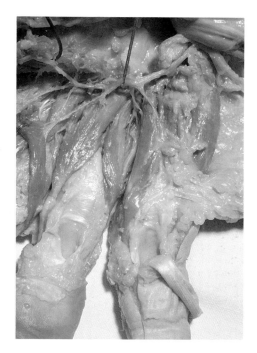

Figure 1.102. The nerve supply of the interosseous muscles arises from the deep branch of the ulnar nerve. The dorsal and palmar components of the dorsal interossei receive separate branches from the ulnar nerve.

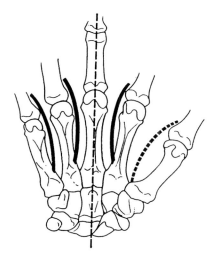
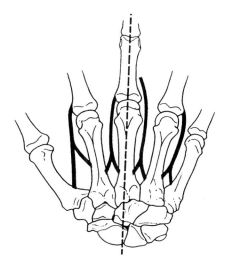

Figure 1.103. Diagram of the palmar interossi, which approximate the fingers: they originate only on the side of the metacarpal facing the axis of the hand. The palmar interosseous of the first interspace, shown here in dotted lines, is not described by all anatomists.

Figure 1.104. Diagram of the dorsal interossi muscles, which open out the fingers. They have a double origin from the two metacarpals that bound the space. They also have a double distal insertion, bony and aponeurotic, except for the first, which inserts on bone alone.

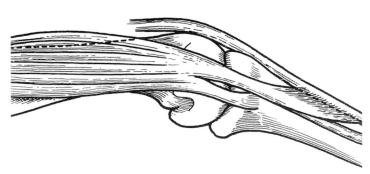

Figure 1.105. The deep insertions of the interosseous muscle into the base of the proximal phalanx and the capsule of the metacarpophalangeal joint.

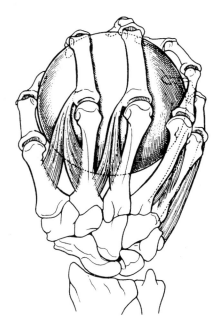

Figure 1.106. The bony insertion on P_1 of the dorsal interossei and hypothenar muscles promotes cupping of the fingers by abduction, rotation, and flexion of the proximal phalanx of each digit.

interosseous hood. The angle of approach of the palmar interosseous at the metacarpophalangeal level is greater than the angle of the dorsal interosseous (Figure 1.107). The interosseous muscles flex the MP joint by means of the interosseous hood.

2 A second group runs more distally over the dorsal aspect of the proximal phalanx. The oblique fibers blend with the central band of the extensor tendon forming the central extensor tendon, and insert into the base of the middle phalanx, which they extend.

3 A third group of distal fibers blends with the fibers coming laterally from the lumbrical and runs into the lateral band of the extensor tendon forming the lateral extensor tendon.

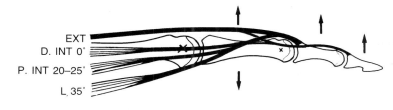

Figure 1.107. The angles of approach of the intrinsic tendons at the metacarpophalangeal level. The angle of approach of the lumbrical (L) is the greatest. (D. INT) dorsal interosseous muscle; (P. INT) palmar interosseous muscle.

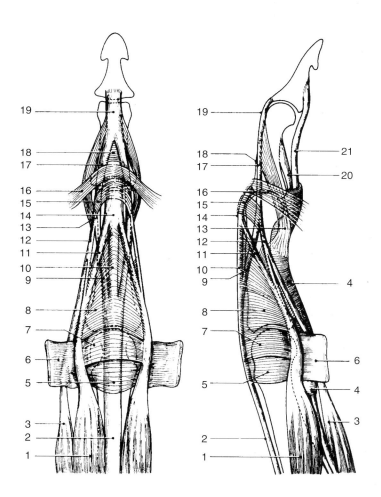

Figure 1.108. The extensor apparatus of the fingers—frontal and lateral views: (1) interosseous muscle; (2) extensor communis tendon; (3) lumbrical muscle; (4) flexor tendon fibrous sheath; (5) sagittal band; (6) intermetacarpal ligament; (7) transverse fibers of interosseous hood; (8) oblique fibers of hood; (9) lateral band of extensor tendon; (10) central or middle band of extensor tendon; (11) central or middle band or interosseous tendon; (12) lateral band of interosseous tendon; (13) oblique retinacular ligament; (14) middle extensor tendon; (15) spiral fibers; (16) transverse retinacular ligament; (17) lateral extensor tendon; (18) triangular ligament (or lamina); (19) terminal extensor tendon.

The two lateral extensor tendons join together on the dorsum of the distal interphalangeal joint, forming the distal extensor tendon, which inserts into the base of the distal phalanx (Figure 1.108). The *lumbricals* are four small fasciculi that arise from the tendons of the flexor profundus in the palm. Each passes to the radial side of the corresponding finger, superficial to the transverse intermetacarpal ligament, and terminates on the lateral extensor tendons. The angle of approach to the dorsal aponeurosis is greater than that of the interossei.

This is the general arrangement. There are different patterns in the insertions of the interossei and lumbrical muscles for each finger, and even for each side of each finger, allowing greater functional individuality. The index and little fingers have quite specialized intrinsic muscles because of their peripheral location. The index finger has the first dorsal interosseus, whose digital insertion is entirely interosseus. The radial aponeurotic wing is formed almost entirely by the first lumbrical. On the little finger, the tendinous wing on the ulnar side is formed by the abductor digiti minimi.

Actions of the intrinsic muscles

Interosseous muscles

The interosseous muscles produce lateral movements of fingers through their insertions on the lateral aspect of the base of the proximal phalanges. If they are paralyzed, it considerably diminishes these movements. Slight lateral movement persists, owing to the proximal convergence of the long extensor tendons.

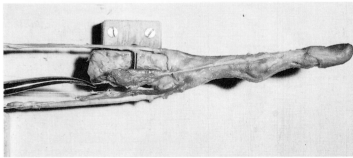

A

Figure 1.109. Traction on the interosseous muscles with the metacarpophalangeal joint in (A) extension and (B) flexion. When the MP joint is flexed, the interossei muscles cannot extend the distal phalanges.

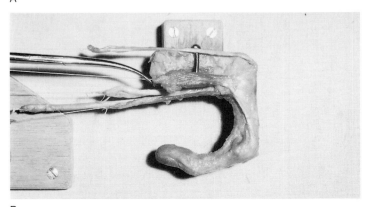

B

The interosseous muscles also play an essential role in flexion–extension movements of the phalanges. Schematically, they flex the proximal phalanx and extend the two distal phalanges. These movements depend on the metacarpophalangeal (MP) joint position. When this joint is in extension, the interosseous hood covers the MP articular space. The oblique fibers of the interossei are put into tension and extend the distal phalanges. In MP joint flexion, the hood is pulled distal to the articular space and the force of the interossei is applied to the back of the proximal phalanx, thus reinforcing its flexion. They lose their extensor action on the distal phalanges (Figure 1.109). Although the actions of the interossei are dependent on the position of the MP joint, they are independent of wrist movement.

Lumbrical muscles

The lumbricals are longer than the interossei, giving them a greater contractile potential, though their volume is much less than that of the palmar interossei. Unlike the interosseous muscles, the lumbrical muscles are able to extend the two distal phalanges whether the MP joint is in extension or flexion (Figure 1.110).

The integrity of the lumbricals at the level of the index and long fingers, in cases of isolated paralysis of the ulnar nerve, is sufficient to prevent development of the claw deformity. However, this deformity is latently present even though it is not

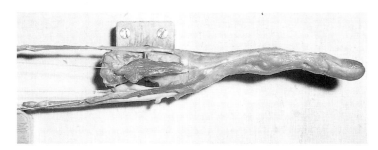

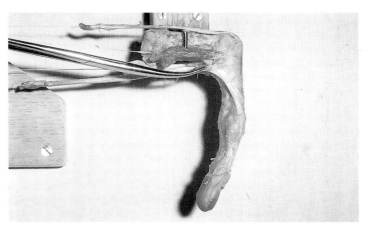

Figure 1.110. Lumbrical muscle action. Note that with the metacarpophalangeal joint in flexion, the lumbrical is able to extend the distal joints.

exhibited. During a strong grip between the thumb, index, and long fingers, the MP joint has a tendency to hyperextend while the interphalangeal (IP) joints are hyperflexed (hyperflexion sign of Mannerfelt). This latent deformation is evident when the patient is asked to flex the index and long finger MP joints while maintaining the IP joints in extension ("lumbrical plus" position). Slight pressure on the volar aspect of the proximal phalanx will cause immediate flexion of the proximal IP (PIP) joint. These patients are hindered in their ability to grasp small objects with precision and strength, although movements of the index and long fingers made without effort appear normal.

However, the lumbricals appear primarily to be interphalangeal extensors, following which (and only then) they could possibly act as metacarpophalangeal flexors (Backhouse, 1968). The action of these small slender muscles between the flexor profundus tendons and the extensor apparatus is subtle: they participate in extension of the distal phalanges by pulling distally on the flexor profundus tendon when this muscle is at rest. As has been shown by Long (1975), this permits a reduction of the viscoelastic resistance of the flexor profundus and indirectly facilitates the action of the common extensor on the distal phalanges. Contraction of the lumbrical muscles, whose relatively free play is little impaired by attachments to the dorsal hood, also contributes directly to the extension of the distal phalanges, regardless of the position of the metacarpophalangeal joint, whether the proximal phalanx is extended or flexed.

By contrast, the interosseous muscles have a decreasing extensor effect at the IP joints as flexion of the MP joint increases. This explains why, despite their feebleness, lumbrical muscles can form an "active diagonal system" between the flexors and extensors at the proximal part of the finger. To take a comparison from the field of electronics, one can say that they have a "transistor effect" (Kapandji).

Thus these muscles, which have the same innervation as the corresponding flexor profundus, play a co-ordinating role between the extensor and flexor systems. Rabischong (1963) demonstrated the richness of the sensory receptors at their level; thus these small, weak muscles are true proprioceptive organs.

Action of extrinsic and intrinsic muscles on the equilibrium of the proximal phalanx

Mechanical analyses show that the forces of the extensor digitorum communis (EDC) and of the flexor superficialis (FS) on the middle phalanx have a component that produces extension of the proximal phalanx. It is this force that the intrinsic muscles (lumbrical and interossei) normally oppose. When these are paralyzed, no force exists to prevent the proximal phalanx from swinging into hyperextension. Inversely, this hyperextension is seen only if the EDC and FS are active (Figure 1.111).

The long extensor, which exhausts its action at the level of its proximal insertions, has no effect on the distal phalanges. MP joint hyperextension is prevented initially by the volar plate of the joint, but capsular resistance progressively yields and the

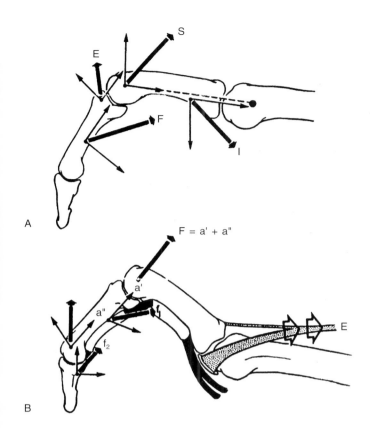

Figure 1.111. (A) Mechanical explanation of the claw-hand deformity. Force (E) of the extensor communis contributes to carrying the proximal phalanx into hyperextension. The force of the flexors also produces extension in the proximal phalanx. Force (f) of the flexor superficialis (FS) has an axial component (a'). Force (f_2) of the flexor profundus has an axial component that, as it is transmitted to the head of the middle phalanx, can be broken down into an axial force (a''), and an extension force on the middle phalanx counteracted by the flexion component of (f_1). The sum of (a') and (a'') represents the total force of extension acting on the middle phalanx (F). (B) Force (E) of the extensor communis and force (F) of the (FS) each has an axial component: the sum (S) of these is applied to the head of the proximal phalanx over which it extended. Force (I) of the intrinsic muscles counteracts this extension force at the proximal phalanx.

deformity will worsen. The claw is a progressive deformity that accentuates with the stretching of the palmar tissue. The claw does not represent the inevitable stigma of every ulnar paralysis, but is rather a secondary deformity that occurs with distal ulnar paralysis.

The extensor aponeurosis
The expansions of the extensor tendons and of the intrinsic muscles on the dorsal aspect of the finger form a veritable fibrous plexus, the extensor aponeurosis, which is activated at various levels by the tendons of the long extensors, the palmar or dorsal interosseous muscles, and the lumbricals. It is also anchored by fixed fibrous structures, such as the oblique retinacular ligaments, which act like a tenodesis (Figure 1.112).

The movements of the two interphalangeal joints are thus bound by the common aponeurotic expansion and by the retinacular ligaments. The proximal and distal interphalangeal joints can normally only move in the same direction simultaneously; they form a functional unit, the interphalangeal system.

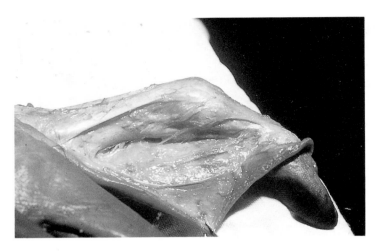

Figure 1.112. The oblique retinacular ligaments.

Distal gliding

Because of the non-elastic structure of the extensor aponeurotic expansion, the lengthening that must occur when the fingers are flexed is achieved by a gliding movement in two directions, laterally and distally.

The distal gliding is especially important at the level of the metacarpophalangeal joints. It is made possible and later checked by the peculiarities of the proximal insertions of the long extensor. The sagittal bands, attached into the volar plates of the metacarpophalangeal joints, are directed obliquely forward and distally when the joint is extended (see Figure 1.96). Their dorsal attachments are then proximal to the joint; in full flexion they cover the joint. The extensor tendon is attached to the base of the proximal phalanx by means of a long thin insertion which is relaxed during flexion of the interphalangeal joints and taut during extension (see Figure 1.118).

The interosseous hood is displaced distally during flexion. This gliding movement extends about 16 mm at the level of the long finger. The hood covers the metacarpal head in extension but slides distal to the joint in flexion. This gliding has important physiological results.

The position of the MP joint determines the application of the forces of the interossei:

1 In extension of the MP joint, the contraction of the interossei is transmitted by the lateral extensor tendons and contributes to the extension of the distal phalanx (see Figure 1.81).

2 In flexion of the MP joint, the interosseous hood slides distal to the joint. The contraction of the interossei tightens the hood against the dorsum of the proximal phalanx and increases the flexion (Figure 1.113). However, sometimes certain distal bundles (the equivalents of the lumbricals) are capable of extending the distal phalanges even if the metacarpophalangeal joint is flexed, because they are relatively free from the hood.

3 In this position with complete extension of the fingers, with the exception of the middle or ring fingers which are flexed at the metacarpophalangeal and proximal interphalangeal joints, the extensor apparatus of the flexed fingers glides distally. The

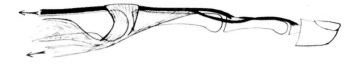

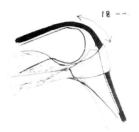

Figure 1.113. In flexion of the MP joint, the interosseous hood slides distally. The contraction of the interossei tightens the hood against the dorsum of the proximal phalanx.

Figure 1.114. Floating distal phalanx.

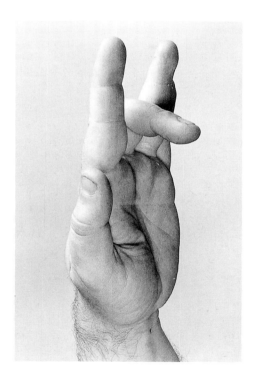

extensors fail, therefore, to control the extension of the distal phalanx from this position. The flexor profundus also is neutralized by the "quadriga (four-horse chariot) effect" described by Verdan (1960) and the distal phalanx is "floating" (Figure 1.114). The effect can be due to a non-differentiation in the muscular mass of the flexor digitorum profundus, to flexor interdigital tendinous connections, and/or to double origins from the two adjacent tendons of lumbrical muscles.

101

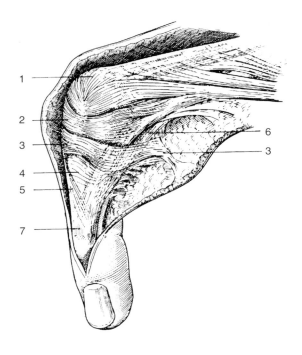

Figure 1.115. Diagram showing anatomical features of the extensor apparatus: (1) insertion of the middle extensor tendon on the base of the middle phalanx; (2) spiral fibers; (3) transverse retinacular ligament, which is inserted laterally in the dermis; (4) triangular lamina; (5) lateral extensor tendon; (6) oblique retinacular ligament; (7) terminal extensor tendon.

Lateral gliding

On the dorsolateral aspect of the PIP joint, the two lateral bands of the interosseous tendons receive lateral bands from the extensor communis to become the lateral extensor tendons. Both these fiber bands glide along the posterolateral aspect of the joint during flexion movements; the gliding is closely checked by several fibrous structures— the triangular ligament, the spiral fibers of the extensor apparatus, and the retinacular ligaments.

Fibrous structures of the extensor apparatus

Triangular ligament

The triangular ligament or lamina comprises the transverse fibers arising from the medial borders of the lateral extensor tendons at the level of the middle phalanx (see Figure 1.115). They form a fine triangular membrane at the apex of which the two lateral tendons unite.

Spiral fibers

The spiral fibers are more proximal and curl from the lateral extensor tendons to the central tendon over the proximal interphalangeal joint. These fibers were described by Hauck in 1923 and then by Baumann and Patry in 1943, but lately they have been

102

confused with the other transverse structures of this region, the transverse lamina and the transverse retinacular ligament. Their action has been more recently defined by Gaul (1971) and by van Zwieten (1980). The spiral fibers are continuations of the long extensor tendon and the interosseous tendons. They branch off the lateral margins of the lateral tendons at the distal third of the proximal phalanx and run distally and medially, spiraling over the dorsal surfaces of the lateral tendons. They are arranged in two flat sheets, which join together in midline at the level of the distal part of the central tendon. These fibers prevent lateral displacement of the lateral extensor tendons.

Oblique retinacular ligament

The oblique retinacular ligament was identified by Weitbrecht (in 1742) under the name of "retinaculum tendinis longi" (Kaplan, 1965) and has been described by Landsmeer (1949), who defined its function. This fibrous bundle extends symmetrically on either side of the proximal interphalangeal joint and has no muscular connection. Part of it inserts on the volar aspect of the lateral surface of the distal third of the proximal phalanx and part inserts on the fibrous flexor tendon sheath. Running distally and dorsally, it crosses obliquely the lateral aspect of the proximal interphalangeal joint. It progressively approaches the lateral extensor tendons, which it joins in the distal half of the middle phalanx. The fibers mingle with the fibers of the two lateral extensor tendons and form the distal extensor tendon, inserting into the base of the distal phalanx.

These ligaments co-ordinate the movements of the interphalangeal joints (Figure 116). In fact, these ligaments, which cross diagonally the axis of rotation of the proximal interphalangeal joint, are placed under tension by flexion of the distal interphalangeal joint and cause simultaneous flexion of the proximal interphalangeal joint. The ligaments are also placed under tension by extension of the proximal interphalangeal joint (caused by the central extensor tendon), which in turn causes extension of the distal interphalangeal joint.

This mechanical action of the oblique retinacular ligament tested on cadaver (Tubiana and Valentin, 1964) has been challenged by Harris and Rutledge (1972), as the structure and extent vary from one finger to another in the same hand and even on each side of a particular finger. If the functional value of these ligaments is probably variable and limited in normal fingers, their role becomes evident under pathological circumstances; when thickened and contracted they contribute to fixation of a boutonnière deformity. The same applies to the transverse retinacular ligament (Figure 1.117).

Transverse retinacular ligament

The transverse retinacular ligament is non-tendinous but moves superficially and runs in the subcutaneous and subfascial spaces around the proximal interphalangeal joint. These fibers are attached to the skin and the subcutaneous layers as well as to the extensor apparatus, and form a thin fibrous lamella on the lateral and dorsal surfaces of the extensor apparatus to which they adhere on either side of the joint.

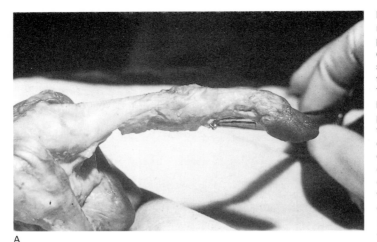

A

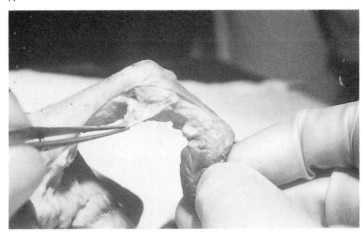

B

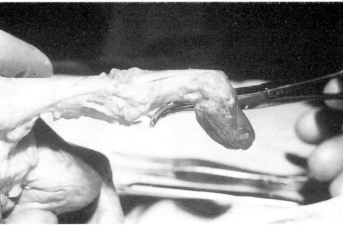

C

Figure 1.116. The oblique retinacular ligaments cross the proximal interphalangeal joint obliquely going from the fibrous sheath of the flexor tendons to the lateral extensor tendons. They coordinate extension between the proximal and distal phalangeal articulations. When the distal insertions of the oblique retinacular ligament are divided (A and B), the tenodesis effect is abolished. Thus, extension of the middle phalanx will not be followed by extension of the distal phalanx (C).
(A) The distal phalanx is extended 45° when the middle phalanx is put in extension.
(B) The oblique retinacular ligaments are divided. (C) The middle phalanx is extended but the distal phalanx remains totally flexed.

A
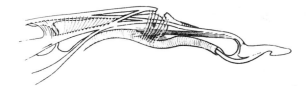

Figure 1.117. Boutonnière deformity. (A) Initially, the deformity is reducible. (B) Fixed boutonnière deformity—contracture of the fibrous structures (retinacular ligaments, volar plate, ligaments) prevents correction of the deformity.

B
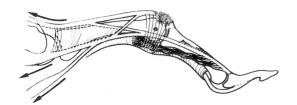

Flexion of the proximal interphalangeal joint causes distal and lateral gliding of the lateral extensor tendons. This results in a reduction in tension within the lateral and terminal extensor tendons and allows the distal interphalangeal joint to be flexed by the flexor profundus. The lateral displacement is controlled by the lateral transverse structures. The triangular lamina can have only an accessory role because it is thin and is situated distally. The transverse retinacular ligament is an even more fragile structure and can have such an action only when it is sclerosed and thickened in pathological situations, as in the boutonnière deformity.

It is the spiral fibers that normally play the essential role in the control of and co-ordination between the lateral tendons, by virtue of their obliquity, their length, their location in relation to the proximal interphalangeal joint, and their combined attachment to the lateral tendons and the central tendon. The mechanism of these displacements has been well demonstrated by van Zwieten (1980).

Any disturbance in the delicate balance of forces in the fingers results in a deformity.

Boutonnière deformity (see Figures 1.122 and 2.45)
In the boutonnière deformity, the primary lesion lies in the middle extensor tendon, leading to flexion of the proximal interphalangeal joint and hyperextension of the distal interphalangeal joint.

Swan-neck deformity (see Figures 1.122 and 2.43)
In the swan-neck deformity, the proximal interphalangeal joint is in hyperextension and the distal interphalangeal joint in flexion. The deformity can be caused by a variety of factors which have in common excessive traction on the middle extensor tendon inserted into the base of the middle phalanx.

105

Sequences of flexion and extension movements of the phalanges

The extremity of the finger describes in flexion a curve with a progressively diminishing radius, which allows the closing finger to wrap around objects of decreasing diameter.

The basal joint of the finger (the metacarpophalangeal joint) describes, according to Littler, the largest segment (77 per cent) of the arch of flexion; the middle joint, the proximal interphalangeal joint, contributes 20 per cent and the distal interphalangeal joint, only 3 per cent (Figure 1.118).

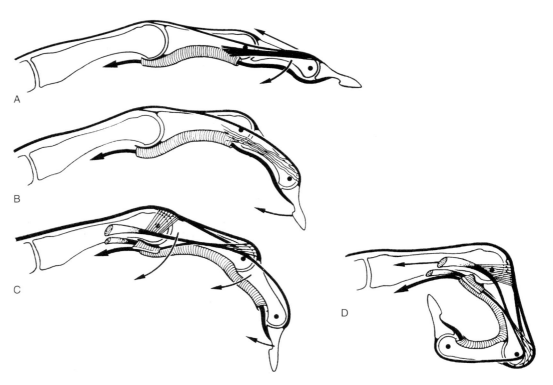

Figure 1.118. The order of flexion of the phalanges is controlled by a complex mechanism. (A) The flexor profundus and extensor digitorum contract simultaneously at the beginning of flexion; the extensor acts as a braking mechanism. The oblique retinacular ligament, which is put under tension by flexion of the distal phalanx, acts as an active tenodesis to initiate flexion of the proximal interphalangeal joint. (B) As the proximal interphalangeal joint flexes, the tension in the oblique retinacular ligament decreases, thereby allowing for more flexion at the distal joint. (C) Flexion of the proximal interphalangeal joint puts the lumbrical and interosseous tendons, which cross obliquely in front of the axis of the metacarpophalangeal joint, under tension, and this initiates flexion of the metacarpophalangeal joint. (D) Flexion of the metacarpophalangeal joint displaces the interosseous hood distally; once distal to the joint, it can act as a flexor of the proximal phalanx. Thus, two structures that cross the joint obliquely at two successive levels have a similar tenodesis effect on the digital kinetic chain. Both are palmar to the axis of flexion proximally and dorsal to the axis distally. An increase in tension in these structures caused by the action of the extrinsic muscles will initiate flexion of the phalanx they cross. This tension can be brought about by two different mechanisms, i.e. flexion of the distal joint or flexion of the proximal joint.

Flexion of the fingers begins normally at the level of the proximal interphalangeal joint, followed by the metacarpophalangeal and distal interphalangeal joints. The distal interphalangeal joint flexes more slowly than the proximal interphalangeal joint, and its flexion is completed only at the end of the movement, locking the grip.

The upsetting of this rhythm of flexion, as in paralysis of the ulnar nerve when the distal phalanx flexes first, strongly impairs the grip, especially of larger objects (see Section 4, Figure 4.21). It is incorrect to assume that the middle phalanx flexes first because the flexor superficialis is the first muscle to contract. The electromyography studies of Long and Brown (1964) demonstrated that during unopposed flexion of the fingers, only the flexor digitorum profundus and the extensor digitorum contract at the onset of the movement. The extensor progressively relaxes afterward, to allow for the flexion of the metacarpophalangeal joint, and acts as a brake throughout the movement of flexion. The flexor superficialis does not contract during unopposed flexion; its action predominates during flexion against resistance. The lumbrical muscles also do not contract during unopposed flexion.

The explanation for these paradoxical phenomena was given by Landsmeer (1949), Landsmeer and Long (1965), Kaplan (1954, 1965), Stack (1962), and Long and Brown (1964). Valentin (1962) studied the rhythm of flexion and extension of the fingers by slow motion films, mechanical models, and cadaver specimens, and the studies confirmed their findings.

As the flexor digitorum profundus contracts, the oblique bands of the retinacular ligaments tighten and cause flexion of the middle phalanx (see Figure 1.118). Because the oblique retinacular ligaments insert into the terminal extensor tendon and cross the lateral aspects of the proximal interphalangeal joint obliquely, they provide a long lever arm that moves the proximal interphalangeal joint more than the distal interphalangeal joint. The extensor, contracting simultaneously with the flexor digitorum profundus, prevents the flexion of the distal interphalangeal joint. The continuous, more rapid flexion of the proximal interphalangeal joint progressively relaxes the tension of the oblique retinacular ligaments and allows complete flexion of the distal interphalangeal joint.

The active flexion of the proximal interphalangeal joint starts the flexion of the metacarpophalangeal joint. This happens because flexion tightens the tendons of the interosseous and lumbrical muscles, and passive flexion occurs as these tendons run in front of the axis of the metacarpophalangeal joint. Then the interosseous muscles can start acting by means of their attachments into the hood. In paralysis of the ulnar nerve, as the viscoelastic resistance of the intrinsic muscles disappears, the action of the extrinsic muscles does not flex the metacarpophalangeal joint; they cause hyperextension of the metacarpophalangeal joint and clawlike flexion of the fingers. In a normal hand, the tenodesis effect of the intrinsic tendons can be overcome by voluntary contraction of the long flexors. The two distal phalanges can be hooked in full flexion while maintaining the metacarpophalangeal joint in extension.

Extension of the fingers starts at the level of the metacarpophalangeal joint. Anatomical studies and electromyography demonstrate that isolated contraction of the extensor

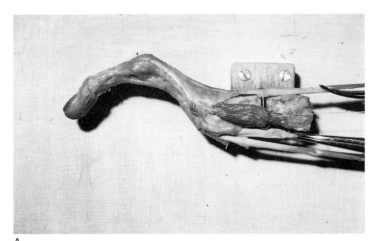

A

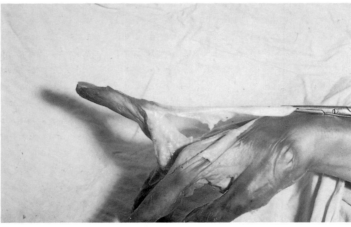

B

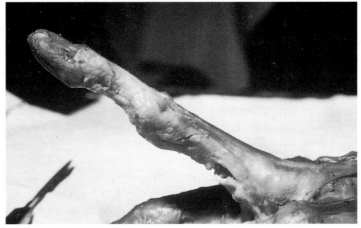

C

Figure 1.119. (A) Traction on the extensor digitorum puts the metacarpophalangeal joint into hyperextension and the interphalangeal joints into flexion. (B) Traction on the extensor communis if its proximal insertions are divided (sagittals bands) will put the interphalangeal joints into full extension. (C) If the flexors are divided, traction on the extensor digitorum will extend all the joints.

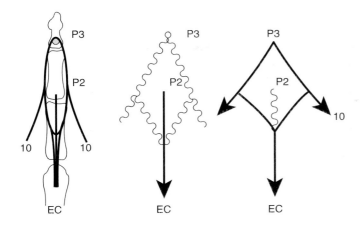

Figure 1.120. Extension of the distal phalanx. As the tendons of the interossei pull on the angles of the extensor apparatus the diamond shape becomes broader and shorter.

results in a clawlike position and not a complete extension of the digital chain. The extensor digitorum exhausts its action at the level of the metacarpophalangeal joint, which it hyperextends by means of its proximal insertions, the sagittal bands (Figure 1.119). Division of the sagittal bands allows the extensors to fully extend the interphalangeal joints, together with the metacarpophalangeal joint. The viscoelastic resistance of the long flexors increases in hyperextension of the metacarpophalangeal joint and flexes the distal phalanges. Contraction of the lumbrical suppresses this resistance and corrects the claw position.

Extension of the proximal interphalangeal joint by traction of the middle band of the extensor tenses the oblique band of the retinacular ligament and starts the extension of the distal phalanx. The movement is completed by the combined actions of the extensor communis and the intrinsic muscles. Viewed from the dorsal aspect Stack (1962) has noted that the extensor apparatus can be seen to form a diamond shape at the level of the DIP joint. The tendons of the interossei are attached to the lateral angles of the diamond. As they pull on these angles, the diamond shape becomes broader and shorter (Figure 1.120).

In cases of paralysis or division of the flexor tendons, traction on the extensor tendon causes complete extension of the fingers, but in a sequence contrary to the normal one: the distal interphalangeal joint extends first, followed by the proximal interphalangeal and metacarpophalangeal joints. Thus, the braking action of the flexors controls the sequence of the extension of the phalanges.

Conclusion

Each of the two systems, the long extensors and the intrinsic muscles, can extend the interphalangeal articulations, provided the muscles and tendons move freely and the metacarpophalangeal articulations cannot be thrown into hyperextension. This "stabilization" of the metacarpophalangeal articulation is normally the result of the action of

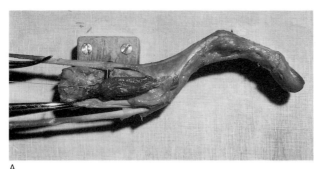

Figure 1.121. The Bouvier test: prevention of hyperextension of the metacarpophalangeal joint allows extension of the distal phalanges by tension on the EDC.

A

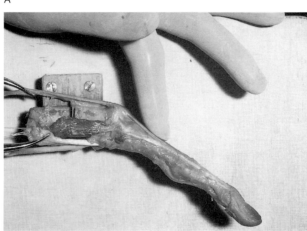

B

the interosseous muscles. Should they be paralyzed, the long extensors act unopposed at the level of their proximal insertions (the sagittal bands and the inconstant insertion on the base of the proximal phalanx) and hyperextend the metacarpophalangeal articulations. This precludes any further action in the interphalangeal joints. Holding the metacarpophalangeal joints in slight flexion, as described by Bouvier in 1851 (Figure 1.121), allows extension of the distal phalanges. Complete extension of the phalanges is produced if hyperextension of the proximal phalanx is prevented or if the two flexor tendons are divided. Then, it is only possible to extend all the phalanges with traction on the long extensor.

Various surgical procedures can prevent hyperextension of the metacarpophalangeal joints—tendon transfers, tenodesis, and capsulodesis—so that the long extensors can be allowed to extend the distal phalanges. Correction of the muscular imbalance is not sufficient to re-establish function after paralysis of the intrinsic muscles of the fingers. Besides correcting the deformities, the reconstruction of prehension requires tendon transfers strong enough to ensure useful flexion of the metacarpophalangeal joints and good abduction of the index finger to resist the pressure of the thumb.

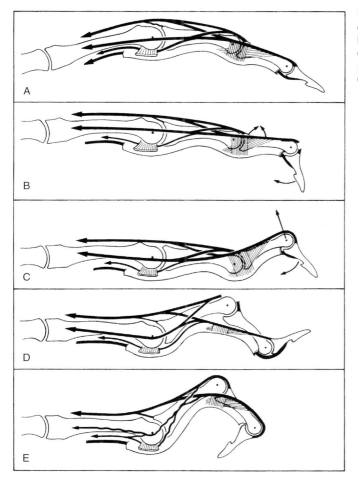

Figure 1.122. The digital kinetic chain and its deformities. (A) Normal balance of the chain. (B) Mallet deformity. (C) Swan-neck deformity. (D) Boutonnière deformity. (E) Claw deformity.

The three phalanges have a large freedom of movement. However, they constitute an interdependent kinetic osteoarticular chain: lesions of the extensor apparatus at one level may alter the balance of the whole finger, and so characteristic deformities occur (e.g. the mallet finger, boutonnière deformity, swan-neck deformity, and claw hand (Figure 1.122) (see *Examination of the musculotendinous apparatus*, page 207).

Movements of the thumb

The wide range of motion of the column of the thumb allows opposition to the palm and to the other digits. This very special movement, which contributes to the uniqueness of man's hand, is the result of:

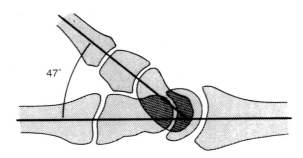

Figure 1.123. The carpometacarpal ray of the thumb is anterior to the plane of the other metacarpals and makes an angle of about 47 degrees with the second ray.

- the forward tilt of the radial carpometacarpal column (Figure 1.123);
- the configuration of the trapeziometacarpal, metacarpophalangeal, and interphalangeal articular surfaces;
- muscular traction; and
- control by ligaments. The dorsal ligaments of the trapeziometacarpal joint form a unit with the thenar muscles that partially determines the movement of the first metacarpal (Zancolli, 1977).

The three articulations of this chain have different sectors of mobility. The more proximal they are, the more directions of mobility they have.

The interphalangeal articulation

The interphalangeal articulation is a trochlear type of articulation, allowing mainly flexion and extension; the flexion is accompanied by a slight degree of rotation in pronation. A lack of extension of greater than 15 degrees is functionally more disabling than lack of flexion.

The metacarpophalangeal articulation

The metacarpophalangeal articulation is of a condylar type. In addition, it is capable of small lateral movements, especially to the radial side. Flexion is always accompanied by radial deviation and pronation, thus stretching the ulnar metacarpophalangeal ligament. This helps to ensure stability of this articulation, which is more important than movement from a functional viewpoint.

Trapeziometacarpal joint

The distal articular surface of the trapezium is usually likened to a saddle whose concave curvature lies in a dorsopalmar direction: the corresponding surface on the base of the first metacarpal presents a grooved surface in the radioulnar direction. In reality these surfaces are asymmetrical. The longitudinal crest of the trapezium as well as its transverse groove are curved as if to sit on a "scoliotic" horse (Kuczynski, 1974) (Figure 1.124).

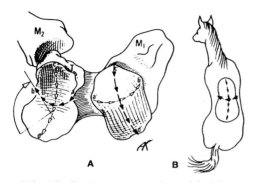

Figure 1.124. The articular surfaces of the joint between trapezium and metacarpal. (A) The surfaces of the trapezium (T) and the first metacarpal (M) are asymmetrical (an open joint). The ridge (cd) and the groove (ab) of the trapezial surface are curved (the change in direction of the groove is 90 degrees). Thus, the ridge (a'b') of the first metacarpal slides in the groove of the trapezium, causing a change in the orientation of the first metacarpal. Thus flexion is necessarily accompanied by pronation and extension by supination. (B) The "scoliotic horse": assuming the saddle is sufficiently soft to mold itself exactly to the horse's back, then the ridge and groove thus obtained will curve inwards in exactly the same manner as does the trapezium.

The trapeziometacarpal joint has two longitudinal axes and two degrees of freedom and is best likened to a universal joint. In such a joint, successive or simultaneous movements produce a conjoined rotation (MacConaill, 1946) of the mobile segment (the first metacarpal) around its longitudinal axis. The longitudinal rotation is largely responsible for changing the orientation of the thumb pulp, which is in pronation when the thumb is in opposition and in supination when the thumb is in retroposition. The shape of the articular surface does not make for good stability except in anteposition and pronation (the thumb ray is brought in front of the plane of the palm) when the two surfaces are congruent. The necessary stability is provided by a complex ligamentous system which does not limit mobility. It essentially consists of a strong ulnar ligament from the base of the first metacarpal to the second metacarpal and to the trapezoid (it is this ligament that resists in a Bennett fracture), and a couple of oblique ligaments (anterior and posterior), which were described by Haines (1944) and whose role was accurately defined by a Caffinière (1970) and Pieron (1973) (Figure 1.125).

The oblique ligaments tighten and thus become efficient as stabilizers in complete pronation of the thumb, i.e. in the position of the thumb–digital grip.

The radial side of the joint has a much weaker ligament. Thus, there is an intrinsic instability at the level where the pressure is very high; this pressure is proportional to the force of the grip at the distal end of the thumb and to the length of the lever arm (Figure 1.126).

Cooney and Chao (1977) found that the joint compression forces during simple pinch averaged 3.0 kg of force at the interphalangeal joint, 5.4 kg at the metacarpophalangeal joint, and 12.0 kg at the carpometacarpal joint. Compression forces of up to 120 kg may occur at the carpometacarpal joint during strong grasp. Stability here is dynamically provided by a single structure, the tendon of the abductor pollicis longus, which has stabilizing function only when the first metacarpal is abducted. In adduction, the long abductor increases the risk of subluxation of this joint.

This design of the trapeziometacarpal joint accounts for the functional efficiency of the joint. It also explains the frequent pathological subluxations occurring after trauma, in rheumatoid arthritis, and after trapeziometacarpal joint implants.

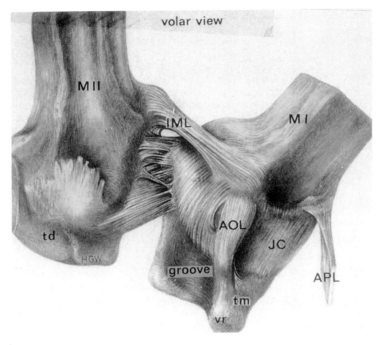

A

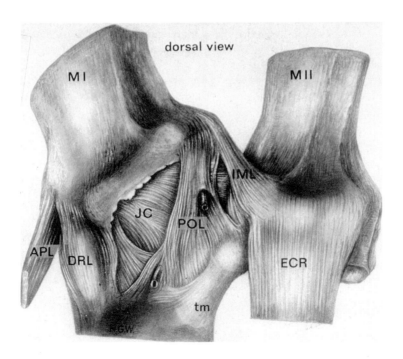

B

Figure 1.125. (A) Volar view of the right first carpometacarpal joint: on the left the metacarpal II (MII); on the right side the trapezium and metacarpal I (MI). (B) Dorsal view of the right first carpometacarpal joint and the arrangement of the ligaments and joint capsule (JC).

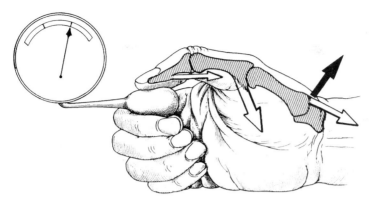

Figure 1.126. The strength of grip at the distal phalanx of the thumb depends on the stability of the thumb column and the force of the adductor muscles. The two muscles that provide most of the power in grip are the flexor pollicis longus and the adductor pollicis. The flexor pollicis longus works as an adductor and a flexor of the metacarpophalangeal joint when the interphalangeal joint is stabilized in extension. The adductor pollicis plays a very important role in the strength of grip. This is noted especially in ulnar nerve palsies in which there is a considerable loss of force. The stability of the thumb column is provided by the capsuloligamentous structures as well as by muscles, essentially the adductor pollicis and the flexor pollicis brevis at the metacarpophalangeal joint, and by the abductor pollicis longus at the trapeziometacarpal joint when the first metacarpal is abducted. In terminal grip a significant compression force is exerted at the trapeziometacarpal joint. Cooney and Chao (1977) showed this to be 12 kg, with a terminal force of 1 kg. Thus, it is easy to understand that the tendency for radial subluxation of the base of the first metacarpal (black arrow) is much greater when the first metacarpal is adducted.

The movements of the three articulations of this functional unit, which make up the thumb ray, are partially able to compensate for each other in flexion–adduction or extension–abduction. However, bringing the thumb ray in front of the plane of the palm (anteposition) is a movement of the first metacarpal that is unique to that carpometacarpal joint.

The movements of the thumb have been the object of numerous analyses, at times controversial. They will be discussed in Section 2.2, pp. 193–99.

Intrinsic and extrinsic muscles of the thumb

Movements of the thumb are produced by two groups of muscles consisting of the extrinsics, which are the long muscles of the thumb, and the intrinsics (Figures 1.127 and 1.128).

It is essential to remember that in the thumb, the intrinsic muscles are stronger than those of the extrinsics (Table 1.5), which is the opposite of the situation in the fingers. The strength of these muscles was evaluated by Fahrer in 1981 (1981b). The adductor has a force greater than that of all three lateral thenar muscles together. These muscles are innervated by the three principal nerves of the upper extremity—the radial,

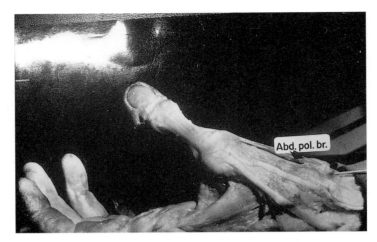

Figure 1.127. Anatomical preparation showing the lateral aspect of the thumb and first commissure; the thumb is in anteposition.

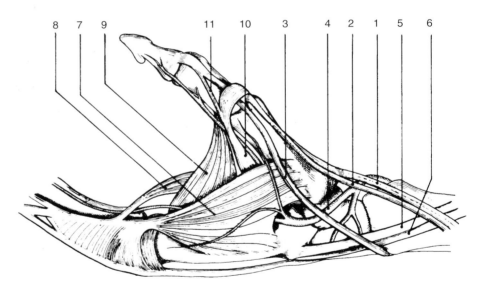

Figure 1.128. Lateral view of the thumb and first commissure with the thumb in anteposition. The tendons of the posterior extrinsic muscles can be distinguished: laterally the abductor pollicis longus (1) and the extensor pollicis brevis (2) and medially the extensor pollicis longus (3). These tendons define the anatomical snuffbox through which pass the radial artery (4) and the tendons of the extensores carpi radialis longus (5) and brevis (6). The intrinsic muscles are also shown. The first dorsal interosseous (7) inserts essentially on the base of the first phalanx; the radial side of the dorsal interosseous aponeurosis is often reinforced by the fibers of the first lumbrical (8), which is more developed than the others. Note the two components—transverse (9) and oblique (10)—of the adductor pollicis inserting on the internal sesamoid as well as on the base of the first phalanx. The adductor sends a dorsal slip (11) to the extensor apparatus, thus playing a role in extension of the distal phalanx of the thumb.

Muscle	Muscular work
Extrinsic muscles	
Flexor pollicis longus (FPL)	1.2 kg.m
Extensor pollicis longus (EPL)	0.3 kg.m
Abductor pollicis longus (APL)	0.5 kg.m
Extensor pollicis brevis (EPB)	0.1 kg.m
Intrinsic muscles	
Abductor pollicis brevis (APB)	0.5 kg.m
Opponens pollicis (OP)	0.4 kg.m
Plexor pollicis brevis (FPB)	0.5 kg.m
Adductor pollicis (AP)	1.5 kg.m

Table 1.5. Value of the thumb muscles

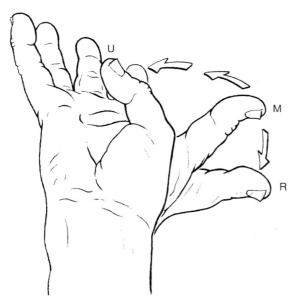

Figure 1.129. Motor innervation of the thumb. The three main nerves of the upper extremity contribute to thumb movements—the radial nerve (R) for extension and retroposition, the ulnar nerve (U) for adduction, and the median nerve (M) for anteposition and opposition.

the median, and the ulnar nerves—which participate jointly and successively in opposition of the thumb (Figure 1.129).

The actions of the muscles can be thought of as follows:

• the three long posterior muscles (C7 root), innervated by the radial nerve, stabilize the thumb column like shrouds and permit opening of the thumb–finger pinch, the indispensable prelude to opposition; then, after opposition, they bring the thumb back to its starting point;

117

- the lateral thenar muscles (T1 root), innervated by the median nerve, produce rotation of the thumb away from the palm;
- the adductor pollicis (T1 root), innervated by the ulnar nerve, pulls the first metacarpal toward the second and third metacarpals, producing closure of the pinch and giving power to the grip.

The motor territory of the radial nerve is fairly constant, but the same is not true for the median and ulnar nerves. A better knowledge of the action of each muscle will help us to understand the effect of selective paralyses.

Flexor pollicis longus
The flexor pollicis longus (C8) is the only extrinsic muscle of the thumb that is innervated by the median nerve. It flexes at the distal phalanx and contributes to flexion of the proximal phalanx. It plays an important role both in precision pinch, which requires movement of the distal phalanx, and in power grip. Its action is not that of an adductor, as Duchenne (1867) showed, and it has only a minor direct effect on the trapeziometacarpal joint. Indirectly, however, it reinforces the adductor power of the extensor pollicis longus by placing it under tension.

Extensors of the thumb
The extensor mechanism of the phalanges of the thumb is simpler than that of the digits, since there are only two instead of three phalanges. Each phalanx has a clearly defined extrinsic extensor tendon: the long and short thumb extensors. As in the fingers, the intrinsic muscles of the thumb also contribute (by means of the dorsal expansion of the abductor pollicis brevis and of the adductor) to phalangeal extension, but only for the distal phalanx (see Figure 1.135).

The extensor pollicis longus (EPL), which is much weaker than the flexor, helps to extend the two phalanges of the thumb. it also exerts significant action on the first metacarpal, which it brings into retroposition, adduction, and supination. Fick (1911) named it the "extensor pollicis adducens." Without the opposing action of the lateral thenar muscles, extension of the second phalanx under the effect of the EPL would produce retroposition of the metacarpal and would prevent opposition. When the lateral thenar muscles are paralyzed, this antagonistic action of the EPL impedes the re-establishment of anteposition by a surgical transfer and sometimes necessitates the rerouting of the EPL tendon outside Lister's tubercle. Its contribution to adduction of the thumb plays an important compensatory role in cases of paralysis of the adductor, but with the effect of supination on the column of the thumb.

The extensor pollicis brevis (EPB) extends the metacarpophalangeal joint when the interphalangeal joint is flexed, and thus plays a part in the precision grip. It is also a radial abductor of the first metacarpal.

Abductor pollicis longus
The abductor pollicis longus (APL), whose tendon is slightly more palmar, has a more pronounced effect of anteposition. It is actually a palmar abductor, bringing the first

metacarpal anterior. The APL also plays a role in stabilizing the trapeziometacarpal joint and acts as an antagonist of the adductor, essential for the power grip. Furthermore, it is a radial stabilizer of the wrist and an antagonist of the extensor carpi ulnaris.

Accessory tendons of APL are frequent. They seem to play a part in cases of osteoarthrosis of the first carpometacarpal joint (Zancolli and Cozzi, 1992). These authors classified the sites of distal insertions of the accessory tendons in arthrosis of the thumb as follows:

• insertion into the thenar muscles (opponens and abductor pollicis brevis (APB)) forming a digastric muscle in 82 per cent;
• insertion into the radial side of the metacarpal basis, forming a "double APL tendon" in 10 per cent;
• insertion into both the thenar muscles and the metacarpal basis in 8 per cent.

The difference in the incidence of accessory tendons of the APL between osteoarthritic patients and cadaveric hands (which are not necessarily osteoarthritic) supports the view that the presence of accessory tendons with insertions distal to the basal joint increases the internal compressive forces in the thumb joints. Results obtained by early excision in trapeziometacarpal osteoarthritis seem satisfactory (Zancolli and Cozzi, 1992).

First dorsal interosseous and palmaris longus

The first dorsal interosseous, sometimes called the abductor indicis, has a long origin along the medial aspect of the first metacarpal. It is attached to the radial side of the proximal phalanx of the index finger. It plays an important role in the thumb–index pinch.

The palmaris longus is sometimes considered a muscle of the thumb (Kaplan, 1954). Its lateral tendon, which extends to the APB, causes anteposition, as shown by Fahrer and Tubiana (1976).

The thenar muscles

The thenar muscles form a cone surrounding the first metacarpal, whose apex is centered at the metacarpophalangeal joint. These muscles enter successively into action from lateral to medial in the movement of opposition. They may be divided according to their distal termination into two groups: external and internal (Cruveilhier, 1843) (Figure 1.130):

1 The external thenar (thenar proper) or external sesamoid muscles (abductor pollicis brevis, opponens, and flexor pollicis brevis), innervated by the median nerve, cause circumduction of the thumb at a distance from the palm: they are pronators.
2 The internal thenar (the oblique and transverse heads of the adductor as well as the first palmar interosseous muscle) or internal sesamoids, innervated by the ulnar nerve, bring the thumb metacarpal toward the index metacarpal, and at the end of opposition reinforce the grip: they are supinators.

The three lateral thenar muscles are arranged in two planes. The *abductor pollicis brevis* (APB), the most superficial, has its fibers nearly parallel to the first metacarpal

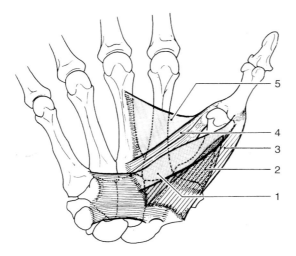

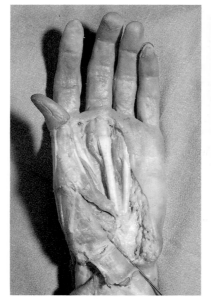

Figure 1.130. Intrinsic musculature of the thumb. On the outside are the (external) thenar muscles or external sesamoid muscles: (1) flexor pollicis brevis; (2) opponens pollicis (coarse stippling); (3) abductor pollicis brevis (hatched). On the inside are the "internal thenar muscles" or internal sesamoid muscles: (4) oblique head of the adductor; (5) transverse head of adductor.

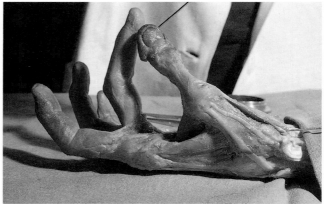

Figure 1.131. The abductor pollicis brevis produces anteposition of the first metacarpal, pronation and lateral deviation of the proximal phalanx, and contributes to the extension of the distal phalanx, but not to the adduction of the thumb ray.

(Figure 1.131). It is the strongest muscle of anteposition. It also pronates and causes lateral deviation of the proximal phalanx, and it contributes to extension of the distal phalanx. Duchenne (1867) called it the opposing phalangeal muscle of the thumb, because by its action the tip of the thumb can reach the distal phalanges of the fingers.

The deeper *opponens pollicis* (OP) acts only on the first metacarpal, which it anteposes, adducts, and pronates (Figure 1.132), because it does not have a phalangeal

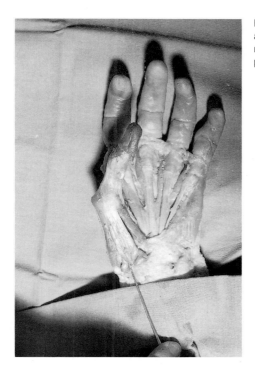

Figure 1.132. The opponens produces anteposition and pronation of the first metacarpal. There is no action on the proximal phalanx.

insertion. Thus, it is the only "opposing muscle" of the first metacarpal. Its almost transverse fibers provide a very effective action. Thus, along with the APL, it is a stabilizing muscle of the trapeziometacarpal joint.

The *flexor pollicis brevis* (FPB) (Figure 1.133), situated on the same plane as the opponens but medial to it, runs a more oblique course. It is therefore a weaker muscle for anteposition than the APB, and a stronger adductor than the opponens. It also contributes to the flexion of the proximal phalanx. It permits the thumb to contact the middle phalanx of the fingers.

The medial thenar muscles, essentially the oblique and transverse heads of the *adductor pollicis*, insert on the medial sesamoid and ulnar aspect of the base of the proximal phalanx of the thumb. They approximate the first metacarpal to the second and third metacarpals, and also produce inward rotation into supination (Figure 1.134), which is the opposite action to that of the lateral thenar muscles. In addition, the oblique head of the adductor sends a dorsal expansion to the EPL (Figure 1.135), thus contributing to extension in the distal phalanx of the thumb. This dorsal expansion is symmetric with that of the APB on the radial side.

The *first palmar interosseous* (Henle, 1868) is very slender. It originates at the trapezium and at the base of the first metacarpal, and inserts on the medial sesamoid. It now is usually considered the most lateral head of the oblique adductor.

121

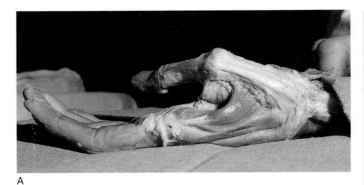

A

Figure 1.133. Flexor pollicis brevis (FPB). (A) The FPB produces less anteposition than the abductor pollicis brevis (APB). (B) More adduction results from the FPB than from either the APB or the opponens. Flexion and pronation of the proximal phalanx also occur.

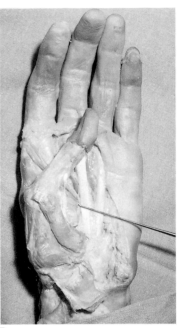

B

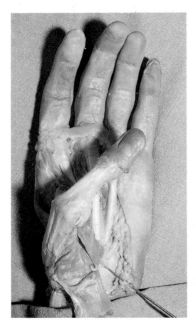

Figure 1.134. Adductor pollicis. The adductor brings the first metacarpal to the second and third metacarpals with rotation in supination.

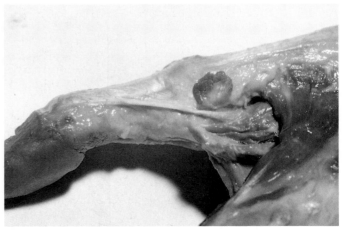

Figure 1.135. The expansion of the oblique head of the adductor pollicis to the extensor pollicis longus contributes to extension of the distal phalanx.

Innervation of the thenar muscles

Between the lateral thenar muscles innervated by the median nerve and the medial thenars innervated by the ulnar nerve, the deep head of the FPB forms a true transitional zone. It frequently receives a double innervation. In most cases, it is the ulnar territory that spills over. Thus, in a patient with a median nerve palsy, the movement of opposition is still possible if the ulnar nerve supplies the two heads of the FPB. The muscle can be seen and felt contracting medial to the fossa created by the atrophy of the APB and OP.

This finding is far from rare; in the author's experience, it occurs in one third of cases. A similar or higher proportion is found in the reports of Highet (1943) and Rowntree (1959). Although movement of opposition is reduced by half in both ante-position and pronation, this may be misleading, especially if there is motorsensory dissociation. The existence of such a movement risks misdiagnosis of a median nerve palsy if the absence of contraction in the APB and the OP is not sought systematically. Likewise, in isolated paralyses of the ulnar nerve, the presence of opposition due to the lateral thenars may cause a misdiagnosis of paralysis of the thumb if one does not look for atrophy of the first web and other signs of ulnar palsy.

Clinical diagnosis may be difficult when there are anastomoses between the median and ulnar nerves. In the forearm, the Martin–Gruber anastomosis is not unusual, and Mannerfelt (1966) has suggested that it is present in six out of 40 cases after selective blocking of the ulnar nerve, with maintenance of innervation of the first dorsal interosseous and/or the adductor. The Riche–Cannieu anastomosis in the palm between the terminal branches of the median and ulnar nerves can provide mixed innervation of the adductor in certain cases.

The hypothenar eminence

Placed in the ulnar aspect of the palm, the hypothenar eminence represents the heel of the hand.

A strong fibrous shell forms the subcorial layer immediately under the hypothenar skin (Landsmeer 1968), Fahrer 1977). Large lobules of semifluid fat are found deep to the fibrous shell. The subcutaneous hypothenar space communicates proximally with the proximal aspect of the forearm.

The tendon of the flexor carpi ulnaris inserts on the pisiform bone and sends several fibrous expansions: the ligamentum carpi volare into the flexor retinaculum, forming the roof of "Guyon's loge (space)" (Figure 1.136), expansions to the piso-hamate and piso-metacarpal ligaments and direct tendinous fibers into the dermis of the hypothenar eminence (Figures 1.137 and 1.138).

The muscles of the hypothenar form three layers:

- a subcutaneous muscle, the palmaris brevis muscle, innervated by the superficial branch of the ulnar nerve,
- a layer formed by two muscles: the abductor digiti minimi medially and the flexor digiti minimi brevis laterally. Between them, a gap traversed by the deep branches of the ulnar nerve and artery.

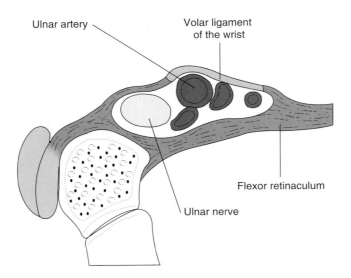

Ulnar artery

Volar ligament
of the wrist

Flexor retinaculum

Ulnar nerve

Figure 1.136. The "Guyon space" (or canal). Section through the pisiform bone.

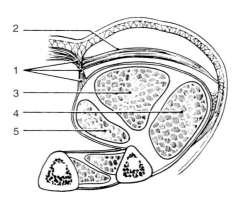

2

1

3

4

5

Figure 1.137. Section through the hypothenar: (1) lateral longitudinal septum; (2) palmaris brevis; (3) flexor digiti minimi brevis; (4) abductor digiti minimi; (5) opponens digiti minimi.

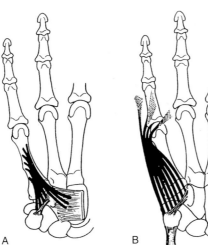
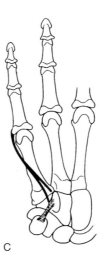

Figure 1.138. Hypothenar muscles. (A) Flexor digiti minimi brevis; (B) abductor digiti minimi; (C) opponens digiti minimi.

A B C

- The deep layer is represented by the opponens digiti minimi.

The nerve supply of these three muscles is from the deep ulnar nerve.

The flexor and abductor digiti minimi can flex and fifth MP joint. The opponens can flex and laterally rotate the fifth metacarpal. The abductor digiti minimi is a strong abductor of the little finger. It can also laterally rotate the fifth MP joint and extend the PIP joint. This muscle can be used as a transfer into the thumb (Littler and Cooley, 1963).

Functional value of the digits

Study of the skeleton and its musculature shows that each digit has an individual and specific functional value. The value of each digit depends on several factors, of which the most important are its strength, its mobility, and its relations with the other digits and in particular with the thumb.

In assessing the disability resulting from the loss of a digit, one must consider the possibilities of substitution of its action by neighboring digits as well as the consequences of this loss on the mechanics of the other digits and on the hand in general. The individual value of each digit must also be estimated in its relation to the hand (dominant or not) and to the occupation and hobbies of the patient. For example, the fifth digit of the non-dominant hand, which finds the far note on his instrument, is of exceptional value to the violinist (Figure 1.139).

Thumb

The thumb is the most important digit because of its mobility and force and because of the privileged and irreplaceable relations it has with the other digits, allowing it to

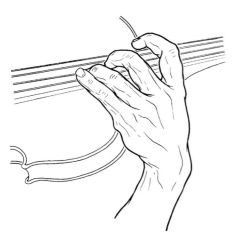

Figure 1.139. Flexion and adduction of the wrist by the flexor carpi ulnaris in the left hand of a violinist. When playing high notes, the violinist must bring his fingers up to the vicinity of the bridge by putting his wrist into flexion–adduction through the action of the flexor carpi ulnaris. When the flexor carpi ulnaris is paralyzed, as was that of Duchenne's famous violinist patient, who presented with "progressive fatty-muscular atrophy," the left hand can no longer reach the very high notes even though wrist flexion is possible through the action of the two radial wrist flexors.

oppose all of them and the palm. Yet one must remember that the exceptional functional value of the thumb comes from the mobility of its metacarpal and its intrinsic musculature, which is stronger than the extrinsic muscles. A contracted web space fixing the first metacarpal in retroposition converts a thumb with only phalangeal mobility into a particularly poorly functioning short digit.

Index finger

The index finger is often considered the most important digit after the thumb because of its strength, its ability to abduct, the relative independence of its musculature, and especially its closeness to the thumb. This proximity enables it to play an essential role in lateral pinch as well as in distal precision handling. The deficit in power that results from amputation of the index finger is usually evaluated at about 20 per cent for digitopalmar lateral grip and supination grip. Power grip, in pronation, is considerably weakened (approximately 50 per cent [Murray et al, 1977]).

In the absence of the index finger, the pronation grip of the hand lacks stability. The stability of the grip in pronation is influenced more than the grip in supination by the area of contact of an object with the hand. The width of the grip extends from the hypothenar eminence and the gripping ulnar fingers, which constitute the internal fulcrum, to the proximal phalanx of the index finger, which is the external fulcrum of movement. It is therefore necessary, in cases of injury to the index finger, to conserve the proximal phalanx when possible in manual workers.

Middle finger

The middle finger has more strength than the index finger in flexion. It is the longest digit, and its median position enables it to participate in grips of power and grips of precision, conferring on it a great functional value. Moreover, its loss leaves the center of the hand with a defect that may cause disorders by the gradual convergence of the neighboring digits. An amputation of the middle finger entails a greater esthetic deficit than that of the index finger.

Ring finger

The ring finger has a strength in flexion far inferior to that of the preceding digits. It is rarely used for precision grip but participates especially in the strong digitopalmar grip, and its action is coupled with that of the fifth digit. Its loss leaves the least functional deficit of any of the fingers.

Little finger

The fifth or little finger has the least strength in flexion because of its small size and the weak flexion strength of its distal phalanges. However, its loss leaves a deficiency out of proportion to its small dimension. The functional importance of the fifth digit, often poorly appreciated, stems from several factors. Its peripheral position confers on it a special role in power grip. Its expansile capacity of abduction augments in effect the capacity of the hand. In digitopalmar grip the fifth digit, as the most ulnar, presses the object or the handle of the tool against the hypothenar eminence. Its viselike action is considerably reinforced by its metacarpal's ability to move forward 20 to 25 degrees, and its strength is reinforced by the powerful hypothenar muscles which flex the first phalanx (see Figures 1.137 and 1.138). As with the thumb, the functional value of the fifth finger can be appreciated only in association with its metacarpal. The fifth ray taken in its entirety probably has the greatest functional value after the thumb ray.

1.4 SKIN COVER

The cutaneous covering of the hand has an exceptional importance because of its physical qualities, its sensory properties, and its microcirculation. Indeed, its characteristics cannot be dissociated from the motor and sensory properties of the hand.

The extent of the cutaneous surface in relation to the volume of the hand is not equaled anywhere else in the body. There is a relationship comparable to that of the brain, whose surface is proportionately much larger than its total volume. The measurements reported by Morel Fatio (1985) as well as by Barreiro and Valdecasas (1981) are very close. Both found that a volume of 1 cm^3 in the digit corresponds to a skin surface area of 2.5 cm^2, whereas in the forearm the value drops to 0.5 cm^2 according to Morel Fatio and to 0.4 cm^2 according to Barreiro.

The integument of the palmar region and of the back of the hand displays a remarkable functional adaptation and, in this respect there is an evident difference between the palmar and dorsal skin: both anatomically and functionally they are different from and independent of each other. The dorsal skin, which is fine and supple, is not used as a resting or sensory surface, and its chief virtue is that it does not impede free articular mobility in flexion. By contrast, the palmar skin is thick, tough, and resistant to pressure; it stabilizes the grip and, particularly at the pulps, has important sensory functions.

The palmar skin

Histological structure

The histological architecture of the palmar skin is similar to that of skin elsewhere, but it has additional features that are functionally relevant.

The epidermis

The epidermis is made up of four elastic layers in addition to the stratum lucidum (Figure 1.140). Starting with the deepest and moving superficially, they are as follows:

The basal layer

The basal layer consists of a unicellular stratum of basal cells mingled with melanocytes. Cell multiplication occurs during periods of skin regeneration. Its deep aspect rests on the basement membrane, a fine acellular structure marking the dermoepidermal junction, to which it is attached by means of protoplasmic prolongations known as hemidesmosomes. The basement membrane itself is anchored to the superficial layer of the dermis by collagen or retinacular fibrils, which indirectly "fasten" the dermis to the epidermis.

The Malpighian layer

The Malpighian layer (or Malpighian body) consists of a thick multicellular layer of polygonal cells that become flatter as they approach the surface. They are united by

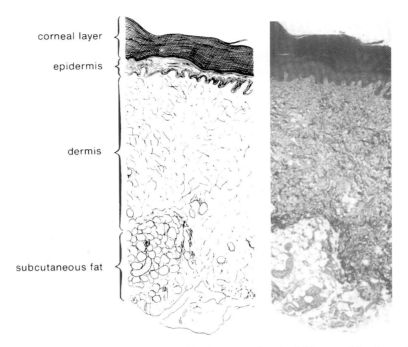

corneal layer

epidermis

dermis

subcutaneous fat

Figure 1.140. Section of palmar skin demonstrating the thickness of the horny layer in relation to the epidermis as well as the thickness and density of the dermis.

intercellular bridges or desmosomes. As with the cells of the basal layer, their cytoplasm is rich in tonofibrils made up of a keratin precursor. This layer is also a site of cellular multiplication and plays a significant part in skin regeneration.

The granular layer

The granular layer is two to three cells thick, and its thickness is further enhanced by active keratinization. The cells take the shape of flattened lozenges and contain numerous cytoplasmic granules of the lipoproteinaceous substance, keratohyalin.

The horny layer

The horny layer (stratum corneum) is made up of flattened cells transformed by keratinization with no detectable intercellular spaces; they are recognizable at the light microscopic level as they have no nuclei or only vestigial nuclei.

The stratum lucidum

The stratum lucidum, situated between the granular and horny layers, is a feature of palmar and plantar skin. It is two or three cells thick, and the cells are flattened, anuclear, homogeneous, translucid and rich in an oily substance, eleidin.

The dermis

The dermis is a connective tissue whose structure is an intertwining of collagen, elastic, and reticular fibers. Within this fibrillar network are scattered a few cells, together with blood vessels and nerve endings.

The superficial layer

The superficial layer is in close contact with the epidermis. On section, the irregular junction line is characterized by alternating dermal protrusions (dermal papillae or papillary ridges) and epidermal protrusions (the epidermal ridges). This type of dermis therefore is known as papillary dermis.

In the superficial papillary zone, the connective fibers form a meshwork, and these fibers tend to follow the axis of the papillae. As we have seen, the reticular fibers, together with the elastic fibers, anchor the epidermis to the dermis. Vascularization here consists of capillaries arising from superficial plexuses and following the axis of the papillae. Sensory nerve endings found in this layer are primarily Merkel's subepidermal discs and the intrapapillary Meissner corpuscles.

The reticular dermis

In a deeper plane lies the reticular dermis. The collagen fibers are thicker and more abundant, and the numerous elastic fibers form an undulating pattern. The orientation of the fibers is mostly in a line parallel to the surface of the skin. Running up from the deeper layers are the fibrous cones, bundles of collagen fibers that unite the dermis to the underlying fascial planes and through which run the vessels and nerves from the subcutaneous layer.

The superficial vascular plexus lies between the superficial and middle layers of the dermis, whereas the deep plexus lies between the dermis and subcutaneous cellular tissue.

Characteristic features of palmar skin

The papillary structure

The junction line between the palmar dermis and epidermis, characterized by alternating dermal and epidermal ridges, indicates that the palmar skin is of the papillary type. The papillary ridges, far from being erased by the superficial epidermis, are actually enhanced, especially by the horny layer. The dermis is said to be delomorphic, its macroscopic relief appearing superficially as ridges that contribute to the dermatoglyphic patterns. The pores of the sweat glands open at the "summits" of these ridges.

Mechanical resistance

Mechanical resistance is a highly important physical feature of skin. It is the result primarily of a particularly thick middle dermis, which is itself securely anchored to the deeper planes by the fibrous cones. It is reinforced by the thickness of the epidermis, all of whose layers show signs of activity. One of the most important factors is the thick horny layer, which has some unusual structural and physiological features.

The horny layer

In the hand the thickness of the horny layer ranges from 0.5 to 2 mm compared with 0.02 mm in other areas. The horny layer is made up of a thick layer of cells whose framework remains visible; this is the site of type A keratinization and contains a filamentous network that presumably favors hydration. The important horny layer can be replaced in its entirety within 20 days without the appearance of a "stratum desqua-mante" visible elsewhere in the skin.

The horny layer has a high hydration potential, which increases its thickness and contributes to its strength and suppleness. This imbibition is maintained by a lipid surface film, which, in the absence of the sebaceous system, originates in the lipids eliminated from the superficial cells. The hydration source is twofold—insensible perspiration, as elsewhere in the body, and a special arrangement of the sweating system.

The cutaneous adnexa

The palm does not possess a pilosebaceous system, but it has an abundance of exocrine sweat glands (400 per cm²). These are characterized by unusually long excretory channels by reason of the thickness of the skin and horny layer and also because they run a spiral course through the epidermis. This arrangement, which facilitates imbibition in the horny layer, is also responsible for the complications of hyperhydrosis.

True physiological, visible perspiration of thermal origin is relatively poor in normal subjects, but it can be modified by various factors (e.g. emotion, pain, smoking). Palmar sweating takes the form of almost continuous insensible secretion, although individual glands show sporadic activity which alternates with that of their neighbors. This insensible perspiration, which is probably absorbed before it reaches the surface, maintains the hydration of the horny layer.

The pores open at the crest of the epidermal ridges and aid in maintaining their moistening and suppleness. In this indirect way the sweating mechanism plays a part in promoting sensation.

Macroscopic appearance of palmar skin

The palm of the hand is characterized by a system of cutaneous folds, which are present from birth and have physiological significance.

Fingerprints

The cutaneous striations that make up the fingerprints form the essential part of dermato-glyphics (Figure 1.141). They reflect the arrangement of the papillary ridges of the underlying dermis whose outline is enhanced by the thickness of the stratum corneum.

Their specific distribution over the pulps is of well-known medicolegal importance, but they are in fact present all over the palmar skin. Their overall orientation is predominantly transverse; at the pulps they form a typical concentric pattern, whereas in the midpalmar area they tend to run longitudinally and obliquely.

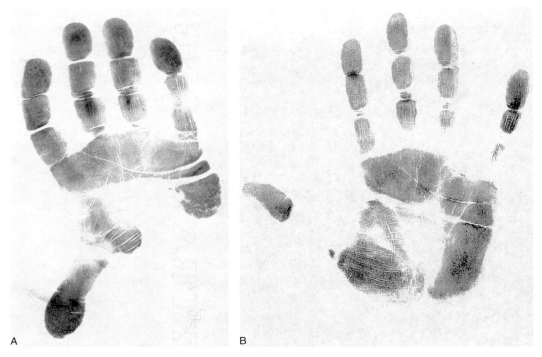

A   B

Figure 1.141. (A) Palmar print taken from a cylindrical tool handle (diameter, 4.4 cm). Note the predominance of pulp prints, especially of the cubital fingers locking the grip, and of the hypothenar eminence. (B) Palmar print, hand flat. Note the concentric arrangement of the pulp prints and the hypothenar print and the transverse organization of the striae on the distal part of the palm. Note also Lange's lines, which form fine longitudinal or transverse striations.

These striae are particularly well developed in cutaneous areas involved in the grasping of objects, and conversely they are much less evident in skin areas not usually concerned with prehension. They are particularly in evidence, therefore, on the ulnar aspect of the distal phalanx of the thumb and the radial border of the three ulnar fingers. They are also prominent in the skin covering the proximal part of the hypothenar eminence, which is important in the grasping of tool handles.

These striae play an important part in the retention of an object during the act of gripping by preventing the object from sliding over the skin. The concentric arrangement of the striae at the pulp ensures the presence of a group of striae perpendicular to the force exerted, whatever its direction. Finally, they have a tactile function by reason of the distribution of Meissner's corpuscles (see "The dermis", page 143). Thus the skin participates in the prehensive function of the hand. This differentiation of the palmar skin makes it difficult to restore with skin grafts from another area.

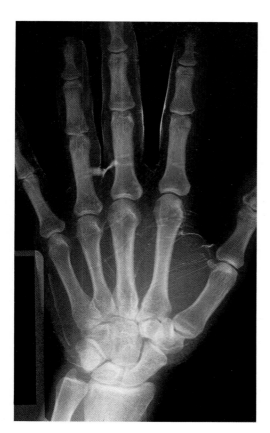

Figure 1.142. Projection of cutaneous folds in relation to the skeleton.

The skin creases

On the palmar aspect of the hand is a system that is primarily composed of transverse creases whose configuration forms the basis of palmistry, or chiromancy. With the exception of the so-called opposition crease, which forms the boundary of the thenar eminence, these creases correspond to the lines along which the skin is folded when the hand is closed; hence the name "flexion creases". In the fingers the flexion creases indicate a line of adherence between skin and fascia with no intervening adipose tissue. In the palm the proximal and distal palmar creases mark the dermal terminations of numerous longitudinal fibers of the palmar fascia. The opposition crease of the thumb coincides with the lateral border of the central fascial triangle of the palm; it marks the boundary between the fixed central palmar skin and the mobile thenar skin that moves with the column of the thumb.

The palmar creases, which are often used as landmarks, do not in fact overlie the joints whose flexion induces them to fold (Figure 1.142). Only the middle digit creases coincide with the proximal interphalangeal joints; the distal crease lies just distal to the distal interphalangeal joint, and the proximal crease lies almost halfway down the proximal phalanx.

133

In the palm the distal palmar crease, which lies in the ulnar half, runs just proximal to the medial metacarpophalangeal joint lines; the more radial proximal crease lies well above these joints.

Lange's lines

As in other zones of mobile skin, the hand shows a fine system of lines of tension, independent of the skin creases, which correspond to Lange's lines.

Relations between the skin and deeper planes: the palmar fat pads

Unlike its dorsal counterpart, the palmar skin is anchored to the underlying fascial planes by a system of fibrous tracts. As we have seen, this union results from close approximation along the lines of cutaneous stasis. The skin also adheres closely to the aponeurosis in the mid-palmar area, a triangle whose boundaries are the opposition crease of the thumb, the lateral border of the hypothenar eminence, and distally the two transverse palmar creases.

In all other areas, the deep aspect of the skin is separated from the superficial palmar fascia by a layer of fatty tissue, which is itself divided into compartments by the fibrous septa already mentioned. The result is a system of fat pads, which are malleable even though they are tethered to the skin above and the aponeurotic plane below (Figure 1.143). Three such pads or cushions are recognizable:

1 The thenar pad lines only that part of the thenar eminence nearest the palm; the proximal and lateral parts of the thenar region are almost fat-free.
2 The hypothenar pad is broader and thicker; it lines the hypothenar muscles and spills over the ulnar border of the hand, giving it its rounded outline. Proximally, the two pads are connected by an adipose band, which stretches in front of the flexor retinaculum.
3 The metacarpophalangeal pad sits transversely over the base of the fingers from the ulnar to the radial border of the hand. It is thicker over the interdigital spaces than over the flexor tendons and is bounded proximally by the transverse palmar creases. Distally it lines the interdigital palmar ligament at the commissure but is absent under the proximal digital flexion creases.

Each phalanx presents a similar system of fat pads between the digital flexion creases. The pulp also has its lobulated palmar pad, but here the fibrous septa join the periosteum of the distal phalanx to the deep aspect of the dermis.

These pads have great functional significance because they are essential to prehension. The lobulated structure under a tough dermis (an arrangement similar to that found in the plantar pads of quadrupeds) provides cushion-like resistance to pressure. In addition, their malleability enables the hand to mold itself around objects without the skeleton's being directly involved. They increase the surface available for contact and thus improve retention during grip.

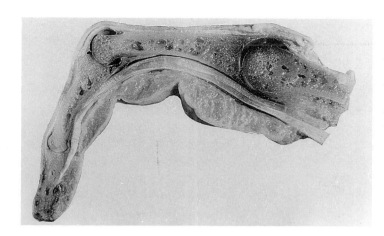

Figure 1.143. Section of the hand and finger showing the subcutaneous palmar fat pads. The metacarpophalangeal and phalangeal pads can be seen. Their structure is similar to that of the pulp, allowing the finger to mold its palmar surface to the object to be gripped.

The most characteristic feature of palmar skin is its tethering to the deeper planes. This is achieved by direct adherence at the lines of stasis and by the fibrous septa that cross the fat pads. This fixation prevents the skin from gliding over the underlying tissues and allows direct transmission of the gripping effort without any risk of skidding. It makes an important contribution to the stability of the grip. The palmaris brevis, which tethers the hypothenar skin to the deeper planes, can be regarded as a complement of this system of cutaneous stabilization. The palmaris longus, flexor carpi ulnaris, and abductor pollicis brevis act similarly through their skin insertions.

The dorsal skin

Histological structure

The histological features of the dorsal skin are not unlike those of its palmar counterpart. It has a papillary dermis, but the papillary ridges do not show on the surface because they are neutralized by the epidermis (adelomorphic dermis). The latter is thin and is lined by a horny layer that is only 0.02 mm thick.

The dermis is also thinner and less resistant; it has only loose connections with the deeper planes, over which it can move freely. Unlike the palm, however, it possesses a normal pilosebaceous system.

Finally, owing to the thinness of the epidermis and the dearth of connective and elastic tissue elements in the dermis, the dorsal skin becomes fragile in old age and has a greater vulnerability to factors causing cutaneous atrophy, such as steroid therapy.

Skin mobility

The dorsal skin owes its suppleness and mobility to its histological structure. Its relative thinness makes it more stretchable, and its loose connections with the deeper planes

135

allow free gliding and full flexion at the digital joints. Indeed, flexion of the fingers produces a significant lengthening of the dorsal skin. Thus, in the middle finger, the distance between the wrist and the ungual fold shows an average increase of 3 cm as the finger goes from extension to full flexion (range: 2.1–3.6 cm). Flexion at the metacarpophalangeal joint alone requires an average skin lengthening of 1.25 cm (range 1–2 cm). The gain in length does not occur solely at the metacarpophalangeal skin; a variable but significant gain occurs as a result of gliding and stretching over the hand and wrist.

This mobility is the result in large part of the loose arrangement of the subcutaneous cellular tissue. When this tissue is distended by edema, the stretching and gliding are considerably reduced during flexion; hence, the posture in extension of the metacarpophalangeal joints in edema of the hand.

Flexion of the proximal interphalangeal joint may occur at the expense of the segment of loose skin immediately above the joint (proximally and distally the integument is more strongly anchored to the digital fascia). This segment is well delinated by deep dorsal creases and can on its own provide a gain in length that is fairly constant, between 0.7 and 0.9 cm.

The dorsopalmar septa

The dorsal and palmar areas of skin are independent because of a system of adhesions that anchors their common boundary to the underlying plane. This anchoring is well marked on the ulnar border of the palm and even more so at the lateral borders of the fingers.

In the proximal part of the first phalanx, fixation occurs almost in a straight line in the plane of the commissural crest: it takes the form of small fibrils arranged in the shape of a fan that unite the deep aspect of the skin and the digital fascia.

More distally, and especially opposite the middle and distal phalanges, the adhesion band is more tightly packed and lies just posterior to the palmar collateral neurovascular bundle on the lateral side. It corresponds to the reinforcement in the digital fascia known as the digital band and to the point of attachment of the osteocutaneous ligaments. These deep attachments stabilize the skin in relation to the skeleton and prevent the integument from sliding freely over the motor system like the finger of a glove.

Blood supply of the skin

The cutaneous circulation of the hand has special anatomical and physiological features that are related to its distal situation far from the cardiac impulse, and to its constant exposure to thermal and postural variation.

The general pattern is not different from that found elsewhere (Salmon, 1936): muscular arteries running into arterioles forming a plexus superficial to the aponeurosis,

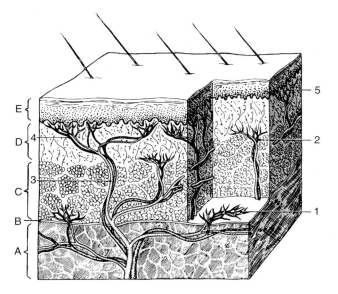

Figure 1.144. Circulation of the skin. (A) Muscle; (B) aponeurosis; (C) subdermis; (D) dermis; (E) epidermis. (1) Plexus superficial to the aponeurosis; (2) subdermal plexus; (3) perforating arteries; (4) dermal plexus; (5) subpapillary plexus.

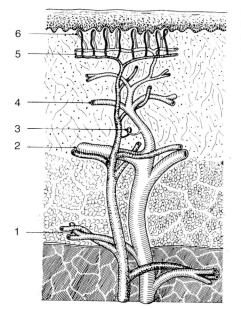

Figure 1.145. Schematic representation of the circulation of the skin. (1) Plexus superficial to the aponeurosis; (2) subdermal plexus; (3) arteriovenous anastomosis; (4) dermal artery; (5) subpapillary plexus; (6) capillary loops.

a dermal plexus and a subpapillary plexus and the return through the venous loops (Figures 1.144 and 1.145). Recent studies of the vascularization of the skin in general has allowed the arterial supply to be classified into three groups:

1 The longitudinal cutaneous arteries, which run part of their course through the subcutaneous tissues.

137

2 The septal arteries, which arise from the main artery and pass through the deep fascia to form a subdermal vascular plexus.

3 The myocutaneous arteries, which arise from the intramuscular arteries and emerge from the muscle belly to supply an area of overlying skin.

Skin flaps

The knowledge of the detailed anatomy of the blood supply has led to advances in the design of skin flaps in the upper limb used for hand reconstruction (Masquelet and Gilbert, 1995) (Figure 1.146).

- Axial pattern flaps are based on longitudinal cutaneous arteries;
- Fascio-cutaneous flaps are based on septal arteries. The main vascular pedicle, the deep fascia and the intermuscular septum must be included;
- Myocutaneous flaps are based on the vascular pedicle of the muscle.

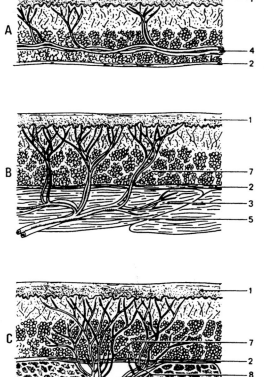

Figure 1.146. Classification of arterialized skin flaps. (A) Axial pattern flap; (B) myocutaneous flap; (C) fasciocutaneous flap; (1) epidermis; (2) fascia; (3) muscle; (4) axial artery running subcutaneously; (5) vascular pedicle of muscle; (6) vascular pedicle giving rise to fasciocutaneous perforators; (7) cutaneous perforators; (8) fasciocutaneous perforator.

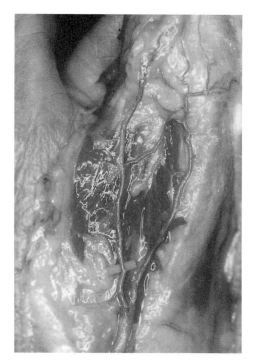

Figure 1.147. The deep and superficial dorsal IM arteries. The deep artery runs along the diaphysis of the second metacarpal.

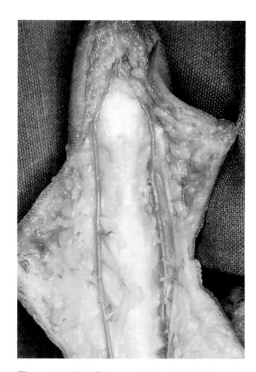

Figure 1.148. Palmar collateral digital arteries.

In the hand (*see* "Arterial supply of the hand", pages 247–56), interest in the vascular anatomy has been spurred by the possibilities of microsurgical reconstruction. The dorsal aspect of the first webspace is supplied by two arteries (Figure 1.147): the deep dorsal intermetacarpal artery which runs along the diaphysis of the second metacarpal and vascularizes the base of this bone; and the superficial dorsal intermetacarpal artery which supplies the skin overlying the proximal phalanx and the metacarpophalangeal joint of the index finger. This skin can be raised with its artery (Foucher's Kite flaps, Foucher, 1985). These two arteries have anastomoses at the metacarpal head, providing reversed flow vascularization to a bone graft taken on the second metacarpal (Brunelli, 1991) used for revascularization of carpal bones.

Deep anastomoses between the other dorsal intermetacarpal arteries and the proximal arterial system allow dorsal intermetacarpal flaps and dorsal webspace flaps.

In the fingers, the blood supply comes predominantly from the two palmar collateral digital arteries (Figure 1.148). They give cutaneous branches for the palmar digital skin and also give cutaneous branches for the dorsal skin. They present digital anastomoses arcades in the pulp and in the nail matrix (Figures 1.149 and 1.150) and also anastomoses in the digital part of the proximal and middle phalanx, under the flexor tendons. This

139

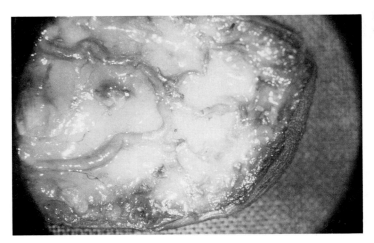

Figure 1.149. Digital anastomoses arcade in the pulp.

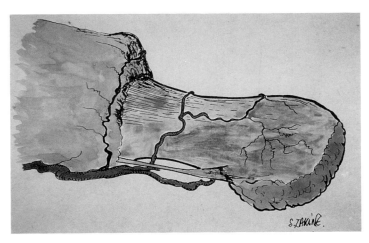

Figure 1.150. Digital anastomoses arcade in the nail matrix.

configuration allows not only heterodigital island flaps (Littler, 1956; Tubiana and Duparc, 1959) but also direct homodigital island flaps and even reversed arterial flow island flaps.

In the thumb, anatomical variations of the vascular system are frequent. The most constant artery on the dorsal aspect of the thumb is the ulnar collateral artery (see page 249).

With all the new procedures of skin cover, surgeons now have an arsenal of techniques, ranging from skin grafts, to composite free flaps, to cover all needs of reconstruction in the upper limb.

Choosing the right cover for each defect is often the main problem.

Thermoregulatory function. The rich vascular supply of the skin of the hand has an important thermoregulatory function (see page 170).

The blood circuit contains a system of shunts between the arterioles, meta-arterioles, and venules as well as more specific structures found mostly in the palm, near the roots

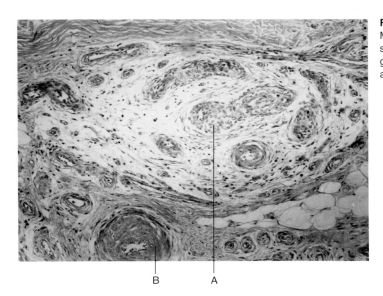

Figure 1.151. Section of Masson's glomus. (A) Capillary surrounded by a casing of glomus cells. (B) Afferent arteriole with muscular wall.

B A

of the nails, and in the pulps. These are direct arteriovenous anastomoses known as Sucquet-Hoyer anastomoses. They consist of spiral vessels that run from the hypodermis to the superficial plexus; on the way the artery loses its elastic fibers and its epithelium becomes more cuboid. The muscle wall thickens and takes on a sheath of epithelium-like cells (regarded by some as muscle cells), and the whole become sheathed by a network of nonmyelinated nerve fibers. This is the complex known as glomus tissue (Figure 1.151). At the summit of the glomus body the arteriole becomes thinner as it enters the subpapillary plexus. This interesting shunt system appears to play a part in local heat regulation.

Capillary circulation

A remarkable feature of the circulatory system in the hand is the great density of capillaries—64 capillary loops per cm² on the dorsum of the hand (compared with 16 at the cheek) and 44 papillary capillaries per cm² of skin on the hand (compared with 27 at the shoulder and 19 at the cheek).

The variation in capillary pressure, which exists elsewhere in the skin, is much more marked in the hand. The variation is noticeable from one moment to another at the same point, and at the same moment at any two points of the network.

The variations in blood flow are no less remarkable. These can be visualized by capillaroscopy at the base of the nail where the capillaries of the papillae run horizontally and parallel to the surface. The loop can be seen in its entirety. In certain conditions, some degree of sludging may be observed; this phenomenon can also be seen with a reduction of capillary pressure or in the presence of local changes, e.g. in the endothelium or the protein film.

141

Capillary pressure itself depends on a number of factors, including:

- arteriolar tone (arteriolar constriction increases peripheral resistance and reduces capillary pressure);
- venous return (increased venous pressure causes an increase in capillary pressure);
- the position of the hand (pressure can decrease from 40 to 4 cm as the hand is raised from the dependent position); and
- temperature.

It is important to notice that the rate of blood flow is highly variable in the distal extremities where arterial irrigation is most marked. This feature has been studied in the fingers and especially in the pulps, where photoelectric plethysmography has shown that the flow can vary between 0.5 and 100 cm^3 per 100 cm^3 of tissue, a factor of 200:1. There is little doubt that this variation is due to the presence of numerous direct anastomoses.

Skin sensibility

The hand is truly the organ of touch. The palmar skin is equipped with an enormous number of receptors of all kinds, in comparison with the skin of other parts of the body. Bossy has calculated that the lateral femoral cutaneous nerve, which has approximately the same diameter as a collateral nerve of the digits, covers a sensory territory of approximately 600 cm^2 as opposed to 15 cm^2 for the collateral nerve.

The cutaneous biotransducers

From superficial to deep, the sensory receptors change from free nerve endings to encapsulated receptors or "mecanoreceptors" (Figure 1.152).

The palmar skin is a matrix of transducers placed vertically and horizontally. This arrangement allows an understanding of tactile discrimination on the surface and brings into play different layers of receptors in the depths, without creating a discontinuity in perception. Because the number of cutaneous receptors is greater than the number of nerve fibers conveying sensation, a nerve fiber can be connected to several receptors (Mountcastle, 1968).

The epidermis

In the epidermis two structures exist: free nerve endings and Merckel cell complexes (Cauna, 1954).

Free nerve endings are seen in the connective tissue of the papillary structures. These penetrate the epidermis between the Malpighian cells. These may be myelinated or unmyelinated fibers of small diameter. They are most sensitive to pain and temperature stimuli.

The Merckel discs are grouped nerve endings when these fibers have enlarged endings with a number of vesicles and assume the appearance of a disc. These are surrounded

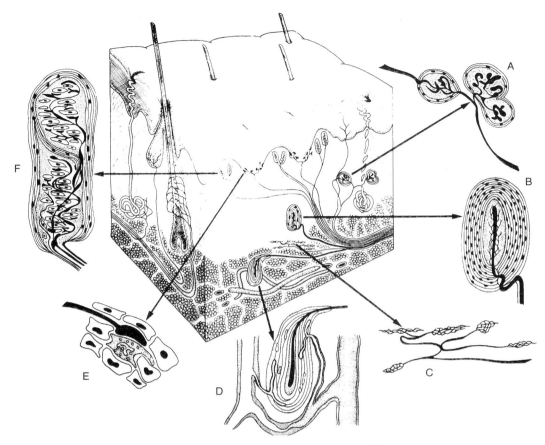

Figure 1.152. Three-dimensional reconstruction of a block of skin. (A) Corpuscles of Golgi-Mazzoni; (B) corpuscles of Vater-Pacini; (C) corpuscles of Ruffini; (D) paravascular corpuscles of Pacini; (E) disk of Merkel; (F) corpuscles of Meissner.

by the Merckel cells, and particularly by their cytoplasmic granules. They are situated at the dermoepidermal junction. They end in large myelinated fibers and are considered to be like the mecanoreceptor with slow adaptation.

The dermis
The dermis contains Meissner, Krause, Ruffini and Pacini corpuscles.

The Meissner's corpuscles are encapsulated receptors covered by a thin layer of connective tissue containing myelinated nerve ramifications and neural cells situated between these neurofibrillary networks. These corpuscles are 100–150 µm in length and are situated in the dermal papillaries. They are particularly numerous in the pulp (350 per cm²). These are connected to myelinated fibers and are considered to be like mecanoreceptors with rapid adaptation.

The sub-papillary dermis

In the sub-papillary dermis, nerve endings are less numerous and one can find simple or branching free nerve endings, and differentiated nerve endings.

Pacinian corpuscles are voluminous and can occasionally be seen without magnification. They are egg shaped with a multilaminated structure inside. This multilaminated structure is the nerve endings. These are connected to large diameter myelinated fibers and are considered mecanoreceptors with rapid adaptation.

The Krause corpuscles are formed by terminal branches surrounded by a connective capsule and are connected to large myelinated fibers. They are considered mecanoreceptors with rapid adaptation.

Ruffini corpuscles are differentiated nerve endings without encapsulation. Their terminal branches join each other to form small swellings. They are considered to be mecanoreceptors with slow adaptation connected to thick myelinated fibers.

Sensation is not of the same value throughout the palm. Certain zones are of special importance—the finger pulps, especially the ulnar half of the thumb pulp and the radial half of the index and middle finger pulps, and the radial border of the index and ulnar border of the little finger (Figure 1.153). It is essential to maintain or restore good sensation in these regions.

Physiology of palmar skin sensation

Palmar skin is unique in many ways, not only because of its wealth of sensory receptors, but also because it is hairless (glabrous), without hair follicles and their accompanying neural apparatus (Jabaley, 1981), and because of its papillary structure.

The anatomy of the papillary ridge has been studied in great detail by Cauna (1954). On its deep surface, the papillary ridge sends two types of longitudinal epidermal folds into the dermis. Those corresponding to the surface grooves are "limiting ridges" and are fixed to the dermis and to the deep fascia. They serve as stabilizers for the entire apparatus. The intermediate ridge lies between the limiting ridges and contains the sweat duct. It descends deeper and is less intimately attached to the dermis. It "floats" freely in the loose connective tissue.

Meissner's corpuscles are concentrated in the dermal papillae, whereas Merckel's discs are situated most frequently at the base of the intermediate ridges.

When the surface of the skin is deformed by a mechanical stimulus, the intermediate ridge acts as a magnifying lever for the transmission of pressure stimuli to the many receptors underneath the ridge. The Meissner's corpuscles, on the other hand, respond maximally only when pressure is applied in the direction of the long axis of the corpuscle. This arrangement contributes to the accuracy of tactile discrimination (Figure 1.154).

It cannot be overstressed that at the time of primary surgery of hand injuries, every effort should be made to preserve viable glabrous skin. Only this skin contains the specialized non-neural cells that lie close to the endings of the first-order sensory afferent neurones.

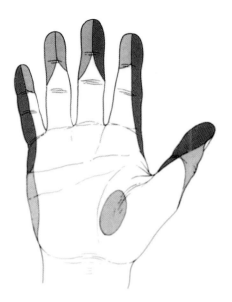

Figure 1.153. The functional zones of grip. In the dark gray areas sensation is most important; in the light gray areas sensation is less important.

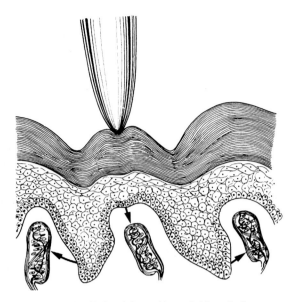

Figure 1.154. Role of the epidermal ridges in the stimulation of Meissner's corpuscles. The lateral resultant of vertical pressure on a papilla and the corpuscle contained in that papilla also stimulates the corpuscles of the adjacent papillae.

Functional cutaneous units

There are "functional cutaneous units" in the hand similar to the ones customarily described in the face. We can schematically distinguish them as follows:

Dorsum of the hand

1 One cutaneous unit extends from the wrist to the proximal interphalangeal joints of the fingers and the interphalangeal joint of the thumb (Figure 1.155).
2 The dorsal covering of the interphalangeal articulations of the digits forms a unique cutaneous unit characterized by a considerable excess of skin when the digits are in extension.
3 The fine tight skin of the dorsal aspect of the middle phalanx forms another unit.
4 The dorsal integument of the distal phalanx is very special because of the nail bed with its matrix.

Palmar surface

The palm forms a cutaneous unit extending from the distal transverse crease of the wrist up to the transverse crease at the base of the digits. The palmar integument may be

145

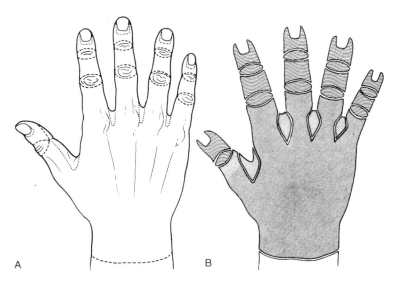

Figure 1.155. The dorsal cutaneous functional units on the dorsum of the hand and digits. In (B) the surface has been projected into a plane.

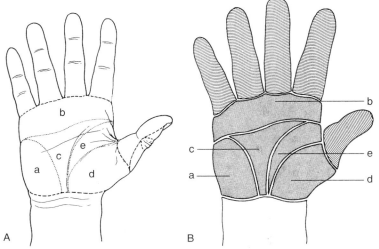

Figure 1.156 The palmar cutaneous functional units. In (B) the surface has been projected into a plane.

subdivided into two separate zones by the oppositional crease of the thumb, which constitutes the oblique axis of the hand (Figure 1.156).

1 The skin of the radial portion, which is relatively well vascularized, covers the thenar eminence and the external part of the palm; it is the mobile portion.

2 The skin of the ulnar and distal portion covers the hypothenar eminence where the skin has poor mobility; the distal part of the palm beyond the transverse distal palmar crease, which is a true hinge just at the level of the metacarpophalangeal articulations; and the central triangular part of the palm, where the skin is fixed and

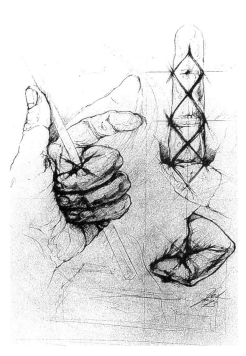

Figure 1.157. The areas of cutaneous contact in the flexed digits (Littler, 1974). These contact regions are diamond shaped when the digit is extended. The sides of the diamond undergo little variation in length during flexion–extension movements, and any incision made along their lines will not retract. When the digits are flexed against the palm, the radial digits whose palmar integument is innervated by the median nerve touch the skin of the thenar eminence, which is also innervated by the median nerve. The ulnar digits whose palmar integument is innervated by the ulnar nerve touch the skin of the palm innervated by the ulnar nerve. When a fist is formed, the palmar face of the thumb innervated by the median nerve comes into contact with the dorsal skin of the middle phalanges of the index and middle fingers, also innervated by the median nerve.

poorly vascularized, covering almost directly the superficial palmar aponeurosis, which inserts into it.

The integument of the palmar face of the digits may be subdivided into phalangeal units. These units are separated by the digital flexion folds: three for the digits and two for the thumb. When a digit is completely flexed, the integument of the adjacent phalanges comes into contact in the zones of the flexion creases, establishing areas of cutaneous contact in the form of a diamond (Littler, 1974). The sides of this diamond do not undergo variations in length during the movements of flexion and extension, and incisions made along their level present a minimal chance of retraction (Figure 1.157). The advantages are multiple, the exposure obtained is excellent, the dorsal branches of the skin being in the form of a Y–V advancement.

The web spaces are formed from the union of two nonsymmetrical cutaneous surfaces (Figure 1.158). The dorsal slope has a gradual incline and its supple skin is not adherent to the subjacent region. The palmar surface is flat and precipitously interrupted, and the skin is densely adherent to the commissural skeleton. This commissural skeleton is formed by the interdigital palmar (natatory) ligament between the fingers and by the distal transverse ligament at the level of the thumb web (by far the deepest and the most mobile). Incisions must take into account the contour of these cutaneous units or of their subdivisions.

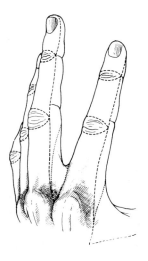

Figure 1.158. Dorsal view of the first and second commissures. The dorsum of the web slopes gently and the skin is supple and non-adherent.

Skin incisions in the hand

In the hand, the siting and the design of skin incisions is extremely important. A misplaced incision can lead to an unsightly tender contracted scar. The design of every skin incision must take into account the structure and mobility of the area it crosses, the relation to deeper structure, the blood supply to the skin, the sensory nerve distribution, previous wounds and cosmetic considerations.

In order to minimize hypertrophic scar formation the incisions should be made in areas of relative immobility; they should never cross a flexion crease vertically but should be broken by an angled or a Z-plasty. For the exposure of volar structures in the digits, the incision should be made either in the midlateral line or in a zigzag fashion (Figure 1.159). In the palm, transverse incisions should be parallel to the palmar creases. Longitudinal digito-palmar incisions should be angled as they cross the palmar creases (Figure 1.160). On the dorsum of the hand, curved incisions skirting the margins of the hand are used (Figure 1.161). The incisions used for exposure of all the MP joints is often a transverse one (Figure 1.162).

The pulps

Palmar skin on the distal phalanges is highly specialized tissue: it makes up the pulps of the fingers, which are really sensory organs (Figure 1.163). The importance of this aspect of the functions of the hand has already been mentioned. In addition to their many sensory endings, the pulps also have an important prehensile function. Their structure is perfectly adapted for grasping, and the papillary crests and the sweat glands ensure good adhesion. The subcutaneous tissue is thick and malleable and is formed by fatty tissues separated by fibrous septa which create small fibrous fat-filled compartments. The septa provide a union between the dermis and periosteum, and this acts to limit the gliding of skin over bone. The pulp is fixed against the bone and nail which provides added support for the fingertip.

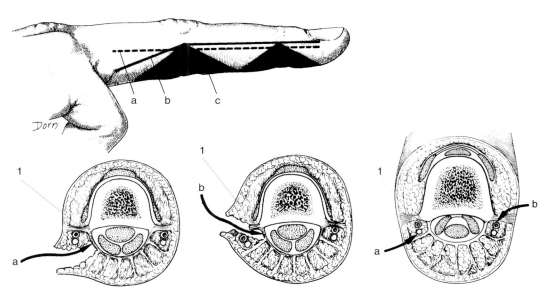

Figure 1.159. For exposure of volar structures the incision should be made parallel to the midlateral line (a), or midaxial, dorsal to Cleland's ligament (b), or in a zigzag fashion (c). (1) Cleland's ligament.

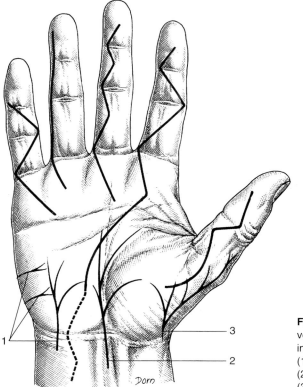

Figure 1.160. Longitudinal, midlateral and volar zigzag incisions. The cutaneous nerves in the palm must not be damaged.
(1) Sensory branches of ulnar nerve;
(2) palmar cutaneous branch of median nerve;
(3) sensory branches of radial nerve.

149

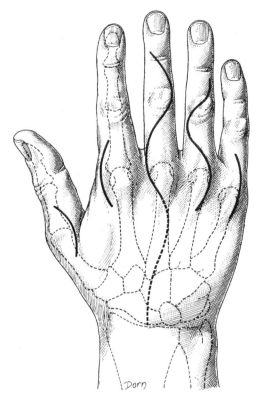

Figure 1.161. Curved incisions are used on the dorsum of the hand.

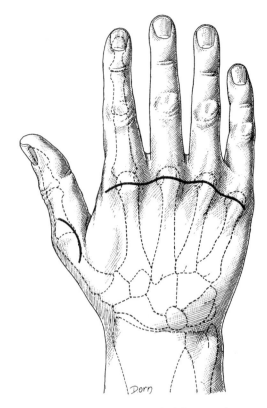

Figure 1.162. A transverse incision may be used for exposure of all the MP joints.

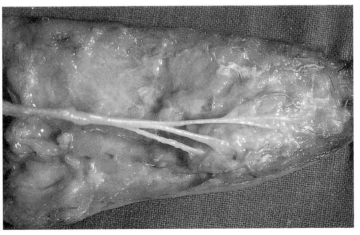

Figure 1.163. Division of the palmar collateral nerve.

The finger nails

The nails in man have lost their defensive role of clawing. Their breadth on the dorsum of the distal phalanx adds support for the pulp, allowing a more precise grip to pick up small objects, and enhances pulp sensibility.

A standardized nomenclature has been suggested by Zook (1981). The perionychium is formed by the nail bed and the tissue around the sides and base of the nail (parony-chium). The proximal end of the nail is enfolded into a depression on the finger (the nail fold). The skin over the dorsum of the nail fold is known as the nail wall. The thin membrane extending from the nail wall a short distance on to the dorsum of the nail is the eponychium. Between it and the nail is a stratified, cornified material known as the nail vest or cuticle (Figure 1.164).

The lunula is the convex white area seen at the base of the nail. The nail separates the dorsal roof from the ventral floor of the nail fold. The nail bed (germinal matrix, sterile matrix) is all the soft tissue between the nail and the periosteum of the distal phalanx.

The hyponychium is the keratinized skin between the distal nail and finger tip.

Two arterial arches, which are in fact an anastomosis between the lateral arteries of the finger, pass just above the periosteum of the distal phalanx and supply the nail bed. One arch is parallel to the lunula and one to the free edge of the nail (see Figure 1.150).

As Hueston (1973) has noted, the areas of constant functional contact in the regions of each hand have a common innervation. Thus, the pulp of the radial fingers, innervated by the median nerve, comes into contact in the palm with the integument of the thenar eminence, innervated by the palmar cutaneous branch of the median nerve; and the ulnar or internal fingers come into contact with the palmar skin innervated by the ulnar nerve. Likewise, the pulp of the thumb, when making a fist, closes on the dorsal surface of the distal phalanges of the middle and index fingers, coming into contact with the integument innervated by the very same median nerve (see Figure 1.157).

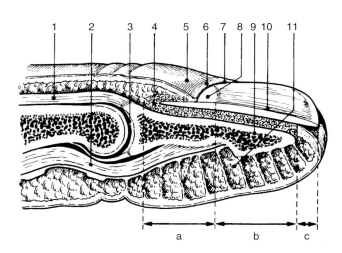

Figure 1.164. Longitudinal section of the distal phalanx showing the disproportionate thickness of the anterior and posterior covering layers; a = nail matrix, b = nail bed, c = hyponychium, 1 = extensor tendon, 2 = flexor tendon, 3 = distal interphalangeal articulation, 4 = nail fold, 5 = distal portion of nail fold, 6 and 7 = eponychium, 8 = lunula, 9 = distal phalanx, 10 = nail shelf, 11 = pulp.

151

Planning skin cover of the hand and forearm

The surgeon has to bear in mind the dimensions of the different skin units if he has to replace these by skin grafts or flaps. According to Kelleher et al (1985), the necessary skin to cover the thumb distal to the metacarpophalangeal joint is about 9 cm wide and 8 cm long. Skin loss of thumb and first metacarpal is 13 cm wide and 12 cm long (Figure 1.165 and Table 1.6).

The skin cover of both the palmar and dorsal surfaces of the hand is 12 cm by 10 cm. The skin covering each finger is 7 cm by 10 cm on both the palmar and dorsal aspects, and for skin grafting or flaps for both sides of the hand and digits requires a skin of 20 cm by 20 cm. Skin grafting or flaps for one aspect of the forearm from wrist to elbow requires skin of 30 cm by 15 cm; both aspects of the forearm requires skin of 30 cm by 30 cm.

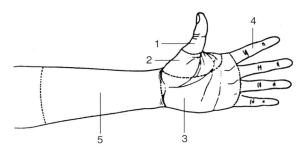

Figure 1.165. Superficial graft or skin flap used to cover a defect. 1, The thumb from the base of the metacarpophalangeal joint: 9 × 8 cm; 2, The first ray: 1 + 2 = 13 × 12 cm; 3, The palm of the hand: 12 × 10 cm; 4, The integument of the finger: 7 × 10 cm; 5, The anterior surface of the forearm: 30 × 15 cm.

	Width (cm)	Length (cm)
1. Thumb skin distal to metacarpophalangeal joint	9	8
2. Thumb skin distal to thenar crease and dorsal line of index metacarpal	13	12
3. Skin for palmar side of hand from thenar crease and midradial border to midulnar border, and from volar crease of wrist to proximal digital crease	12	10
4. Skin for dorsal side of hand, midradial to midulnar border, and volar crease of wrist to dorsal web space	12	10
5. Skin for entire surface of a single digit	7	10
6. Skin for both sides of hands and digits	20	20
7. Skin for volar surface of forearm	28	15
8. Skin for dorsal surface of forearm	28	15
9. Skin for entire volar and dorsal surface of forearm	30	30

Table 1.6. Area requirements for upper limb flaps. (From Kelleher et al, 1985.)

Skin incisions

The design of every skin incision in the hand must take into account the structure and mobility of the area it crosses, the relation to deeper structures, the blood supply to the skin of the palm, the sensory nerve distribution to the area being exposed, and previous wounds or scars. In order to minimize hypertrophic scar formation and contracture, the incisions should be made in areas of relative immobility, such as along the lateral midline of the fingers along the flexion creases of the palm, or along the diagonals that traverse the volar surface of the fingers between the flexion creases. Ideally they should remain within the limits of the functional cutaneous units that we have described or their subdivisions (see Figure 1.156).

The incisions must never cross the flexion creases vertically. Scars under longitudinal tension tend to contract and become hypertrophic. Similar precautions must be taken at the web spaces: an incision parallel to the commissure will lead to a transverse scar contracture, which will prevent abduction of the fingers.

Vascular and nerve supply

One must take into account the blood and nerve supply to the skin when planning incisions. The skin of the fingers is usually richly vascularized, but this supply depends essentially on the two vulnerable digital arteries at the base of the finger.

The blood supply of the palmar skin is not of an even distribution, and although there are three well vascularized areas, namely, the thenar and hypothenar eminences and the area distal to the palmar crease, there is in the center of the palm a poorly vascularized triangle with its apex pointing proximally (Figure 1.166). Extensive undermining should be avoided in the central palmar skin, especially if circulatory problems already exist. Necrosis of palmar flaps after dissection for Dupuytren's contracture is a serious risk in this area.

The dorsal skin of the fingers and hand is mobile but thin; it is reasonably well vascularized. Narrow and acute angled flaps should be avoided. It should be kept in mind that the main venous and lymphatic channels lie on the dorsal aspect of the hand and the fingers. These should be preserved in planning and carrying out surgical exposures in this area.

Sensation

It is of paramount importance to respect and preserve the sensibility of the skin of the fingers and to avoid placing incisions in regions where pressure is commonly applied.

In the palm, the nerves are protected by the overlying aponeurosis, but on the dorsum and palmar aspects of the wrist, and on the dorsum of the hand and fingers, the nerves are superficial and very much at risk if an incision is made without due care. One must know the site of the sensory nerves most susceptible to iatrogenic injuries.

Palmar cutaneous branch of the median nerve

The sensory nerve most susceptible to iatrogenic injury is the palmar cutaneous branch of the median nerve. Its diameter is about 0.8 mm. The nerve originates on the radial border of the median nerve 5 to 6 cm above the distal transverse flexion crease of the wrist, and courses alongside the median nerve for 2–3 cm.

It follows the course of the flexor carpi radialis tendon, and when this tendon enters its own compartment of the flexor retinaculum, the nerve than passes between the two layers of the forearm fascia, which provide it with its own short tunnel just ulnar to the flexor carpi radialis tendon.

It passes through the superficial layer of this fascia at the bifurcation of the palmaris longus into the root of the palmar aponeurosis and the tendon giving origin to the superficial portion of the abductor pollicis brevis (Fahrer and Tubiana, 1976). After only 5–10 mm, the palmar cutaneous branch of the median nerve divides into three terminal branches, which cross the mid-palmar aponeurosis to supply the deep layers of the dermis (see Figure 1.166).

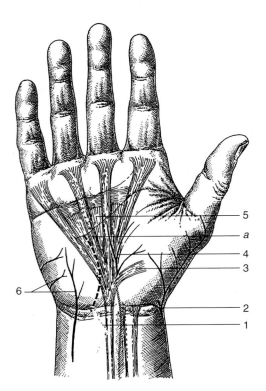

Figure 1.166. (1) Palmaris longus; (2) superficial branch of radial nerve: cutaneous branches; (3) radial division of palmaris longus tendon; (4) palmar cutaneous branch of median nerve; (5) palmar aponeurosis; (6) cutaneous branches of ulnar nerve; *a* incision for carpal tunnel decompression.

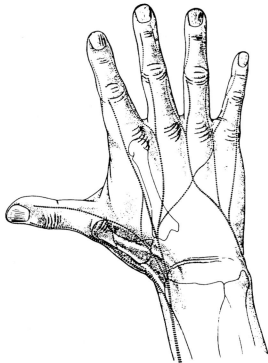

Figure 1.167. Cutaneous nerves on the dorsum of the hand.

To avoid the palmar cutaneous branch of the median nerve and its branches, which constitute the most frequent source of palmar neuromas, the forearm incision must be ulnar to the palmaris longus tendon.

Palmar cutaneous branches of the ulnar nerve

The main branch arises, according to descriptions in the standard textbooks, from the cutaneous branch of the ulnar nerve, originating in the forearm a few centimeters above the origin of the dorsal branch. This cutaneous branch runs against the palmar aspect of the nerve up to the level of the wrist, where it becomes superficial, crossing into the hypothenar eminence palmar to the palmaris brevis muscle.

In fact, such an arrangement is unusual. The palmar cutaneous branch originates at a variable level and was replaced in 16 of 21 cases by branches from the superficial division of the ulnar nerve or from its dorsal division (Engber and Gmeiner, 1980). These ulnar branches are distributed between the pisiform and the distal palmar crease.

The dorsal branch of the ulnar nerve

The nerve arises from the medial aspect of the ulnar nerve at an average distance of 6.4 cm from the distal aspect of the head of the ulna and 8.3 cm from the proximal border of the pisiform (Botte et al, 1990). The nerve passes dorsal to the flexor carpi ulnaris and pierces the deep fascia. It becomes subcutaneous on the medial aspect of the forearm at a mean distance of 5 cm from the proximal edge of the pisiform. Proximal to the wrist, the nerve provides two to three branches. With the forearm supinated, the nerve branches pass along the medial aspect of the head of the ulna, then on the dorsal aspect of the triquetrum. With the forearm pronated, the nerve branches displace slightly ulnarly.

Dorsal cutaneous branch of the radial nerve

The terminal sensory branch of the radial nerve (Figure 1.167) passes deep to the flattened tendon of the brachioradialis and becomes superficial about 4 cm proximal to the radiocarpal joint line. It crosses superficially, from radial to ulnar, the tendons of the abductor pollicis longus and extensor pollicis brevis. The nerve divides into a lateral branch, the dorsal collateral lateral of the thumb, and a medial branch that supplies the index and middle fingers. The course of the nerve is along a line drawn from the dorsolateral border of the radius, which is easily palpable, toward the angle formed by the proximal junction of the first and second metacarpals. The medial branch follows this line and divides just distal to the angle of the first and second metacarpals. The dorsal collateral nerve of the thumb follows the radial border of the extensor pollicis brevis tendon. This branch gives the palmar cutaneous branch of the radial nerve, which follows the tendon of the abductor pollicis longus and anastomoses with or substitutes for the external branch of the palmar cutaneous branch of the median nerve.

155

1.5 FUNCTIONS OF THE HAND

The functions of the hand are multiple, though the most important are the sensory function of touch and the function of prehension. The hand has numerous other functions that play essential roles in our lives—functions of expression through gesture, visceral functions in carrying food to the mouth, emotional and sexual functions in caressing, an aggressive function in the closed fist or the ulnar border of the hand for defense or offense, functions relating to body care, and a thermoregulatory function.

The hand as an organ of information

We often have a tendency to consider only the motor functions of the hand, since this is what the surgeon most frequently endeavors to repair. However, it is impossible to dissociate sensibility and motor function in the hand; it is their association that makes the hand an important organ of information and accomplishment. What confers on the hand its exceptional sensory value is not only the great number of sensitive corpuscles of its cutaneous covering, but also the way it can augment its capacity for obtaining information by means of its voluntary maneuvers of methodical exploration, i.e. by manipulation and palpation. Thus the whole of the hand is a sensory organ (Figure 1.168). Furthermore, it is a sensory organ of particular efficiency. The other sensory organs are fixed to the axial body, whereas the hand can actively move toward an object one wants to know better. It also participates in the education of sight by correlating in three dimensions.

Let us now study briefly the mechanism of this organ of information. There are, as mentioned previously, many varieties of sensibility. These have been the subject of several classifications according to topographical site (Bell, 1833), the nature of the stimuli (Sherrington, 1896), and the hierarchy of sensibility (Head, 1920), from the elementary "protopathic" sensibility to the complex "epicritic" sensibility. Practically, neurologists classify sensibilities according to topography as either superficial or deep.

Superficial sensation
Superficial (exteroceptive) sensation provides information regarding external stimuli of the skin receptors. It is either fine and discriminative ("epicritic") or gross ("protopathic"). It has an essential role in informing and in "discrimination of intensities or qualities and particularly of local specifications" (Head, 1920). It also has a protective role and thus brings about a regional response of defense, the most immediate and least controlled of which is the withdrawal reflex.

Deep sensation
The deep sensation of the hand provides information regarding the position of the skeleton and muscles. Superficial and deep sensation theoretically involves separate neural

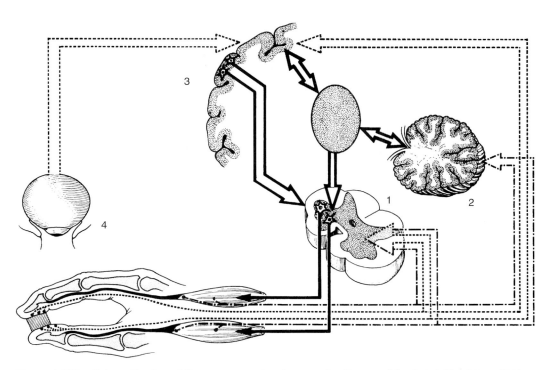

Figure 1.168. Schematic view of the sensory and motor neural pathways of the hand. The heavy lines indicate the motor pathways and the fine dotted lines indicate the superficial sensory or exteroceptive pathways. The dashes indicate the deep sensory or proprioceptive pathways. There are several synapses—in (1) the medulla, (2) the cerebellum and the subcortical region, and (3) the cortical region— thus permitting different medullary and subcortical reflex circuits as well as conscious control. Ocular control (4) is necessary when sensation is absent or insufficient. The knowledge obtained from sensory input or "tactile gnosis" demands cortical participation.

pathways to the central nervous system, which decodes the information at different levels. The distinction between these two types of sensation has been increasingly criticized. It is arbitrary to equate superficial sensibility and exteroceptive sensibility; i.e., stimuli are external. It becomes incorrect when we associate deep sensibility with proprioception, in which the subject creates stimuli himself. In fact, there are proprioceptive corpuscles incorporated in and stimulated by the activity of the parts that contain them, such as bones, muscles, tendons, and joints.

Von Frey (1924) has shown that the functions classically attributed to the deep sensibilities were also assumed by superficial receptors. As he has noted, deep and superficial sensibility refers only to the topographical and anatomical locations of some receptors and does not prove the existence of any determinated functions. The skin also plays a role in proprioception. As shown by Moberg (1972), the cutaneous receptors, stimulated by deformations of the skin, play an essential role in the hand in perception of changes in position and in regulation of motor function. Thus, the cutaneous discriminative test of Weber, useful in appreciating tactile recognition, is also useful in appreciating proprioception.

Tact and touch

"Tact" is passive; "touch" is active and voluntary. Indeed the skin of the rest of the body is capable of immediately recognizing contact, but it is more often being touched than actively touching. "The hand alone can be defined as the true organ of touch," says Brun (1963), "for it alone explores or feels and thus adds to the sense of touch, activity which confers on it a unique talent. . . Only the hand is at the same time touching and being touched." All activities of sensory investigation require the participation of motor organs. Thieffry (1973) wrote:

> We are inclined to imagine that the cells of the retina, the auditory cells of the inner ear, the receptors in the skin, are themselves sufficient to give us the senses of sight, hearing and touch. Reduced to themselves, they give us only vision, hearing and tact. They only realize their full potential with the addition of sensory-motor organs which permit the adjustment to the information content that gives optimal reception.
>
> Thus, to have optimal visual perception by the retina, we must also use the oculomotor muscles of the orbit, which, by virtue of their movements, enable the eye to scan every part of the image presented. With the hand it is not only a matter of several proprioceptive receptors attached to a hidden sensory apparatus. . . This complex sensory motor system has a greater concentration of both superficial and deep receptors than any other part of the body and this is particularly well adapted to psychomotor activity.

When the hand acts voluntarily and modifies its relations with an object to gain more information concerning this object, contact becomes touch. Superficial sensation is precise, not diffuse, and allows "the discrimination of intensities or qualities" (Head, 1920). However, contact with a surface by digital touch is not sufficient for the precise appreciation of the weight, volume, or three dimensional size of the object examined. Palpation and manipulation add information by means of a "stereometric survey." Thus, the hand in its sensory capacity proceeds by stages to explore an object—contact, digital touch, and manual palpation. Touch and palpation together give us knowledge ("gnosis") about an object. This "tactile gnosis" provides the third dimension and educates the eye to appreciate the object's contours.

Stereognosis

Stereognosis, a term used primarily by Hoffmann (1884) to indicate the recognition of the geometrical surfaces of an object (*stereos* in Greek means "solid"), is now used to describe the recognition of any object by touch. Stereognosis is not a function exclusively of the hands. Other parts of the body have stereognosis ability, but with many regional differences. In fact, stereognosis is the sum of partial perceptions. Perception varies from region to region. According to Delay (1935):

> Recognition of forms which is so important for stereognosis depends on spacial perceptions. Recognition of the tridimensional form needs an anatomical system allowing segmentary appreciations, done perfectly in the hands by opposition of the thumb and index [finger]. Without segmentary opposition, appreciation of volume and thickness is impossible. The influence of exercise is considerable and plays a great part in the superiority of manual stereognosis. Thus patients with infantile cerebral hemiplegia who do not exercise their paralytic hands have virtually no stereognosis. On the contrary, blind people develop a greatly increased stereognosis. In the normal adult, regions which have a limited stereognosis ability can be vastly improved by practice.

For example, after a Krukenberg operation we have observed that values in the Weber discriminative test at the distal end of the pincers progressively decrease from 4 cm to less than 1 cm, provided the patient uses the pincers. We also know the value of sensory re-education after repairs of peripheral nerves (Wynn Parry, 1966).

In the past, touch and tactile sensibility have been regarded as the same. Slowly, progress in neurophysiology has allowed us to dissociate the different sensibilities. Touch involves the appreciation of all this information at the level of the cortex. The contribution of elementary sensibilities is indispensable to the intellectual act of recognizing an object.

In our sensory appreciation of an object we do not usually use stereognosis; we proceed by the easier and more rapid means of total symbolic perception, which precedes analysis of the characteristics of the object. This method of symbolic perception, writes Delay (1952), is "the understanding which guides us in the mental reconstruction of an object, just as in the formation of speech we progress from the idea to the phrase and from the phrase to the word." Thus we distinguish two processes in tactile recognition: immediate symbolic perception, "which is not hindered by detail," and analytic perception, which usually only supplements the fundamental information given by symbolic perception.

We see from this short account the essential role that the hands play in the recognition of the external world. Our hands work with the other sensory organs, particularly the eyes; by touch and grasping, we complete the perception of appearances. Focillon (1947) wrote:

> Perception of the world requires a sort of tactile flair. Eyesight extends along the length of the universe. The hand appreciates the reality of an object by its weight, by the texture—rough or smooth, and separates from the background with which its visual image appears to merge. The action of the hand recognizes both intervals of space and solidity in the object it holds. Surface, volume, density and weight are not optical phenomena. It is in the hollow of the palm and between the fingers that man instantly assesses these characteristics. Space is not gauged by

sight but rather by hand and foot, which impart an indefinable appreciation and without which recognition remains like a delightful landscape of a dark chamber—inconsistent, flat, elusive and chimerical.

The hand as an organ of accomplishment

If we exclude walking, the majority of movements involve the hands. The upper limb has lost its locomotor function in man, except on rare occasions, and, freed by the adoption of the upright posture, the hand has become free to diversify its activities. In *The Animal Parts* (IV, 10), Aristotle wrote:

> Those who say that man is not well conceived, and that he is less well endowed than the animals, are wrong. Animals each have only one mode of defense and this they cannot change. . . . Man, by contrast, has numerous means of defense at his disposal, and it is always possible for him to change tactics and choose a different weapon when he wishes. The hand can become a claw, a fist, a horn or spear or sword or any other weapon or tool. It can be everything because it has the ability to grasp anything and hold anything.

Compared with other highly specialized organs of execution in animals, the hand is very versatile. It is both a means of expression and a variety of instruments, "a device that can, in turn, strike, receive and give, feed, take an oath, beat a musical rhythm, read for the blind, speak for the mute, reach to a friend, stop a foe, and become a hammer, pincer, alphabet. . ." (Valery, 1938).

The hand is more than just a corporal instrument. "The hand is a natural tool with the ability to fashion artificial tools" (Brun, 1963). The situation is completely different in the animal, in which the tool is an integral part of the body and "individual creativity is impossible" (Piveteau, 1955). The action of the corporal instrument of an animal is programed and is always repeated in the same manner. By contrast, "man has the liberty of his freed hands. . . . to the tool or the machine is delegated, to a greater or lesser extent, the execution of a program of concerted action" (Thieffry, 1973).

Functions of the hand

It is impossible to describe the innumerable functional adaptations of the normal hand in expressing, palpating, grasping, pushing, carrying, counting, and manipulating objects that differ widely in form, consistency, and weight. One may categorize its functions schematically according to the degree of mobility demanded of the hand:

1 The passive function, in which the hand remains immobile—flat, cupped, opened with the fingers extended for carrying, scooping, pointing, and pushing. It is the proximal part of the limb that must be mobilized to place the hand in the required position.

2 The percussive function of tapping fingers, clapping hands, or pounding fists. The distal articulations are immobile; the motion starts from the metacarpophalangeal articulations, the wrist, or more proximally.

3 Functions requiring a great deal of mobility of the hand, such as expressive gestures that are of symbolic significance, as in the language of mime, or prehensible gestures, ranging from the simplest ordinary grip to maneuvers of intricate complexity requiring collaboration between both hands.

Numerous schematic classifications of positions adopted by the fingers and thumb during prehension have been suggested, but these have tended to describe prehension only in mechanical terms, when in fact it is a much more complex action, bringing into play consciousness, sensation, and motor function.

Grip and prehension

In the animal world a variety of organs are adapted for prehension. According to Rabischong (1971), they may be divided into four types: organs that pinch, encircle, push, and adhere. Usually an animal can utilize only one of these forms of prehension. Man, owing to the multiple possibilities and malleability of his hands, can reproduce all types of pinch, from simple lateral pinch between two digits to thumb–finger opposition, and of encirclement, from the simple hook to digitopalmar grip. He can also use his two upper limbs for grips between the arms and the body.

Each mode of prehension in an animal is guided by a specialized system used to obtain information—the visual apparatus of a bird or the olfactory apparatus in quadrupeds, which in turn may be specially adapted, as in an elephant's trunk. Man also possesses a specific system of information and control incorporated in the hand: touch. Being able to use different types of grips, man must choose and adapt his mode of prehension not only to the object seized but also to the purpose of the grip.

To take is not simply to grasp. Like touch, prehension is intentional. This implies an awareness of utilization, and this is why prehension differs fundamentally from grip. Unfortunately there is currently much confusion between the two terms.

Prehension may be defined as all the functions that are put into play when an object is grasped by the hands—intent, permanent sensory control, and a mechanism of grip. Grip is the manual mechanical component of prehension. (*See* "Nature and power of the common grips" pages 326–7 and "Grasp and prehension" pages 343–4.)

Phases of prehension

Prehension is accomplished in several stages, as described by Rabischong (1971): approach, grip, and release of grip.

Two parameters must be known in order to determine the trajectory of the hand toward an object: direction and distance. Three methods of approach are possible.

The approach via sight is the most precise; the visual apparatus immediately provides the coordinates for direction and distance. It is possible to control only one hand—not both—at a time by visual means. Visual control is essential for hand function when there is no sensibility, when the two point discrimination is more than 12 mm, or when the patient has a prosthesis (Moberg, 1978a). The absence of visual control necessitates the second approach, the approach via palpation. In the third approach—via memory—the gift of memory may guide the hand toward an object.

The choice of the type of grip is preselected; the hand then adapts to the form of the object.

Grip consists of three stages (Figure 1.169):

- opening of the hand,
- closing of the digits in order to grasp the object, and finally
- regulation of the force of grip.

Opening of the hand requires the simultaneous action of the long extensors and intrinsic muscles. The extent is proportional to the volume of the object grasped.

Positioning of the mobile elements of the hand in order to grasp an object and adapt to its form consists of a variety of combinations.

Napier (1966) has noted that the diversity of movement of the hand is more apparent than real, if one forgets the multiplicity of grasped objects and remembers only the attitudes of the hand. The functional activities of prehension may be thus divided into power grips, in which the digits maintain the object against the palm, and the thumb may or may not participate, and precision grips, in which the palm may or may not participate. These two forms of grip depend less on the form of the object than on the reason for which the object was grasped.

Thus, when an orthopedic surgeon drives a Küntscher nail into a femur, he holds the handle of the hammer forcefully with his whole hand. The digits are flexed as tightly

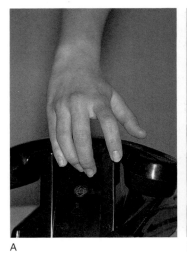 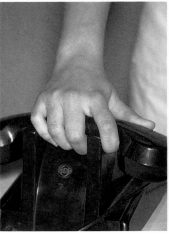 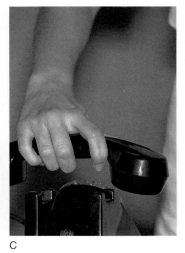

A   B   C

Figure 1.169. The three stages of grip: (A) opening of the hand; (B) closing of the digits; (C) regulation of the force of grip.

162

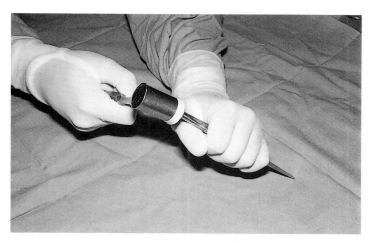

Figure 1.170. In power grip, the right wrist is in ulnar deviation. The adducted thumb encloses the fingers and reinforces the grip. Movement occurs at the shoulder, elbow, and wrist. The left hand grips the chisel with the wrist fixed in extension. (See also Figure 1.63.)

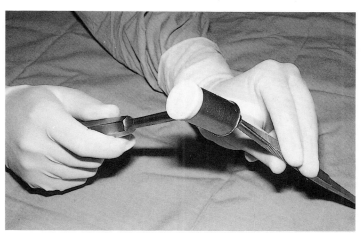

Figure 1.171. In precision grip, the control of the object exerted by the hand is more extensive. The right hand holds the handle of the hammer by combining two types of grip—terminolateral grip between the thumb and the index finger and digitopalmar grip for the ulnar fingers. The thumb is in complete extension, and control of grip of the hammer extends over a wide area of the hand with more precision than that in Figure 1.170. Movements occur at the wrist. The left hand holds the chisel with precision by means of a multiple pulp grip between the fingers and the thumb.

as possible in slight ulnar deviation; the wrist is fixed in extension, in midposition between supination and pronation, and also in slight ulnar deviation; and the thumb is adducted and rolled over the fingers to strengthen the grip and lock it (Figure 1.170). If, however, the surgeon wants to use a chisel with precision on a bony surface, the same hammer is taken with only slight deviation of the wrist, the radial fingers are less flexed than the ulnar fingers, the index finger is in slight external rotation, and the thumb is along the axis of the handle (Figure 1.171). The wrist, while still in midposition between supination and pronation, now has movement from radial deviation to ulnar deviation as the surgeon strikes the chisel. As the hand gains more control of an object, precision of grip is greatly increased (Figure 1.172).

The thumb is indispensable for grip precision. It provides both stability and control of direction, which are necessary for precision movements. The thumb is also useful in

163

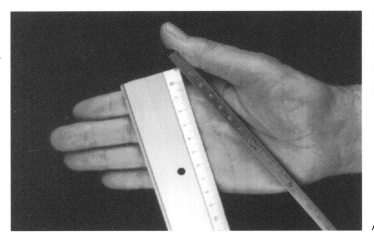

A

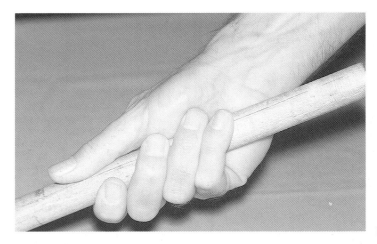

B

Figure 1.172. Grip of an object along the oblique palmar axis, or palmar groove, involves a longer area of contact and thus more control than grip along the transverse palmar axis.

controlling the power of the grip, forming a buttress that resists the pressure of the object that is held together by the pressure of the other fingers.

The thumb is not indispensable for all forms of power grip. Certain grips require only a simple hook formed by the fingers (Figure 1.173), which is controlled by the powerful digital long flexor and extensor muscles. They have more stamina than the intrinsic muscles, which control flexion of the metacarpophalangeal joints and adduction of the thumb, but tire easily. Thus, with fatigue, full closure of the hand around an object is transformed into a hook of the interphalangeal joints, and precision is lost (Figure 1.174). The intrinsic muscles assume increased importance when agility and precision are necessary; when the stress is on power, the extrinsic muscles become more important.

Landsmeer (1962) describes "precision handling," which requires continual adaptation between the thumb and the fingers without participation of the palm

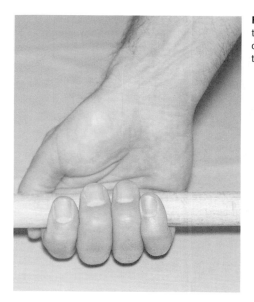

Figure 1.173. In digitopalmar grip, flexion movements at the metacarpophalangeal and interphalangeal joints can complement each other. In this type of hook grip the thumb is not used.

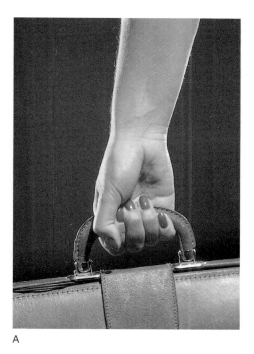

A

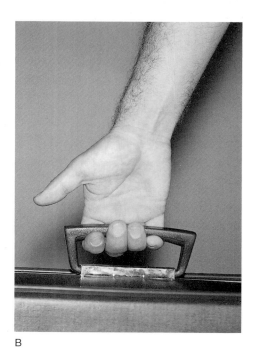

B

Figure 1.174. (A) Full closure of the hand around an object, involving the thumb. (B) With fatigue, the grip becomes a hook of the interphalangeal joints and precision is lost.

165

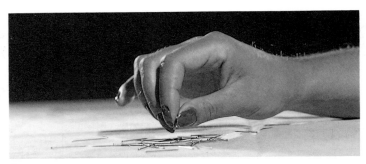

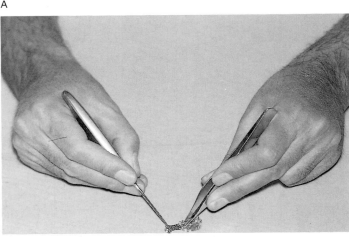

A

B

Figure 1.175. Precision handling: (A) involving the thumb and index finger; (B) tripod precision handling.

(Figure 1.175); this has a dynamic significance, whereas "precision grip" implies more stasis of activity.

Regulation of the force of grip is essential. The force must be varied according to the weight, fragility, surface characteristics, and utilization of the object. Precise and continuous sensory information is indispensable for safety in preventing premature release or excess pressure. The anesthetic hands of patients with Hansen's disease (leprosy), for example, have lost their capacity to receive sensory safety signals and are constantly subjected to wounds caused by excessive pressure.

Opening the hand releases the grip. It is of interest that the various functions of the digits can be related to the pattern of the nerve supply. Flexion and sensation of the ulnar digits, important in the digitopalmar power grip, depend on the ulnar nerve, whereas flexion and sensation of the radial digits, important in precision grip, are controlled chiefly by the median nerve. Also the muscles of the thumb required for opposition are innervated by both the median and ulnar nerves. Opening of the hand depends on the radial nerve.

Many lesions, traumatic as well as other types, can alter prehension with all its forms of grip. We cannot hope by surgical means to restore prehension with all its central

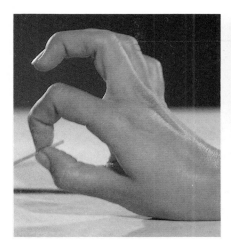

Figure 1.176. Terminal pinch.

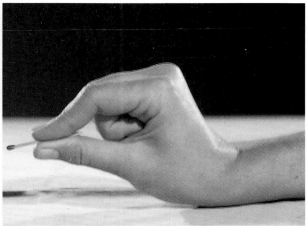

Figure 1.177. Subterminal or pulpar pinch.

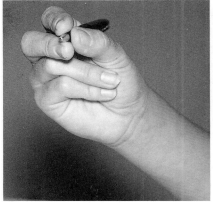

A

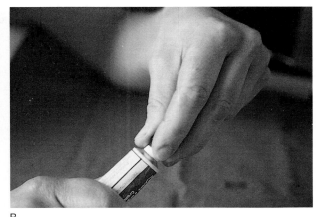

B

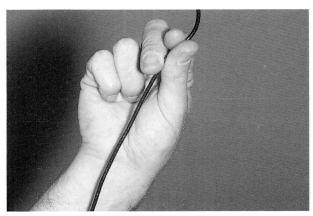

C

Figure 1.178. Adding a third digit to the grip brings more precision.

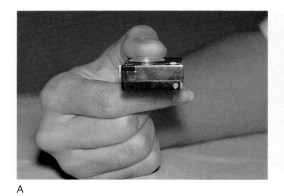
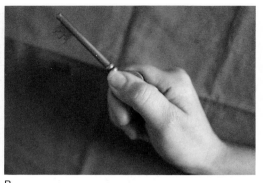

A   B

Figure 1.179. Thumb-finger grip. One of the most useful forms of this mechanism is lateral pinch between the thumb and lateral border of the index finger. This is also the easiest to reconstruct surgically.

and peripheral components. This would imply the restoration of the many sources of sensory information and control that regulate functions, the re-establishment of the numerous voluntary motor circuits at all levels of the nervous system, the reconstruction of normal muscular and articular action, as well as provision of a cutaneous covering having sensory properties. We try to make the best of the local possibilities in order to re-establish sensibility in the prehensile zones and insure a sufficient degree of mobility for the two essential forms of grip:

1 Digitopalmar grip for grasping depends essentially on the movements of the fingers opposing the palm.
2 Thumb–finger pinch requires, as a minimum, active contact between the thumb and a digit, requiring the mobility of the thumb and an opposing finger, usually the index. The pinch can be terminal, the distal phalange flexed (Figure 1.176) or subterminal pulpar, with the distal phalanges extended (Figure 1.177). The adjunction of a third digit to the grip brings more precision (Figure 1.178). The lateral pinch requires only the mobility of the thumb ray (Figure 1.179). The size of the object gripped depends on the size of the web spaces and the lengths of the rays of the digits, especially the thumb and little finger (Figure 1.180).

These concepts are relevant to hand reconstruction and also to prosthesis design.

Nutritional and expressive functions

The hand and the mouth

Just as the hand as an organ of information is complementary to the eye, the hand as an organ of action has numerous interactions with the mouth. The act of grasping, common to both man and animals, makes use of the jaw or the hand. The hand and

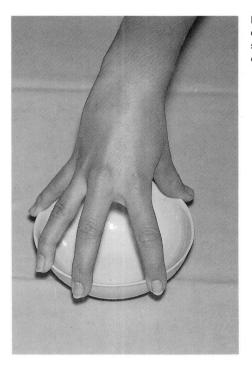

Figure 1.180. The gripping of large objects depends on the size of the web spaces and the lengths of the digits, especially the thumb and little finger.

the mouth collaborate for the nutritional function. Placed at the extremity of the upper limb, the hand is functionally organized to take food, prepare it, and then carry it to the mouth by means of a special motion of the upper extremity—flexion of the elbow and supination of the forearm.

The hand and speech

The mouth and the hand have other subtle connections. After liberating themselves partially from their close nutritional collaboration, the hand first became a tool and then learned how to use tools, while the mouth contributed to sounds and then to words, yet always working together with the hand. Gestures with the hand have helped shape language by contributing a rhythm, by mimicking the oratorical action. The hand, along with speech, mirrors our emotions.

Leroi-Gourhan (1964) in his work, *Gesture and Speech*, analyzed the paleontologic evolution of the motor area, including two complementary territories—the facial and the manual. As one goes up the animal scale one finds an increase in the motor area related to the activities of the mouth and the hand. These are located in the precentral gyrus. In man there is a remarkable increase in the area corresponding to the tongue, the lips, the larynx, the pharynx, the fingers, and the thumb. Eighty per cent of the motor cortex is devoted to the function of the upper limb and the mouth (Figure 1.181).

Other functions of the hand

Body care

Among the many functions of the hand is its role in personal hygiene. All parts of the body are accessible to each hand under normal conditions. Impairment of this upper limb function, which makes it impossible to reach the perineum or to brush the hair, makes the patient dependent upon others and has serious psychological consequences.

The hand and sexuality

The hand, which evolved between the oral and sexual poles, plays an important role in sexual life, especially in human contact. Caress heightens perception; the malleable hand adapts itself to the caressed form. Tetraplegic patients questioned by Moberg (1975) preferred to conserve a supple hand for human contacts rather than undergo arthrodesis, which might have made possible better motor function. It is easy to understand the frequent psychological repercussions that result from injuries to this organ, which is so essential in our relationships with others.

Thermoregulatory role

The rich vascular network of the hand, as well as the relatively large surface of the integument, gives the hand an important thermoregulatory role. The importance is increased by the fact that usually the hands and the face are the only exposed areas of the body surface. Thermal regulation is controlled not only by the large radiation surface of the hands but also by the abundance of sweat glands. We all have experienced "sweaty palms" during times of emotional stress. This is an example of the central nervous system influence on the neurovascular regulatory role.

Physiological studies have revealed important differences in the distribution of blood between the forearm, the palm of the hand, and the digits and that the hand is greatly overperfused with regard to its metabolic needs (Burton, 1939). In the forearm, 80 per cent of the blood flow is directed to muscle, a small proportion to bone, and the rest to skin. In the palm of the hand it is divided equally between muscle and skin, whereas in the digits the flow is primarily to the skin because muscle is absent. The blood flow in the digits can increase to 100 times the minimum value; the minimum value for the fingers is the value resulting during the intense vasoconstriction following exposure to cold, and is 5–10 ml per minute per 100 ml of tissue. It is estimated that less than 10 per cent of the blood flow is required for nutrition and that more than 90 per cent is required for thermoregulation (Montagna and Fellis, 1961).

One of the characteristics of the vascular system of the hand is the abundance of arteriovenous anastomoses, which, by a short-circuit mechanism, control heat loss. This mechanism is regulated by the glomus bodies, which, by opening the shunts, increase cutaneous circulation but decrease capillary perfusion (see Section 1.4, page 141).

Regulation of circulation

All these observations emphasize the importance of the system of autonomous regulation that prevails in the skin everywhere, especially in the extremities and the hands. It is responsible for the maintenance of adequate muscle tone in the arteriocapillary network.

This regulator mechanism receives sympathetic discharges of central (hypothalamic) origin every 30 to 40 seconds, resulting in the liberation of norepinephrine (noradrenalin) at the extremities. Regulation is not under voluntary control but is activated by various factors acting through the so-called long axon reflexes. These include pain, emotion, forced inspiration, and smoking, which chiefly influence the distal circulation, probably because of the presence there of numerous arteriovenous anastamoses.

It is generally accepted that vascular tone is reduced during sleep, and this factor would explain the vasodilation normally observed in the hands and feet during that period.

Inhibition of this mechanism under certain conditions can induce antidromic vasodilation (i.e. transmitted against the direction of flow of the normal nerve impulse). This response, which is the reverse of the previous one, has a slow onset (20 to 40 second lag), lasts for 5 to 10 minutes, and appears to be mediated by acetylcholine.

This mechanism is reminiscent of the short-axon reflex, which is also antidromic and induces vasodilation as a result of local stimulation. It is probably important in hand disease. Indeed this type of reflex and its persistence have been incriminated in the spread of causalgia, which is sometimes seen after injury to the peripheral nerves, especially the median nerve.

The hand and the central nervous system

A complex system connects the hand to the central nervous system. The richness of the sensory information and the co-ordination required for the numerous muscles account for the large area of cortical representation as well as all the subcortical cerebellar and pontomedullary circuits that control hand functions.

The cortical territory of the hand was mapped out by Forster (1934), then by Penfield and Boldrey (1937) and Penfield and Rasmussen (1950) using electrical stimulation. The hand occupies nearly one third of the primary motor area, at the junction of the upper and middle thirds. The lower third is occupied by the face. The thumb occupies a particularly wide area and the fingers are all represented individually (Figure 1.181). *Cortical representation is not therefore proportional to the muscle mass active during a movement but is proportional to the precision and dexterity of the movement.*

Since antiquity the relationship between the hand and the mind has been the subject of countless theories and philosophical interpretations. Evolutionists tend to regard comprehension as merely a corollary of the action of talking. Teleologists, however, believe that nature bestowed the hand on human beings because they alone have the

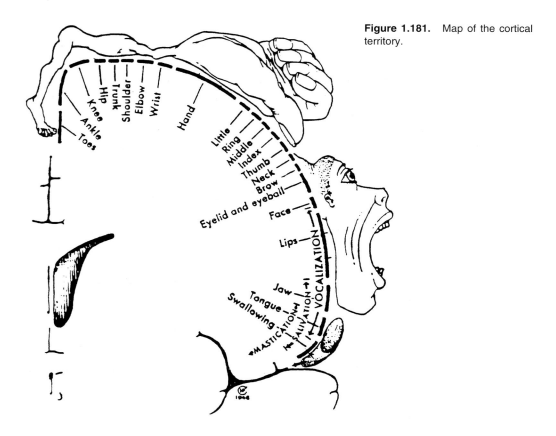

Figure 1.181. Map of the cortical territory.

mission to build and to understand. Thus, Charles Bell, who in 1833 wrote the first treatise on anatomy of the hand, *The Hand, Its Mechanism and Vital Endowments as Evincing Design,* believed that the hand gives to the mind the power of universal domination and constitutes the proof of the existence of God.

Modern philosophers have regarded this multitalented organ as the agent of conscious activity, a distinctive characteristic of man. Focillon (1947) wrote:

> But between the mind and the hand the relationship is not so simple as that of a master to a humble servant... Gestures may continually reflect the inner feelings. [Conversely,] hands have their gifts inscribed in their very shape and design—the gracile hands of the analyst, the long, fine, mobile fingers of the debater, prophetic hands exuding their fluid, spiritual hands expressing grace and character even at rest, and loving hands. The art of physiognomy, once assiduously practised by our elders, would have benefited from greater attention to the hands.

A little schematically, he concludes:

> The mind makes the hand; the hand makes the mind.

172

Automatic function and sublimation of the hands

The basic principle of economy governs the everyday activities of an organism in its relationships once the phase of sensorimotor apprenticeship is over. New connections between the preformed central nervous pathways are established, allowing automatic responses. In addition to conscious control of manual activities, control is exerted at the subconscious level; to use Moberg's comparison (1976), it is "computer control." This automatism manifests itself also in tactile perception, numbed by the monotony of routine actions, so that the grasp of familiar objects under usual circumstances becomes a stereotyped gesture. We emerge from this automatism only when something unusual occurs or a special interest draws our attention to the activities of our hands.

An almost continually conscious grasp is required in manual activities such as the artisan crafts, graphic arts, sculpture, instrumental music, and surgery in which intelligent collaboration between the brain and the hands does not allow for distraction. In certain cases we witness a true sublimation of the hand that allows it, with adequate training, to replace direct vision. It is especially true of the blind, who can read with their hands. In most religions the hand has a special symbolic significance; the laying on of hands signifies almost everywhere a pact or a blessing.

Collaboration of the two hands

The nervous system enables us to know the position of each hand at all times. In spite of a certain functional asymmetry, a cooperation or synchronism exists between the hands as well as a substitution potential that is well illustrated in amputees.

The significance of the hands has varied according to beliefs and epochs. In the Song of Songs each hand has a symbolic complementary value, the left representing strictness and the right, love.

The right hand is usually dominant. Is this only the consequence of our social practices, or is it due to dominance of the left cerebral hemisphere? Does this then challenge the usual morphological symmetry for the other species of animals? It is a theme to which Bichat (1855) referred on many occasions in his *Physiological Research on Life and Death*.

> Differences of the locomotor organs are not, or almost never, natural; they are an obvious sequel of social customs, which by increasing the movements of one side, augment their skill. . . As the habit of working perfects the action, we wrongly conclude the idea of the excess agility of the right member over the left. This remarkable difference in the two symmetrical halves of the body is thus by no means an exception to the general law of harmony of action of the external functions. . . It is always true that this discordance is a social result and that nature from the beginning destined them for harmonious action.

One hundred and fifty years later, Focillon (1947) expressed a similar view:

> The two hands are not a couple of passive identical twins. Neither are they distinguished the one more than the other like the older and the younger or like

173

two girls of unequal talent, one trained in many skills and the other burdened by the monotony of hard manual work. I completely disagree with the concept of the eminent dignity of the right hand. If the left fails, the right hand is placed in an almost sterile isolation. The left—this hand which is unjustly designated as the bad side, the sinister or ominous side, that side from which the dead, or an enemy or a bird should not be seen—is capable of being trained to fulfill all the tasks of the other. Constructed like the other, it has exactly the same aptitudes, which it gives up for the role of helper.

Conclusion

The functional architecture of the hand offers this organ multiple possibilities of adaptation, exploration, expression, and prehension. The hand joins, in the same anatomical structure, the powers of knowledge and action. It is both the origin of very precise information and the irreplaceable executor of the wishes of the brain. The hand is the privileged messenger of thought.

The more we study the hand, the more we marvel at its extraordinary efficiency and the wealth of pathways that connect it to the central nervous system. However, this subtle organ, whose mechanisms we have not yet fully understood, is by necessity exposed and complex. It may be threatened or destroyed by many traumatic or pathological processes.

2 CLINICAL EXAMINATION OF THE TEGUMENTS, THE SKELETON AND THE MUSCULOTENDINOUS APPARATUS

INTRODUCTION

Clinical examination is the essential source of information concerning function and lesions of the hand and wrist. Clinical examination of the hand should have two primary objectives—to detect and assess lesions as accurately as possible (the choice of treatment will be based on this assessment) and to evaluate the adequacy of remaining functions. On this evaluation will depend the decision to operate and the quantification of incapacity. However, function can be appreciated only in the light of other factors, such as the condition of the rest of the limb and that of the contralateral hand and the patient's professional background, which in turn will determine the manual requirements and influence the potential for recovery.

It is probably fair to say that the clinical examination is by far the most important source of information. Radiological, electrical, and thermographic examinations supply complementary information limited to certain structures, but only through the clinical examination can the state of the skin, joints, tendons, and aponeuroses be properly assessed. The same applies, of course, to manual function.

The clinical examination of the hand involves a series of specific examinations to appraise the skin cover, circulation, trophic changes and sweating, bones and joints, muscles and tendons, the overall motor performance of the hand, tactile sensibility, and deep sensibility.

All the information given by clinical examination must provide a basis for further understanding. Each examination should be objective, repeatable and preferably numerical to give the basis for a clear picture of the development of the patient's condition.

The clinical examination must be preceded by a full history from the patient noting timing of any trauma and variation of symptoms. The patient's psychological state must also be noted.

Examination is not complete without noting the patient's dominant hand, the function of the whole upper limb and the function of the opposite limb.

The history should elicit precise functional handicaps of daily life, professional and recreational activities. These handicaps have to be ranked in order of importance, which will be determined by that particular patient.

2.1 EXAMINATION OF THE TEGUMENTS, PALMAR APONEUROTIC LESIONS AND TROPHICITY

Characteristics of normal skin

Thickness and suppleness are assessed by noting callosities on the pressure areas and the thickness of the skin folds, keeping in mind that connections to the deeper planes are normally present in several areas. It is thus possible to distinguish between hands with supple skin and normal mobility and hands with thicker skin and reduced passive mobility. From a practical point of view, the three main implications are that the thick, calloused skin of the manual laborer requires more thorough preoperative preparation; that plastic repair is much less likely to succeed on thickened, less mobile skin; and that the thickness of the epidermis and the horny layer must be taken into account in testing cutaneous sensation.

The availability of skin must be assessed prior to all plastic repairs and mobilizing operations, especially in areas that are usually mobile, e.g. the dorsal aspect of the interphalangeal and metacarpophalangeal joints, the dorsal aspect and crest of the first web space, the dorsal aspect of the phalanges (if one intends to perform a Z-plasty on the palmar aspect of the finger), and the dorsal aspect of the hand.

Signs of skin atrophy must be searched for in patients in whom long-term corticosteroid therapy has been prescribed and those with neurovascular problems. Atrophied skin has about the same appearance as the skin in senile cutaneous degeneration—a shiny appearance, a thinning of the dermis and epidermis, and a loss of elasticity. Reduced thickness and persistence of the skin creases are the characteristic signs. The presence of stellate pseudoscars is a typical change. These alterations limit the scope of plastic repairs and are usually associated with poor skin healing.

Scars and skin contractures

Careful scrutiny of all scars is an essential part of the examination of the skin. Scars can be one of the factors responsible for reducing the mobility of joints and must be taken into account in testing articular mobility. The most common are longitudinal palmar scars that run across the flexion creases; contracture of these scars interferes with extension of the fingers. Dorsal scars, especially where they create adhesions, may reduce the mobility and extensibility of the skin, even in the absence of contracture. Flexion is then affected. Web space scars, by invading the palmar interdigital system, can interfere not only with separation of the fingers but also with flexion at the metacarpophalangeal joints.

Estimating tissue loss

The area of tissue loss that must be covered after release of contractures, alteration of the wound contours, and fashioning of angles to prevent new contractures is always much greater than the area of the wound before preparation.

In planning skin incisions and skin flaps at the outset of any operation, one should take into account every existing scar. Flaps must not be based on a scarred area. In adherent zones, undermining may lead to skin necrosis. Sinuous scars outline flaps whose base must not be divided when the surgeon designs new exposures.

Aponeurotic lesions

These are most often seen in Dupuytren's disease. They may appear as palmar nodules or bands which can be seen and felt in the mid-palmar aponeurosis, the first web space and fingers, where they cause flexion contractures and may also form knuckle pads on the dorsum of the proximal interphalangeal joint.

Assessment of deformity in Dupuytren's disease

An objective method of evaluating the lesions in Dupuytren's disease allows accurate preoperative assessment and indicates the amount of improvement achieved by the operation.

The formula that we use takes into account not only the degree of individual digital flexion but also the distribution of lesions throughout the hand.

The hand is divided into five segments, each consisting of a finger and corresponding palmar zone, which includes the pretendinous band of the palmar aponeurosis to the four medial fingers and its adjacent segment of the palmar aponeurosis. The fascia of the thenar eminence and the first web space are part of the thumb segment. For each of these five segments the distal and palmar aponeurotic lesions are allocated a number corresponding to a certain stage of the disease. Each stage thus represented, corresponds to a progression of 45 degrees of the total of the deformity of each finger. These total deformities are measured by adding together the individual flexion deformities (deficiency of extension) of the three joints—the metacarpophalangeal (MP), proximal interphalangeal (PIP), and distal interphalangeal (DIP) joints. When there is hyperextension of the DIP, the degree of hyperextension is added to the total flexion deformity of the other joints.

Theoretically *for each finger* the range of deformity is from 0 degrees (complete extension) to 200 degrees (contracture of the finger in the palm).

Thus six stages can be distinguished for the four fingers (Table 2.1 and Figure 2.1).

Stage 0 = no lesion
      N = palmar or digital nodule without established flexion deformity
      1 = total flexion deformity between 0° and 45°
      2 = total flexion deformity between 45° and 90°
      3 = total flexion deformity between 90° and 155°
      4 = total flexion deformity exceeding 135°

For the thumb, we assess contractures of the MP and IP joints, then contracture of the first web space. This is evaluated by measuring the angle formed by the axes of the

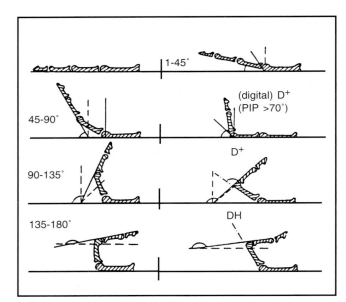

Figure 2.1. Schematic drawing of the different stages of deformty in Dupuytren's disease. Each stage corresponds to a progression of 45 degrees of the total deformation of all the joints of each finger, which may consist of different combinations.

first and second metacarpals where they intersect in the sagittal plane. Normally the angle exceeds 45 degrees, with each stage of the assessment corresponding to a loss of 15 degrees (Figure 2.2). Thus in theory the thumb's range of deformity is from 0 degrees to 160 degrees for the MP and IP joints (Figure 2.3), and from 0 degrees to more than 45 degrees at the level of the web.

For each ray, we distinguish between palmar lesions, indicated by the letter P, and digital lesions, indicated by a letter D. If the lesion includes both the palm and fingers, the number designating the stage is followed by the letters PD. The letter H for hyper-extension, designates advanced cases in which the distal phalanx is fixed in this position.

Each ray of the hand is examined individually, beginning with the thumb, and the stage of the disease is noted. If no lesion exists, a 0 is recorded. An aponeurotic lesion without joint deformity is designated by an N (nodule), followed by P or D according to whether the nodule is palmar or digital.

At the first ray, contractures of the IP and MP joints are indicated by the letter D, and consist of 4 stages corresponding to a progression of 45 degrees just as for the fingers. Then the four possible stages of contracture of the first web are indicated by a number followed by the letter P (see Figures 2.2 and 2.3).

Assessment of the first web contracture:
- stage 0:   more than 45° anteposition of the first metacarpal
- stage 1:   between 45° and 30°
- stage 2:   between 30° and 15°
- stage 3:   less than 15°

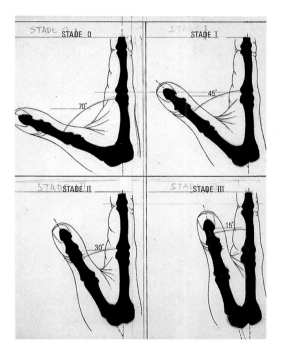

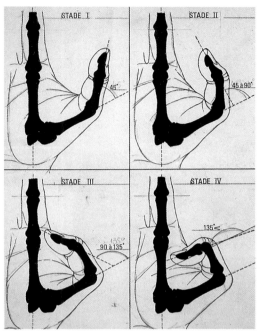

Figure 2.2. Assessment of first web contracture.

Figure 2.3. Assessment of the range of deformity of the first ray.

The lesions of the first ray have particularly important functional consequences, so are evaluated by two numbers.

Both hands are systematically coded each time they are examined. The numbered assessment of each ray allows one to obtain an accurate clinical record of the disease. Among the other advantages it also encourages a full examination of each hand and reveals lesions of the radial half of the hand which often go undetected.

All these elements are recorded beginning with the thumb. Each of the five rays of the hand (the finger corresponding to the palmar zone) is represented in turn by a number (or an N) indicating the stage followed by the appropriate letters. The rays without aponeurotic lesions are indicated by a 0. One can appreciate immediately the number of rays affected, the localization and the severity of the lesions. The presence of a PIP joint contracture of greater than 70 degrees has a severe prognostic importance and is indicated by a '+' after the digital letter (D⁺). Flexion contracture at the MP joints are more easily corrected than at the PIP.

Since the five elements of this evaluation express the spread of the disease, and each number signifying the stage expresses the intensity of the contracture, it becomes possible to indicate the total state by adding the numbers of each ray. It is necessary to

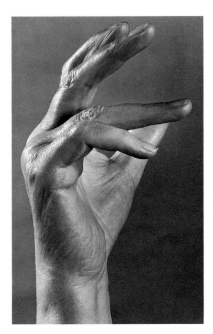

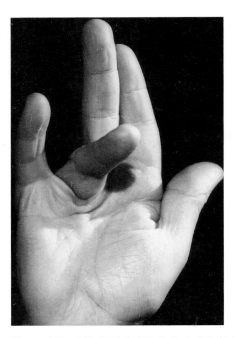

Figure 2.4. RH: 0P-0D, 0, 1, 2, 3. This translates as follows: RH (right hand), 0P-0D (no lesion of thumb ray), 0 (no lesion in index/second ray), 1 (contracture of middle finger less than 45°), 2 (contracture of ring finger (MP + PIP) between 45 and 90°), 3 (total deformity of all joints of little finger ray 110°: MP 60° + PIP 50°). Total evaluation: 1 + 2 + 3 = 6.

Figure 2.5. RH: 3P-0D, NP, 0, 3, 1. RH (right hand), 3P-0D (contracture of first web, less than 15° of anteposition, no contracture of thumb joints), NP (palmar nodule on second ray without deformity of index), 0 (no lesion in third ray), 3 (100° contracture in ring finger: MP 80° + PIP 20°), 1 (20° flexion contracture at PIP of little finger). Total evaluation: 3 + 0.5 (for nodule) + 3 + 1 = 7.5. In spite of severe flexion deformity of the ring finger, the correction will be easy because of its location at the MP joint.

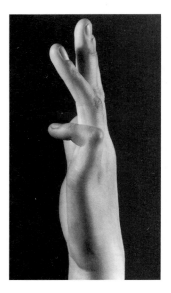

Figure 2.6. LH: 0P-0D, 0, ND, 1, 3+. LH (left hand), 0P-0D, 0 (no lesion in thumb/index rays), NP (digital nodule without deformity in middle finger), 1 (contracture of ring finger less than 45°), 3+ (flexion deformity of 100° at PIP joint of little finger; + indicates flexion deformity of more than 70° of PIP joint). Total evaluation: 0.5 (for nodule N) + 1 + 3 = 4+.5. In spite of a rather low total evaluation, the severe contracture at the PIP joint of the little finger (+) will be difficult to correct.

assign a value to nodules without contractures, so the stage N is evaluated 0.5. One can then represent a hand with Dupuytren's disease by one total number, pre-operatively between 0.5 (one nodule without deformity) and 23 (five digits deformed to stage 4 and the thumb web contracted to stage 3) (Figures 2.4, 2.5 and 2.6).

After intervention, the evaluation is recalculated, giving evidence of the benefits for each finger. A new summary is obtained by adding the figures of the new formula.

The difference between the total pre-operative and post-operative numbers expresses the absolute gain obtained by the operation.

Circulation

Even though the patient may have no specific vascular disease, a careful study of the circulation is essential both preoperatively and postoperatively (Figure 2.7).

Recognition of vascular disease is important for the appreciation of tolerance to a tourniquet, i.e. induced ischemia, and for assessing the likelihood of postoperative edema. Vascular disease also makes necessary a more conservative attitude toward the remaining arterial trunks, especially after severe injuries. The following points merit special consideration in an examination of the circulation:

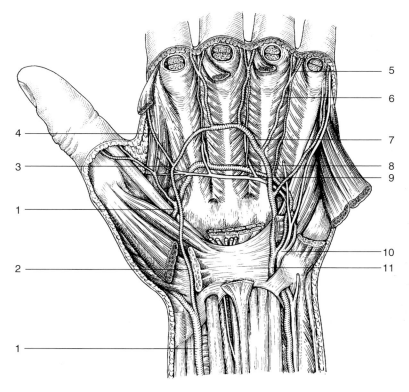

Figure 2.7. Arteries of the hand: (1) radial artery; (2) palmar branch; (3) arteria princeps pollicis; (4) arteria radialis indicis; (5) digital artery; (6) metacarpal artery; (7) superficial palmar arch; (8) deep palmar arch; (9) deep branch of ulnar nerve; (10) ulnar nerve; (11) ulnar artery.

Color. The examiner notes whether the skin is pale, red, or cyanosed.

Distal arteriolar flow. The distal arteriolar flow is measured by the time taken for color to return to the nail bed after pressure.

Pulse. The pulse classically taken at the radial wrist groove is not the only accessible one. The ulnar pulse is usually palpable at the entry to Guyon's canal. The radial artery can also be felt as it exits from the anatomical snuffbox (Figure 2.8) at the proximal part of the dorsal aspect of the first web space; it should remain accessible after a crush injury. The collateral digital arteries can be felt at the base of the finger, just anterior to the dorsopalmar cutaneous line, in patients with supple skin and a strong pulse.

Arterial territories. A simple clinical test aids in deciding whether the radial or the ulnar artery is responsible for the major arterial supply to the hand. This is the Allen test, which is carried out as shown in Figure 2.9a.

The maneuver is then repeated to test for the other artery. Predominance of the radial artery is common.

The digital Allen test is performed in a manner similar to that at the wrist level (Figure 2.9b).

Venous return. The venous return is more difficult to measure. Localized cyanosis is obviously a sign of venous stasis, but edema is the most common feature of an abnormal venous return. Two points are worth stressing here:

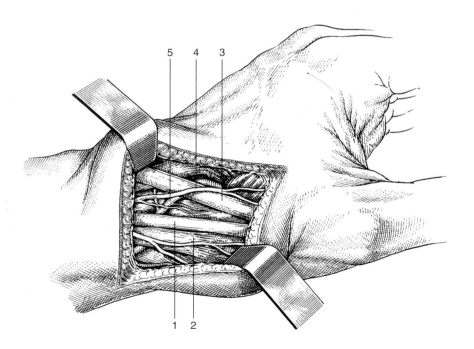

Figure 2.8. Radial artery in the anatomical snuffbox: (1) extensor pollicis brevis; (2) abductor pollicis longus; (3) extensor pollicis longus; (4) superficial branch of radial nerve; (5) radial artery.

1 Edema is most readily demonstrable on the dorsum of the hand. When severe, it is obvious; if less marked, it rounds off the bony contours of the metacarpals. Minimal edema causes the disappearance of the shallow transverse furrows that are normally present in dorsal skin.

2 Edema of the palmar tissues is more easily overlooked. It becomes obvious when it is abundant enough to fill the concavity of the palm between the thenar and hypothenar eminences. More often, there is but slight infiltration of the tissues, which is just palpable and is suggested by limitation of flexion of the fingers.

Complementary examinations. When the hand has a poor circulation, complementary examinations can be performed—*see* Section 3.2, *Investigation of the circulation.*

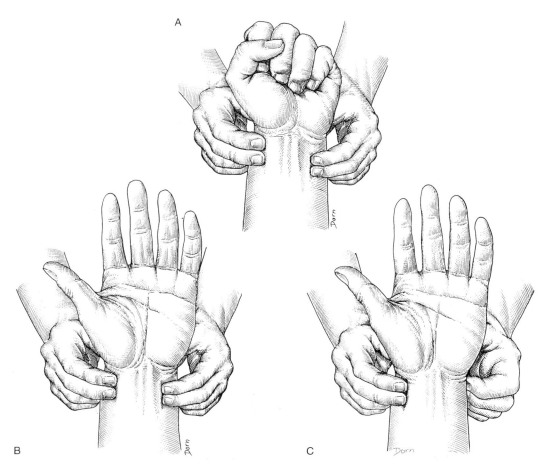

Figure 2.9a. Allen test at the wrist level. The patient is asked to raise and clench his hand to squeeze the blood out of the cutaneous vascular bed. (A) the examiner compresses the radial artery in the radial groove and the ulnar artery in Guyon's canal; (B) the patient opens his hand without hyperextending his fingers. The palm appears exsanguinated; (C) the examiner releases one compression and notes the time taken for the palm to recover its normal color. The maneuver is then repeated to test for the other artery.

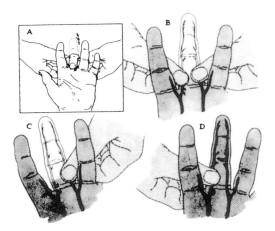

Figure 2.9b. The digital Allen test is performed in a manner similar to that at the wrist level (A and B). Release of one digital artery at a time may reveal a unilateral occlusion, demonstrated in this patient with a post-traumatic radial digital artery thrombosis (C and D).

Trophicity and sweating

Trophic changes are due to vasomotor and neurological factors. To assess trophicity, one should examine not only the skin but also the nails and dorsal hairs as well as the thickness of the soft tissues, especially in the pulp.

The amount and distribution of sweating can provide information about possible vasomotor disturbances (reflex sympathetic dystrophy). Localized differences in sweat secretion indicate the presence of a peripheral nerve lesion.

The nails

Examination of the nails is useful, not so much to detect disease involving the ungual tissue proper but as a guide to atrophic changes and to study of the pinch. The pulp tissue is supported by the nail matrix. Loss of, or damage to, the nail may affect the precision and power of the pinch.

The muscles

Atrophy of the intrinsic muscles is seen in paralyses of the upper limb. A lesion of the median nerve gives rise to atrophy of the abductor pollicis brevis and opponens. This causes a loss of the normal thenar contour, and the resultant depression allows the bone of the first metacarpal to be seen on the radial aspect of the hand.

Flexor pollicis brevis may be preserved if it has a predominant ulnar nerve supply.

In ulnar nerve palsy, atrophy is visible in two muscle groups:

1 The interossi, where atrophy is seen first, followed by depressions of dorsum of the first web space, between the metacarpal bones and on the dorsum of the hand.
2 The hypothenar muscles show atrophy on the ulnar aspect of the palm medial to the 5th metacarpal.

184

2.2 EXAMINATION OF THE BONES AND JOINTS

We shall study at each level (wrist, carpometacarpal joints, digital rays):

- bone morphology and landmarks
- the passive mobility of the joints, which does not depend exclusively on articular freedom. It may be limited by contractures of the skin and soft tissues as well as by obstruction to tendon movement. Loss of mobility in any joint should always be measured by comparison with its contralateral equivalent
- clinical signs in the joints: swelling, effusions and instability.

The wrist

Landmarks

There are distinct bony landmarks at two levels of the dorsal aspect of the wrist. The proximal border consists of the two distal extremities of the forearm bone. From the radial border of the wrist, the radial styloid process can be felt, followed by a distinct drop to the anatomical snuffbox limited radially by the compartment of APL and EPB, and ulnarly by the EPL. The EPL tendon changes direction at Lister's tubercle. Ulnarly to Lister's tubercle, the dorso-ulnar angle of the radius can be felt, then the ulnar head, easily palpable with the forearm pronated. The ulnar styloid can be felt dorsally in supination and more "volarly" in pronation. More distally the wrist corresponds to the carpus. The floor of the anatomical snuffbox is formed by the body of the scaphoid (see Figures 2.35 and 2.36). The proximal pole of scaphoid is palpable just distal to Lister's tubercle with the wrist in flexion. Articulating distally with scaphoid are the trapezium along the axis of the thumb and trapezoid in line with the index finger.

In slight wrist ulnar deviation the scapho-lunate joint can be felt radially to a notch called the "crucifixion notch". Distal to the lunate is capitate and then the carpo-metacarpal joints. In full flexion, the neck of capitate is the most prominent feature of the dorsum of the wrist. Between the capitate and trapezoid is the styloid process of the third metacarpal where ECRB inserts.

On the ulnar border of the wrist, the ulnar styloid process, triquetrum, hamate and base of the fifth metacarpal can be felt in turn. With radial deviation, the luno-trique-tral joint is palpable.

Immediately beyond the ulnar styloid is a notch—the "ulnar snuffbox". It is circum-scribed by the ECU and FCU tendons running posteriorly and anteriorly over the ulna at the wrist. In radial deviation, the floor of this depression is formed by the triquetrum; in ulnar deviation, by the joint between triquetrum and hamate.

Joint mobility

Pronosupination: It should be evaluated with the elbow flexed to prevent shoulder rotation from disguising the range of movement. To eliminate the effect of intracarpal movement it is important to only note the movement of the bistyloid line around the axis of the forearm. Starting with the hand level with the flexed elbow, supination is 90 degrees from neutral and pronation 80 degrees.

Flexion–extension: the relative contribution of the radiocarpal and mediocarpal joints cannot be measured separately without the help of radiology.

Flexion or palmar flexion: the amplitude of palmar flexion is somewhat greater than that of extension, about one third of the amplitude of movement occurring at the intercarpal joints. Movement is measured with the limbs of the goniometer placed on the dorsal aspects of the forearm and third metacarpal, over the convexity of the flexed wrist. Mean flexion as measured by Wynn Parry (1981b) in 100 young males was 75 degrees, with a range of 52 to 93 degrees.

Extension or dorsiflexion: the intercarpal joints provide about half the amplitude of extension. Goniometry is performed with the limbs of the instrument on the palmar aspects of the forearm and the third metacarpal across the palmar convexity of the extended wrist. Wynn Parry's average extension reading (in 100 young males) was 64 degrees, with a range of 42 to 79 degrees.

Abduction and adduction: clinical examination of abduction (radial deviation) and adduction (ulnar deviation) movements in the wrist reveals the contribution of the frontal deviation of the glenoid surface of the radius only if the interstyloid line is examined first. Adduction and abduction occur mostly at the radiocarpal joint and partly at the intercarpal joint; the contribution of each cannot be assessed clinically. Adduction–abduction is measured with the wrist held straight. The goniometer limbs are placed on the dorsal aspects of the forearm and third metacarpal. Mobility in this plane is reduced when the wrist is extended and is virtually absent if the wrist is flexed. Adduction readings show a mean of 29 degrees, with a range of 19 to 35 degrees (Wynn Parry, 1981b). Abduction is normally less – 19 degrees on average (range 11–39 degrees).

Clinical assessment

The understanding of wrist anatomy and carpal mechanics has improved greatly in recent years and is necessary for the diagnosis of some difficult clinical problems. The history of a reproducible maneuver aggravating pain or restraining a particular movement suggests a mechanical cause in a specific area. The association of paresthesia or disturbed sensation may be related to the irritation of the terminal branches of the median, ulnar, radial or posterior interosseous nerves.

Examination

In addition to the normal described movements, a series of special maneuvers are applied. The ligamentous habitus of a given individual must be assessed using information from the normal wrist, because of the wide variation in mobility and laxity.

The individual stressing of the scapholunate joint, the lunotriquetral joint, the triangular fibrocartilage complex, the distal radioulnar joint, the midcarpal joint, and the

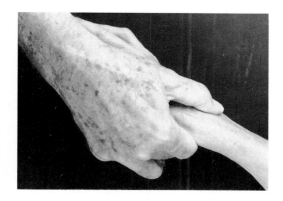

Figure 2.10. Examination of the DRUJ. The hand is held in ulnar deviation, the ulnar head pressed volarward by the examiner's thumb.

Watson test are performed first on the normal side. An identical examination is performed on the symptomatic wrist, and any areas of tenderness, any clicks or clunks associated with the production of any pain are noted.

The distal radioulnar joint
An exaggeration of the normal ulna head prominence is seen in dorsal subluxation or articular effusion. The prominence may be temporarily reduced by direct pressure over the ulna head. In the rheumatoid wrist, this prominence is further exaggerated by a supination deformity of the carpus.

If the hand is held in full ulnar deviation and the ulna head is held forward by the examiner's thumb, significant pain may be precipitated by this movement alone and this suggests DRUJ pathology. However, pain precipitated by pronosupination while the ulna head is pressed volarward and the pisiform pressed dorsally (Figure 2.10) is usually indicative of some form of ulnar impingement or abutment syndrome.

Radio-carpal and intercarpal instability
There are numerous maneuvers evaluating the various ligamentous structures.

The *radio-carpal* and *midcarpal joint/anteroposterior drawer:* one of the examiner's hands holds the patient's hand by the metacarpals to apply axial traction while the other hand stabilizes the patient's forearm. While holding this traction, anteroposterior force is applied and a drawer is elicited at the radio-carpal, then the midcarpal joint (Figure 2.11). The ability to push the midcarpal joint volarward is present to a varying degree in most normal asymptomatic patients. A marked drawer test is a sign of congenital laxity.

The midcarpal joint/the *"pivot shift" test of the mid-carpal joint:* this consists of supinating and volar subluxing the distal row of the carpus. It is performed (Stanley and Saffar, 1994) by placing the patient elbow upon a firm surface, holding the elbow at 90 degrees, putting the hand into a fully supine position and holding the distal forearm firmly (Figure 2.12). The hand is moved into full radial deviation and then the ulnar side of the carpus is forced into further supination and a volar subluxed position. The wrist must not be flexed. The hand, still with the displacing force applied,

187

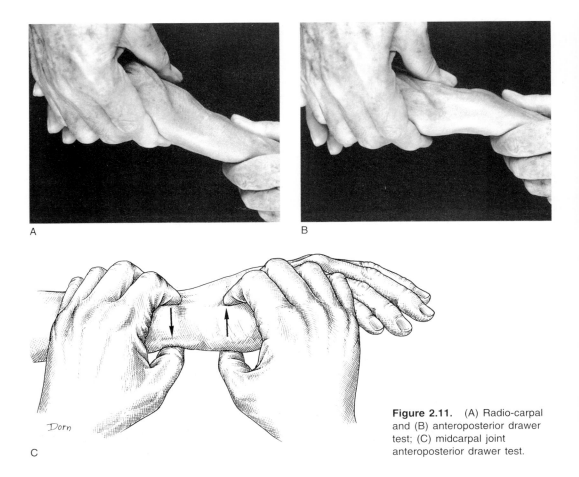

Figure 2.11. (A) Radio-carpal and (B) anteroposterior drawer test; (C) midcarpal joint anteroposterior drawer test.

is gently moved from radial to full ulnar deviation. The normal wrist will notch into a less supinated position as the head of the capitate engages the lunate, because of the restraint of the anterior capsule and triquetrolunate interosseous ligaments. Rupture, attenuation or excess laxity do allow the capitate to drift out of the lunate.

Watson's test (1988), or *scaphoid shift test*, is designed to show scaphoid instability. The examiner puts one hand on the radial border of the distal forearm with the thumb on the palmar aspect of the scaphoid (Figure 2.13), while with the other hand the examiner moves the patient's hand to bring about ulnar then radial deviation of the wrist. The thumb pressure on the scaphoid is maintained, while the wrist is brought into radial deviation. This causes a dorsal subluxation of the scaphoid, accompanied by a painful click.

The *ballotment tests*, or shear tests, consist of demonstrating abnormal movements between adjacent bones by exerting pressure in opposite directions. One may thus show instability of scapholunate joint (Figure 2.14), lunotriquetral joint (Figure 2.15) (Reagan's test) (1984), capitolunate joint or at the distal radioulnar joint.

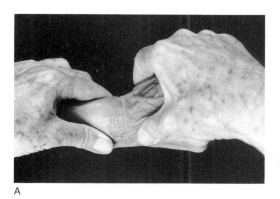
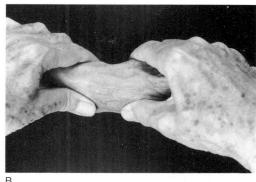

A B

Figure 2.12. (A) The "pivot shift" test involves supinating and volar subluxing the distal carpal row. B) The hand in supination is moved from radial to full ulnar deviation.

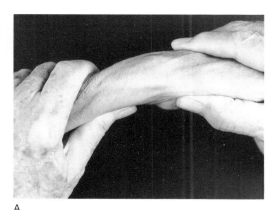
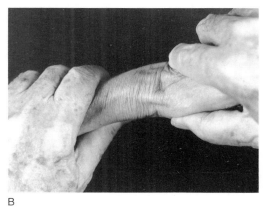

A B

Figure 2.13. Watson's test. (A) One examiner's hand is placed on the radial border of the distal forearm with the thumb maintaining a constant palmar pressure on the scaphoid. (B) With the other hand the examiner moves the patient's hand (in pronation) to create ulnar and radial deviation of the wrist.

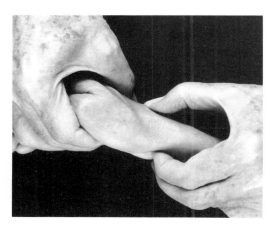

Figure 2.14. The scapholunate ballotment test: Stressing of the scapholunate joint by volar pressure on the tubercle of the scaphoid and dorsal pressure on the lunate. If there is any ligament damage, pressure on these two bones causes a painful shearing of the scapholunate joint.

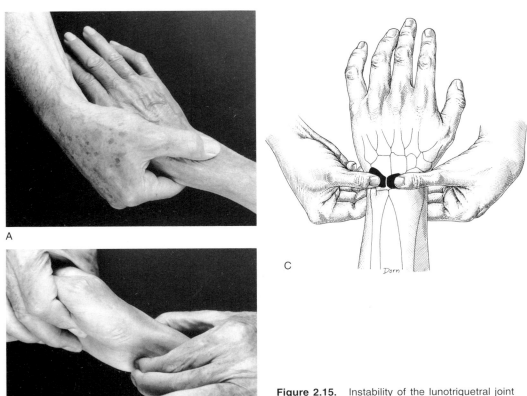

Figure 2.15. Instability of the lunotriquetral joint (Reagan's test). (A) Dorsal view: pressure of the examiner's thumb on the lunate. (B) Volar view: pressure of the examiner's index on the triquetrum. (C) Lunotriquetral shear test: the examiner uses both hands (Masquelet, 1989).

Triquetral hamate instability is demonstrated with the wrist straight with ulnar deviation. After a range of about 20 degrees, it produces a firm block. If one forces a sharp click accompanied by discrete posterior movement of the wrist, the proximal row of the carpus has moved from the VISI position (volar intercalated segment instability) to that of DISI (dorsal intercalated segment instability), thus allowing a complete ulnar deviation of the wrist joint.

Radiographic assessment (see pages 226–35)

The most current measurements used in rheumatoid arthritis are those described by Shapiro (1970), which evaluate the radial deviation of the wrist and the ulnar deviation of the fingers by two angles (Figure 2.16):

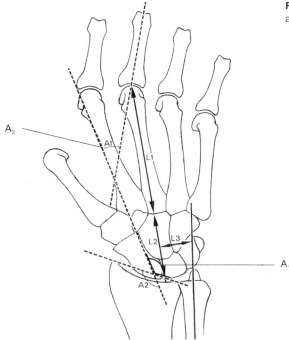

Figure 2.16. Radiographic assessment.

- the A1 angle is formed by the tangent of the inferior aspect of the radius and the radial aspect of the second metacarpal. This angle, indicating "radial angulation" is normally 120 degrees to 125 degrees. It is greater when the wrist is radially deviated
- the A2 angle measures the ulnar deviation of the fingers. It is defined by the angle formed between the tangent of the radial aspect of the second metacarpal and the axis of the proximal phalanx of the middle finger. It becomes pathological when it exceeds 25 degrees.

The ulnar translation of the wrist and its reduction in height are measured according to the criteria of McMurtry et al (1978). These are:

- the length of the third metacarpal (L1)
- the height of the wrist while passing through the center of the head of the capitate (L2) and
- the distance between the center of the head of the capitate and the extended axis of the ulnar epiphysis (L3).

The ratio of L2:L1 is normally 0.54 ± 0.03, decreasing with involvement of the wrist. The L3:L1 ratio is 0.30 ± 0.03; this is reduced with displacement of the wrist in the frontal plane.

The strict lateral view in a neutral position permits the study of sagittal deviations. The wrist tends to sublux anteriorly. Usually, the radial axis extends through the lunate

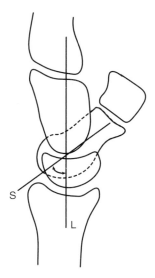

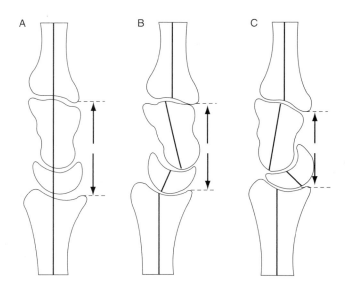

Figure 2.17. The scapho-lunate angle.

Figure 2.18. The carpal bones can be likened to kinetic chains. (A) Thus in the central column the lunate and capitate are intercalary segments, which subject to "zigzag" displacement in cases of imbalance or instability. In (B) the lunate is tilted in flexion (its distal surface points volarly) and the capitate is in extension. (C) The lunate is tilted in extension. In fact, the capitate is stable; the lunate is the site of instability.

axis and the capitate axis (Figure 2.17). The scaphoid makes an angle of 30–60 degrees with this axis as does the dorsal or palmar displacement of the lunate with this same angle. The dorsal or palmar displacement of the lunate explains its instability; it is judged at the level of the distal pole (Figure 2.18). Thus, the DISI or VISI formula (Linscheid and Dobyns, 1971) signifies that the distal joint surface of the lunate is turned in extension (dorsal) or in flexion (volar). In both cases, the scaphoid tends to become horizontal.

Carpometacarpal joints

Landmarks

On the dorsal surface, the tubercle of the base of the second metacarpal marks the carpometacarpal joint line and the insertion of the extensor carpi radialis brevis.

On the ulnar border of the hand behind the relief of the hypothenar eminence the styloid of the fifth metacarpal is situated in the extension of the tendon of extensor carpi ulnaris which brings the wrist into extension and ulnar deviation.

On the radial aspect, the outline of the base of the first metacarpal is palpable in the distal part of the anatomical snuffbox.

Joint mobility

There is normally no clinically detectable mobility at the second and third carpometacarpal joints. Movement at the fourth carpometacarpal joint is limited to only a few degrees in the sagittal plane and, although detectable, it is virtually impossible to measure accurately. The fifth carpometacarpal (metacarpohamate) joint has an appreciable mobility, which is important functionally in adaptation to the transverse arch of the palm and surgically in phalangization of the fifth metacarpal. Movement occurs in an almost sagittal plane, which is slightly oblique toward the axis of the hand. It can be observed clinically on the ulnar side of the hand when the head of the fifth metacarpal is mobilized, and it is measured by reference to the third metacarpal, which is fixed. The overall amplitude is about 20 degrees.

The first carpometacarpal joint

The first metacarpal (trapeziometacarpal) joint is functionally the most important, because it allows movement of the whole column of the thumb. Movements at this joint are so complex that they must be expressed conventionally. It is likely that in the movement considered, peritrapezial mobility does intervene.

Terminology

The complexity of these movements explains the confusion in terminology. Each author justifies his own terminology by advocating a mechanism or making an analogy with the movements of the fingers or with the muscle responsible for the motion. However, such a terminology should also be clear, as universal as possible in its terms, and acceptable to all. We are far from this goal in discussing movements of the thumb.

The difficulty with terminology describing thumb movements arises from two causes. The first is conceptual: some authors describe abduction as any movement of separation of the first metacarpal from the second metacarpal and specify the direction of movement by an adjective, such as radial abduction or palmar abduction. This is the terminology adopted by the International Federation of Societies of Hand Surgery. This definition of each movement by necessity employs two terms.

Another international society, the International Anatomical Society, has adopted the terms abduction and adduction to describe the movements in the sagittal plane and flexion and extension for movements in the frontal planes (Nomina Anatomica, 1960). However, Rabischong (1971) prefers to distinguish the movements of the phalangeal segments from those of the first metacarpal. According to him, the terms flexion and extension should be reserved to designate only movements of the phalanges.

The second difficulty is in the anatomical realm: as demonstrated by Kapandji (1972), the axes of the trapeziometacarpal articulation are oblique in relation to the planes of reference (Figure 2.19). In order to study the movements of this articulation, a special reference system must be used, the trapezial system, which may be measured precisely only by radiography.

With these difficulties in selecting a terminology, authors understandably avoid the use of traditional terms and attempt to define the movements of the thumb according

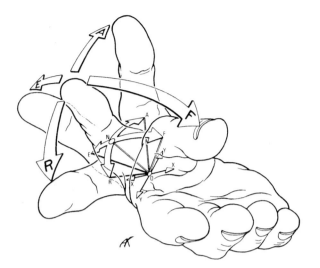

Figure 2.19. The trapezial system of reference. Starting from position 0 (N), the first metacarpal is able to perform two types of pure movement (without any longitudinal rotation occurring): anteposition (A) and retroposition (R) around the metacarpal axis XX′ and flexion (F) and extension (E) around the trapezial axis YY′.

to its trajectory in relation to the index metacarpal. This is the solution adopted by Caffinière (1970) and by Ebskov (1970). In its larger elliptical path, the distal end of the thumb metacarpal realizes a motion of "circumduction"; that is to say, it inscribes a conical segment at the farthest distance from the second metacarpal. In its smaller elliptical path of circumduction, it moves as close as possible to the second metacarpal.

In an effort to be precise, we have to distinguish between terms defining a set position of the thumb metacarpal in space and terms defining the movements.

For terms defining a set position, we will use the two static coordinates proposed by Duparc et al (1971) with the following nomenclature and definitions:

- the angle of separation is the angle formed between the thumb and index metacarpal in the sagittal plane (Figure 2.20); and
- the angle of circumduction (the term we prefer to the term "angle of spatial rotation," which the last-mentioned authors use) is the angle formed between two planes—one plane formed by the thumb and index metacarpal and the other (the reference plane) formed by the index and middle metacarpals (Figure 2.21). The angle can be measured with the back of the hand resting flat on a table. In fact, the first metacarpal cannot be placed in the reference plane because of the anteposition of the trapezium. It is understood that the definition of the position of the first metacarpal with the help of these two angular coordinates can be applied to the thumb only if the phalanges are extended in prolongation of the metacarpal.

Terms defining the movements. In clinical practice these movements do not require the same precision of description, and it seems reasonable to us to continue to use a terminology indicating movements forward, backward, inward, and outward, starting from a theoretical resting position (Figure 2.22).

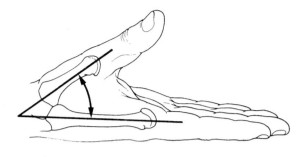

Figure 2.20. The "angle of separation" formed by the intersection of the axes of the first and second metacarpals in a sagittal plane.

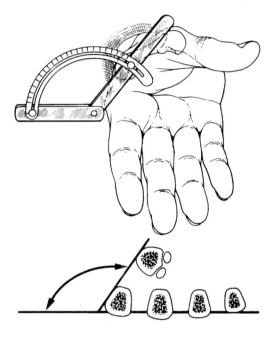

Figure 2.21. The "angle of circumduction" formed by the intersection of two planes, one passing through the second and third metacarpals and the other through the first and second.

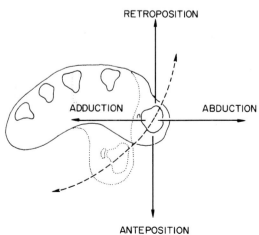

RETROPOSITION

ADDUCTION

ABDUCTION

ANTEPOSITION

Figure 2.22. Terminology used to describe the movements of the thumb metacarpal: anteposition, retroposition, adduction (or flexion–adduction), and abduction (or extension–abduction).

195

The movements are broken down as follows:

- outward movement of the thumb in the plane of the palm: at rest, the first metacarpal lies against the second; it moves away from the second metacarpal during abduction—the opposite happens in adduction (Figure 2.23). The angle of abduction can be measured between the axes of the first and second metacarpals from the dorsal side and is usually 45–70 degrees
- movement of the thumb perpendicular to the palm: at the start of this movement, the first metacarpal lies on the palmar surface of the second metacarpal; in the movement away from that surface, the thumb is placed in anteposition (Figure 2.24). The measurement is taken between the ulnar border of the first metacarpal and the radial border of the second metacarpal; it varies between 40 and 80 degrees
- axial rotation (pronation–supination of the thumb column): this component, which intervenes in movements of the trapeziometacarpal joint during opposition, is difficult to assess clinically. One should watch for the changing orientation of the dorsum of the first metacarpal, and of the nail, during the movement from full abduction to full anteposition. Rotation of the first metacarpal is demonstrated in this way, and rotation of the phalanges is not taken into account.

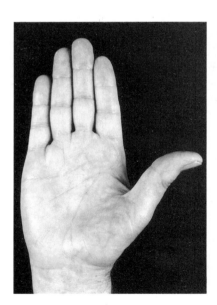

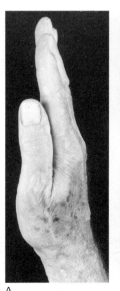

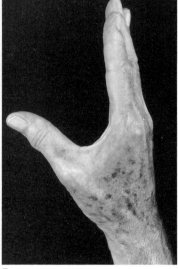

A   B

Figure 2.23. Abduction of the thumb. Maximal separation in the plane of the palm is evaluated clinically by measuring the angle made by the first and second metacarpals.

Figure 2.24. Anteposition of the thumb. Separation of the thumb perpendicular to the plane of the palm can be measured by the angle formed by the first and second metacarpals. Simultaneous axial rotation can be observed, which modifies the orientation of the plane of the nail.

The following corollaries merit consideration:

1 In practice, whatever the origin of the movement, the plane of the second metacarpal represents the extreme limit of displacement of the first metacarpal toward the axis of the hand.
2 A quantitative assessment of the movement of retroposition is of little practical value. It is the movement that carries the first metacarpal from full anteposition to a point behind the plane of the hand. Its amplitude rarely exceeds 10 degrees.

It seems that the terms anteposition and retroposition are clear and useful. We recommend their adoption. However, the terms abduction and adduction, as well as flexion and extension, used alone, may be confusing. Each time we use them we must redefine them. Instead of using them alone, we can group them in the pairs—flexion–adduction and extension–abduction.

The movement carrying the thumb ray into anteposition is accompanied by an internal rotation (pronation) of the thumb ray. The movement of the thumb ray into retroposition is accompanied by an external rotation of the thumb ray (supination). This has been described as "automatic" longitudinal rotation (Kapandji, 1972) or "conjunct rotation" (MacConaill, 1946).

Opposition is a combined movement involving all three segments of the thumb (Figure 2.25): the metacarpal segment moves in anteposition and then in adduction, a movement that is accompanied by an "automatic" longitudinal rotation into pronation (Figure 2.26). The proximal phalanx flexes, pronates, and radially deviates. The distal phalanx flexes to a variable degree, and this flexion is accompanied by a slight pronation adapted to the requirements of the grip. It is evident that the vast movement of opposition requires an expansile, mobile web space and that any contraction of the webbed area (cutaneous, muscular, tendinous, aponeurotic, or capsuloligamentous) will impair the thumb's mobility.

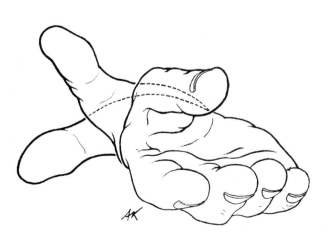

Figure 2.25. Opposition of the thumb is a complex movement of the entire thumb column bringing the pulp of the thumb opposite that of the fingers. It combines anteposition and adduction (or flexion–adduction) of the first metacarpal, flexion of the metacarpophalangeal and interphalangeal joints, and a global movement of rotation of all the skeletal elements into pronation. In this large opposition movement, the tip of the thumb follows a "wide course of opposition," away from the palm, before reaching the little finger. In a "restricted opposition motion," the thumb crawls in the palm and can reach the base of the little finger, but this is not a real opposition movement.

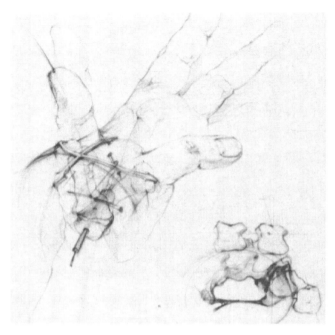

Figure 2.26. The movements of the first metacarpal in anteposition and flexion–adduction are accompanied by an "automatic" longitudinal rotation in pronation.

Kapandji's method for clinical evaluation of thumb opposition

Kapandji (1986) described a method of evaluation of thumb opposition using the hand itself as the reference system. The method is based on the successive thumb–finger pinch during the wide course of opposition. Eleven stages are defined (Figure 2.27).

Stage 0: The tip of the thumb is located on the lateral aspect of the proximal phalanx of the index finger.

Stage 1: The tip of the thumb is in contact with the lateral aspect of the middle phalanx of the index finger.

Stage 2: The tip of the thumb is in contact with the lateral aspect of the distal phalanx of the index finger (Figure 2.28).

Stage 3: Terminal pinch between the thumb and the index finger.

Stage 4: Terminal pinch between the thumb and the middle finger.

Stage 5: Terminal pinch between the thumb and the ring finger.

Stage 6: Terminal pinch between the thumb and the little finger.

Stage 7: The tip of the thumb is in contact with the distal interphalangeal crease of the little finger.

Stage 8: The tip of the thumb is in contact with the proximal interphalangeal crease of the little finger.

Stage 9: The tip of the thumb is in contact with the proximal crease of the little finger.

Stage 10: Finally, the tip of the thumb reaches the distal palmar crease at the base of the little finger.

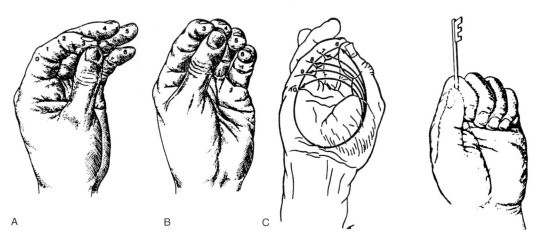

A   B   C

Figure 2.27. Method of evaluating thumb opposition in numerical stages. (A,B) Kapandji's system (1986). (C) Modified version of Kapandji's system.

Figure 2.28. Lateral thumb grip.

This opposition test is considered valid when stage 10 is reached after passing through every stage of the "wide course". In fact, stage 10 may be reached by passing the "restricted opposition motion," with the thumb crawling in the palm.

Swelling, effusions, and instability

Effusions in the small, closely packed carpometacarpal joints are seldom detectable clinically, with the possible exception of the trapeziometacarpal joint.

Instability occurs mainly on the two mobile carpometacarpal joints, the fifth and the thumb. It is caused by traumatic, infectious, nervous, or rheumatoid lesions. Instability of the proximal joint of a digital ray may lead to deformities in the distal joints.

The digital rays

We have to examine the three joints of the rays of each long finger and the two joints of the thumb ray.

Landmarks

The metacarpus not only is easily palpable but is visually identifiable on the whole of the dorsum of the hand. The third metacarpal—the axis of the hand—is a landmark of wrist movements. The styloid process, which projects from its base, is easily palpable and marks the line of the carpometacarpal joints. The relative lengths of the metacarpals can be seen along the line made by the metacarpal heads with the metacarpophalangeal joints flexed (normally the third is the longest metacarpal, followed by

199

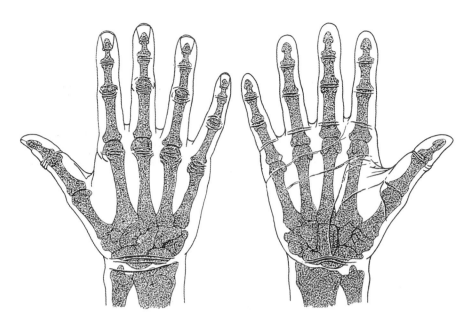

Figure 2.29. Diagram showing the relationship between the skin creases and the position of the metacarpophalangeal joints.

the second, the fourth, and the fifth). Proximal displacement of one of the metacarpal heads indicates a shortening of the corresponding metacarpal. Abnormal rotation after a metacarpal fracture can be diagnosed by observing flexion of the metacarpophalangeal (MP) joints. Malrotation is manifested by ulnar or radial deviation of the corresponding proximal phalanx; the greater the deviation, the more severe the malrotation.

The MP joints are easily accessible on the dorsal and lateral aspects. They are not palpable in the palm, but their position can be derived from the flexion creases. The MP joints lie approximately on a transverse line that begins in the distal palmar crease on the ulnar side and runs into the proximal crease on the radial border (Figure 2.29).

The phalanges and interphalangeal joints are visible and easily palpable on the dorsum and sides of the fingers, with the exception only of the proximal part of the proximal phalanx, which is embedded in the soft tissues of the web space. Deformities at that level, especially in the sagittal plane, are often difficult to detect clinically.

Distally, lateral or anteroposterior deviations of the phalanges are clinically obvious. Defects of axial rotation in a digital segment are demonstrated, as with the metacarpals, by flexing the joint immediately distal: these defects are then confirmed by deviation of the next phalanx (Figure 2.30).

The axes of flexion are so arranged that flexion of all the MP and proximal interphalangeal joints causes the fingers to converge toward the scaphoid. The examiner should note any variation from this.

200

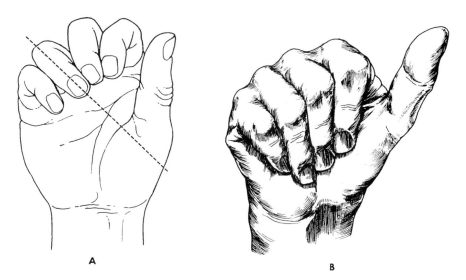

A   B

Figure 2.30. (A) Fracture of the proximal phalanx of the ring finger causing overlapping of the ring finger on the long finger. (B) After reduction, flexion of all fingers into the palm is the only way of demonstrating that rotational displacement has been corrected. The tips of the fingers converge without overriding.

Joint mobility

The metacarpophalangeal joints of the four long fingers

Flexion–extension: flexion–extension is measured by the angle formed with the limbs of the goniometer placed on the dorsal surfaces of the proximal phalanx and its corresponding metacarpal (Figure 2.31).

Glanville (personal communication) has described a simple procedure to determine successive angles of flexion and extension during rehabilitation. It consists of placing on the dorsal aspect of the digit a malleable metal filament that is adapted to the angles of the phalanges. The filament is then removed and used as a template to make a diagram of the state of the mobility. Successive drawings demonstrate progress.

Flexion: flexion is invariably less in the index than in the other fingers. The average is 82 degrees (range 61–96 degrees) (Wynn Parry, 1981). The amplitude is similar for the middle, ring, and little fingers, i.e. a mean value of 88 degrees, ranging from 52 degrees (little finger) to 104 degrees (middle finger) (Wynn Parry, 1981).

Metacarpophalangeal extension: there are great variations in MP extension. Active extension varies between 10 and 20 degrees, but passive extension can reach 90 degrees in loose jointed subjects. Conversely, it may be nil in subjects whose soft tissues are unusually stiff. This point deserves careful study in patients with paralysis of the intrinsic muscles of the fingers (Figure 2.32).

Sideways movements are normally possible at the MP joints. They must be tested with the fingers held straight, because they become impossible (as a result of increased

201

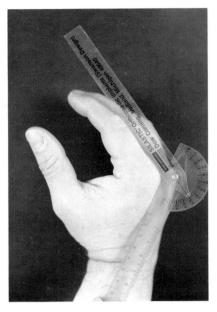

Figure 2.31. Examination of joint amplitude can be carried out by using a goniometer placed on the dorsal aspect of a finger.

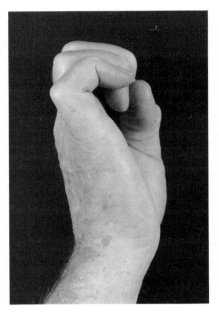

Figure 2.32. In a normal subject, active hyperextension of the metacarpophalangeal joint remains possible when the wrist is dorsiflexed in spite of active interphalangeal flexion.

tension of the collateral ligaments) once the fingers are flexed. In the normal hand, freedom of movement is always greater on the ulnar than on the radial side.

The metacarpophalangeal joint of the thumb
Landmarks: the dorsal and radial aspects are subcutaneous. The medial aspect is palpable on the dorsal aspect of the first web. Its palmar aspect is marked by the proximal flexion crease of the thumb. An effusion of this joint is noted by a fusiform swelling dorsally or laterally.

The movement is less than that of the fingers. No extension is possible except in cases of hypermobile joints. Flexion is about 55 degrees but varies greatly, from as little as 35 degrees to as much as 90 degrees—normal is what the patient has on the opposite side.

Stability: the lateral movements are normally very restricted but again this varies with individuals; the important reference point is the opposite side.

Radial deviation or passive abduction is limited in extension by the tension of the fibrocartilage capsule and collateral ligaments, and in flexion by the tension of the ulnar collateral ligament alone (Figure 2.33). Examination must be conducted in flexion to elicit any loss of lateral stability indicating a ruptured collateral ligament.

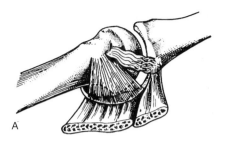
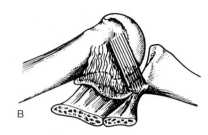

Figure 2.33. (A) Metacarpophalangeal joint of the thumb in extension: the metacarpophalangeal part of the collateral ligament is loose and the metacarpoglenoid part is taut. (B) In flexion, the situation is reversed.

The proximal interphalangeal joints

The proximal interphalangeal joints have only one plane movement, namely, flexion–extension; they are remarkably stable laterally. Mobility is measured by the angle formed by the limbs of the goniometer on the dorsal surfaces of the proximal and middle phalanges.

The range of flexion is usually more than 100 degrees (Wynn Parry's averages for passive flexion range from 104 degrees for the little finger to 114 degrees for the ring finger, 1981). Some individuals have more limited flexion, the lowest figures having been recorded in the index finger. Extension is usually nil at the proximal interphalangeal joints. It is also worth noting that it is the orientation of the axes of flexion at these joints that produces the normal convergence of the fingers toward the scaphoid.

The distal interphalangeal joints

The distal interphalangeal joints move essentially in flexion and extension, but slight side-to-side movement is also usually possible. The range of flexion is normally less than that in the proximal joints (the average is 80 degrees). Some degree of passive extension is normal (about 30 degrees); it is more marked in the index finger.

The interphalangeal joint of the thumb has similar characteristics to the distal interphalangeal joints of the fingers. However, it is capable of active and passive hyperextension—there is only passive hyperextension in the fingers. Flexion of the interphalangeal joint is accompanied by rotation into pronation, which favours opposition of the pulp.

Ulnar movement is greatest in the index finger (mean is 42.7 degrees) and smallest in the ring finger (mean is 24 degrees). Radial movement is greatest in the little finger (average is 29.4 degrees) and least in the middle finger (Hakstian and Tubiana, 1967) (Figure 2.34). Some passive axial rotation is usually possible when the metacarpophalangeal joint is extended.

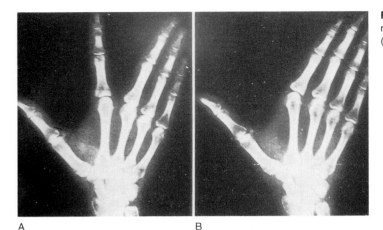

Figure 2.34. (A) Radial movement of the fingers. (B) Ulnar movement.

A   B

Articular swelling, effusions and instability

Swelling arising from the MP joints is manifested mostly on the dorsal side. However, there is also some lateral swelling that fills the adjacent intermetacarpal depressions and tends to obscure the normal projection of the metacarpal heads on the dorsal side of the hand.

Instability of the MP joints of the fingers accentuates the normal ulnar deviation of these joints. The weakness or rupture of the capsuloligamentous structures which stabilize these joints, particularly in rheumatoid arthritis (when the MP joints are distended by proliferative synovium) or after capsulectomies of MP joints in hands in which the intrinsic muscles are paralyzed, results in pathological ulnar deviation.

2.3 EXAMINATION OF THE MUSCULOTENDINOUS APPARATUS

In this section we will deal with direct and indirect function of the tendons; motor function will be discussed in Section 4.2.

Landmarks

Only the extensor tendons are accessible to visual inspection and palpation, owing to the thin dorsal skin on the hand. They are visible with the fingers in active extension and the thumb in abduction (Figure 2.35).

From radial to ulnar they are described (Figure 2.36):

- abductor pollicis longus and extensor pollicis brevis can be seen between the radial styloid proximally and the base of the first metacarpal distally;
- the extensor pollicis longus can also be seen running from the radial styloid to the ulnar side of the base of the first metacarpal. The extensor pollicis longus is best seen with the thumb in active retropulsion;
- the extensor communis and proprius tendons of the fingers lie in the axis of each metacarpal to the level of the proximal phalanx;
- the extensor carpi radialis tendons are only palpable for a short distance proximal to the bases of the second and third metacarpals with the wrist in resisted extension;

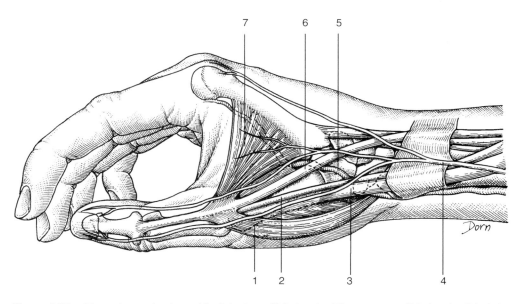

Figure 2.35. The extensor tendons: (1) abductor pollicis brevis; (2) extensor pollicis brevis; (3) abductor pollicis longus; (4) radial nerve (sensory branch); (5) deep branch of radial artery; (6) extensor pollicis longus; (7) adductor pollicis.

205

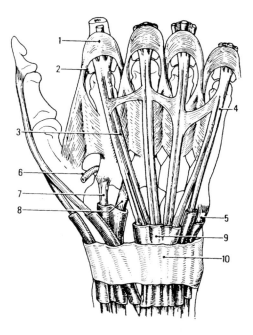

Figure 2.36. Posterior view of the dorsal carpometacarpal region and of the tendinous plane of the wrist. (1) The interosseous hood; (2) bony insertion of the first dorsal interosseous; (3) extensor indicis; (4) extensor digiti minimi; (5) extensor carpi ulnaris; (6) radial artery; (7) extensor carpi radialis longus; (8) extensor carpi radialis brevis; (9) extensor digitorum; (10) extensor retinaculum (dorsal annular ligament of the wrist).

- the extensor carpi ulnaris tendon is palpable during resisted extension and adduction of the wrist, immediately distal to the ulna styloid until the fifth metacarpal. On the palmar aspect the motor tendons of the wrist are also palpable, and the flexor carpi ulnaris is felt in active flexion of the wrist immediately proximal to the pisiform.
- the flexor carpi radialis and palmaris longus tendons are also palpable and visible in resisted flexion of the wrist just proximal to the distal wrist flexion crease.

Assessment of flexion–extension mobility of the digits

Numerous methods of assessment utilized to study the results of tendon surgery on the hand have been described. At present, there is no internationally accepted system of evaluation. Several factors need to be taken into account in any system of evaluation. It is necessary to standardize the method by which these measurements are made, as this will influence the results.

Use of the goniometer

With the wrist in neutral position and the wrist joint in pronation and then in supination, the patient is asked to make a fist and then extend the fingers. One then measures the maximum flexion and extension of the three joints of each finger. The measurements to evaluate flexion of each joint must be made with the closed fist without maintaining the proximal segment of the joint to be measured in extension.

This requirement reflects the fact that less tendon excursion is required to produce middle and distal joint flexion with the metacarpophalangeal (MP) joints held in full extension than with all three joints in composite flexion. The true measurement of flexor tendon performance therefore requires that the patient attempts to actively flex all three joints simultaneously.

The limbs of the goniometer must be short enough not to impede movement. The goniometer is placed on the dorsum of the digit, as it is difficult to place it laterally on the central digits. One measures successively the active and passive mobility.

The sum of the movement of flexion of all three joints is not sufficient. *Flexion of the MP joints depends in part on the intrinsic muscles, whereas flexion of the interphalangeal (IP) joints depends entirely on the long flexor tendons.* The addition of the total range of flexion may give a misleading impression of the results of flexor tendon surgery. However, the evaluation of the movements of the IP joints is insufficient by itself, as the function of the fingers also depends on movements of the MP joints.

The range of movement in the proximal interphalangeal (PIP) joint has the greatest functional value and reflects most accurately the action of the two long flexors. But it is also necessary to take into account to a lesser degree the active mobility of the MP joint and distal interphalangeal (DIP) joint.

Measurement of pulp–palm distances may also be misleading, e.g. when the IP joints have a full range of motion and the MP joints are stiff in extension or one of the IP joints is in fixed flexion.

The postoperative total active motion value must be compared with the preoperative value and may be an indication for tenolysis. It is insufficient, however, to allow evaluation of the function of the finger.

The lack of extension must be evaluated at each joint. However, these measurements must be of functional value to allow meaningful comparison of results. The tables, which consist of a great number of measured angles, are difficult to interpret and difficult to use for comparative statistics, and they do not provide a useful evaluation of the functional state of the digit.

Total active and total passive mobility

The Committee for Evaluation set up by the American Society for Surgery of the Hand (1976) recommended the use of a formula comparing the total passive mobility to the total active mobility:

Total passive mobility = total passive flexion (MP + PIP + DIP) – lack of passive extension (metacarpophalangeal + proximal interphalangeal + distal interphalangeal).

Total active mobility = total active flexion (MP + PIP + DIP) – lack of active extension (MP + PIP + DIP).

This method is simple and has the advantage of being usable in other situations as well as after tendon surgery. However, it lacks precision and implies an equal functional value for each of the three joints.

Buck-Gramcko's method

Buck-Gramcko (1976) proposed a method that takes composite flexion, pulp–palm distance, and extension deficit into consideration. (He pointed out that the measurements should be performed with slight extension of the wrist without supporting the joints in extension.) Measurements were used to obtain the following values:

1 Composite flexion—the sum of the angular measurements of flexion of all three joints.
2 Extension deficit—the sum of the angular measurements of loss of extension of all three joints.
3 Total active motion—the difference between the composite flexion and extension deficits.
4 The flexion deficit—the distance between the finger and the distal palmar crease.

A functional system was then formulated by assigning points to each of these measurements and totaling the values (Tables 2.1 and 2.2).

Distance finger pulp — distal composite flexion crease*	0–2.5 cm.	≥ 200°	6 points
	2.5–4 cm.	≥ 180°	4 points
	4–6 cm.	≥ 150°	2 points
	>6 cm.	< 150°	0 points
Extension deficit		0–30°	3 points
			2 points
		51–70°	1 point
		> 70°	0 points
Total active motion		≥ 160°	6 points
		≥ 140°	4 points
		≥ 120°	2 points
		< 120°	0 points

Classification
  Excellent: 14–15 points
  Good: 11–13 points
  Satisfactory: 7–10 points
  Poor: 0–6 points

*Buck-Gramcko means by "distal composite flexion crease" the fold formed by the distal transverse flexion crease on the ulnar side of the palm and the proximal transverse flexion crease on the radial side.

Table 2.1. Point system and classification for index, middle, ring, and little fingers (Buck-Gramcko)

Flexion in the interphalangeal joint	50–70°	6 points
	30–49°	4 points
	10–29°	2 points
	< 10°	0 points
Extension deficit	0–10°	3 points
	11–20°	2 points
	21–30°	1 point
	> 30°	0 points
Total active motion	≥ 40°	6 points
	30–39°	4 points
	20–29°	2 points
	< 20°	0 points

Classification	
Excellent:	14–15 points
Good:	11–13 points
Satisfactory:	7–10 points
Poor:	0–6 points

Table 2.2. Point system and classification for the thumb (Buck-Gramcko)

Tubiana's method

We have advocated (Tubiana et al, 1979) a method of evaluation of flexor tendon repairs which includes specifically a method of assessment of proximal interphalangeal joint function which reflects specifically the action of the flexor tendons.

This is easily found by determining the relationship between the long axes of the middle phalanx and the metacarpal (Figure 2.37).

A separate assessment of the flexion deficit and the extension deficit is made, after which a composite assessment is used to determine the functional value. The method of assessment proposed in 1979 has been slightly modified and now includes a supplementary grade "normal."

Flexion deficit

The flexion deficit is graded as follows:

Grade I (F1)   Complete active flexion.

Grade II (F2)   The line of the middle phalanx is parallel to the metacarpal with full active flexion, and the distal joint has at least 45 degrees of active flexion.

Grade III (F3)   The middle phalanx forms an angle 0–30 degrees with the metacarpal with full active flexion, and the distal interphalangeal joint has at least 30 degrees of active flexion.

209

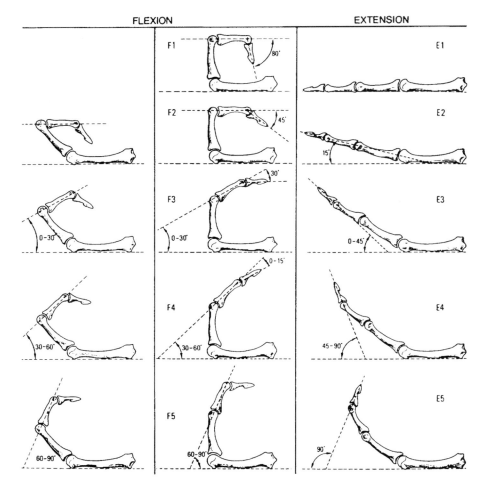

Figure 2.37. The method of evaluation of results that we use takes into account the flexion deficit as represented by the angle between the middle phalanx and the metacarpal (which we consider most important) as well as the different degrees of metacarpophalangeal flexion (note the difference between columns 1 and 2), distal intercarpophalangeal flexion, and extension deficit (column 3).

Grade IV (F4)   The middle phalanx forms an angle of 30–60 degrees with the metacarpal with full active flexion, and the distal interphalangeal joint has at least 15 degrees of active flexion.

Grade V (F5)   The middle phalanx forms an angle of 50–90 degrees with the metacarpal with full active flexion.

If distal interphalangeal joint flexion is less than 45 degrees for grade I, 30 degrees for grade II, or 15 degrees for grade III, the result is dropped one grade.

210

Extension deficit

The extension deficit is estimated by adding the active extension deficit in each of the three joints.

Grade I (E1)   Complete active extension.

Grade II (E2)   The angle between the distal phalanx and the metacarpal is less than 15 degrees.

Grade III (E3)   The angle is less than 45 degrees, with no more than 30 degrees deficit in any one joint.

Grade IV (E4)   The extension deficit is between 45 and 90 degrees and is no more than 45 degrees in any one joint.

Grade V (E5)   The extension deficit is greater than 90 degrees.

If the extension deficit in any joint is more than 15, 30 or 45 degrees, the result is dropped one grade.

Combined assessment

The combined assessment is expressed by utilizing the grades of flexion deficit and extension deficit, for example, F1, E2.

Since a flexion deficit is more important than an extension deficit, a scoring system similar to the one used by Buck-Gramcko (1971) assigning greater weight to active flexion is proposed (Table 2.3).

Active flexion	
Grade I (F1)	7 points
Grade II (F2)	6 points
Grade III (F3)	4 points
Grade IV (F4)	2 points
Grave V (F5)	0 points
Extension deficit	
Grade I (E1) and Grade II (E2)	3 points
Grade III (E3)	2 points
Grade IV (E4)	1 point
Grade V (E5)	0 points
Classification of results	
Perfect	10 points
Very Good	8 to 9 points
Good	7 to 6 points
Fair	5 to 4 points
Poor	3 to 0 points

Table 2.3. Combined assessment of results for the fingers (Tubiana)

We agree with Stark (1977), who stated that the use of such terms as excellent, good, fair, and poor is misleading. However, every author uses these terms to express results. If required, a point system and classification for the index, middle, ring, and little finger could be established by adding active flexion and extension deficit. For example, perfect results would be 10 points, very good results would be 8 to 9 points, good results would be 6 to 7 points, fair results would be 4 to 5 points, and poor results would be 0 to 3 points (Table 2.3).

Evaluation of surgery on the long flexor tendon of the thumb

Evaluation of the results of the flexor tendon surgery in the thumb must be considered from a slightly different perspective. Flexor pollicis longus flexes the distal phalanx, but this action depends in part on the stability of the metacarpophalangeal joint. In normal conditions, the flexion of the joint approaches 90 degrees; however, a good result can be obtained with a lesser degree of flexion, if this flexes within the functional range. On the other hand, the extension deficit of the distal phalanx impedes function more than a lack of extension in another digit. A deficit of more than 15 degrees extension reduces pulp to pulp contact and efficiency of thumb–index pinch.

Flexion deficit

Grade I (F1):   Complete active motion (compared with the opposite side).
Grade II (F2):   The distal interphalangeal joint has at least 60 degrees of active flexion.
Grade III (F3): The distal interphalangeal joint has at least 30 degrees of active flexion.
Grade IV (F4):   The distal interphalangeal joint has less than 30 degrees of active flexion.

Extension deficit

Grade I (E1):   The angle between the proximal and distal phalanges is less than 15 degrees.
Grade II (E2):   The angle between the proximal and distal phalanges is less than 30 degrees.
Grade III (E3): The angle between the proximal and distal phalanges is greater than 30 degrees.

Each of the foregoing values is recorded with the thumb in anteposition so that the final functional assessment is more meaningful (Table 2.4).

Tenosynovitis

Synovitis of the dorsum of the wrist

This is most frequently seen in rheumatoid arthritis and is manifested by swelling.

On the dorsal and ulnar aspect of the wrist, the swelling is due to synovitis of the extensors of the fingers and extensor carpi ulnaris. Occasionally it is seen as a double swelling situated on either side of the retinaculum.

Active flexion	Grade I (F1)	5 points
	Grade II (F2)	3 points
	Grade III (F3)	2 points
	Grade IV (F4)	1 point
Extension deficit	Grade I (E1)	2 points
	Grade II (E2)	1 point
	Grade III (E3)	0 points
Classification of results	Perfect	7 points
	Very Good	5 to 6 points
	Good	4 points
	Fair	3 points
	Poor	2 to 0 points

Table 2.4. Combined assessment of results for the thumb (Tubiana)

On the radiodorsal aspect of the wrist the swelling is due to synovitis around the extensor carpi radialis tendons and the extensor tendons of the thumb, and the swelling lies along the tendinous axis at the level of the anatomical snuff-box.

Tenosynovitis of the first dorsal compartment is more commonly a mechanical tenovaginitis of De Quervain's. This is demonstrated by Finkelstein's test (Finkelstein 1930) which involves passive flexion of the wrist in ulnar deviation, with the thumb held flexed in the palm by the other fingers. This causes pain at the radial styloid by tension on the abductor pollicis longus and extensor pollicis brevis tendons (see p. 224).

Flexor synovitis
When the flexor tendons of the distal forearm are affected the swelling has no clear margin. In the fingers the synovial sheaths lie along the flexor tendons, with their "cul de sac" at the level of the distal palmar crease (Figure 2.38). When infected, pressure at this level is painful for the radial three fingers. In the little finger and thumb the proximal opening of the flexor sheaths lies proximal to the proximal wrist crease. Again pressure here causes severe pain in the presence of infection.

In rheumatoid synovitis, the swelling is less discrete and is elicited by bilateral pressure on the flexor sheath, which is less painful than with infection, and is associated with incomplete flexion and triggering of the fingers.

Tendon excursion, limitations and adhesions

Most of the extrinsic muscles and some of the intrinsic muscles have tendons which cross several joints, so it is possible to tension or relax them by changing the position of these joints. For example, flexion of the wrist joint will relax the flexor tendons.

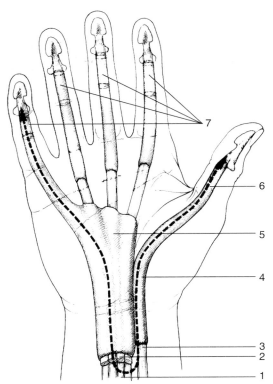

Figure 2.38. Palmar view of the synovial sheath of the flexor tendons: (1) flexor digitorum profundus; (2) flexor digitorum superficialis; (3) flexor pollicis longus; (4) radial bursa; (5) ulnar bursa; (6) sheath of flexor pollicis longus; (7) digital synovial sheaths; arrow: potential connections between radial and ulnar flexor tendon sheaths.

Extension relaxes the extensor system and vice versa. These maneuvers will allow the examiner to:

- judge if the musculotendinous apparatus is normal length or contracted (e.g. flexion of the wrist is necessary for total passive extension of the fingers if a contracture of the flexor tendons exists);
- localize tendon adhesions and to differentiate it from joint stiffness (e.g. dorsal adhesions of the extensors at the metacarpal level will limit flexion of the interphalangeal (IP) joints and will resolve when the metacarpophalangeal (MP) joints are in hyperextension; however, when the lateral ligaments of the proximal interphalangeal (PIP) joints are contracted, the mobility of these joints is not influenced by the position of the MP joints) (Figure 2.39);
- put into tension a muscle to detect a contracture (e.g. extension of the wrist will favour active flexion of the fingers).

Anomalous tendon interconnections

A tendinous interconnection between the flexor pollicis longus and flexor digitorum profundus tendons, usually to the index finger, was described by Linburg and Comstock (1979). The pathognomic sign for this condition is simultaneous index finger IP joint flexion when the thumb is actively flexed across the palm. When index distal joint

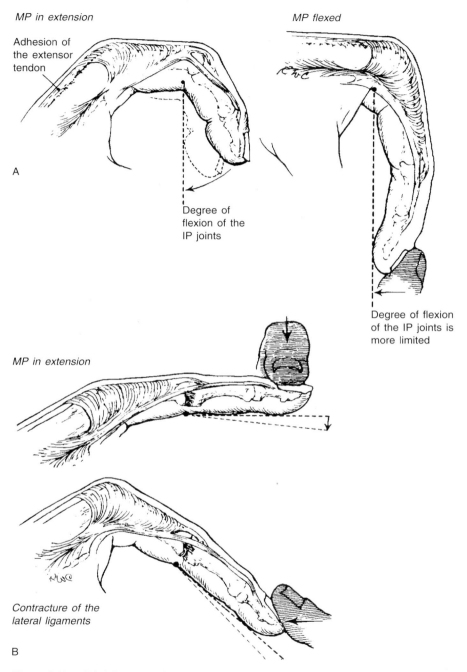

MP in extension

Adhesion of
the extensor
tendon

A

Degree of
flexion of the
IP joints

MP flexed

Degree of flexion
of the IP joints is
more limited

MP in extension

Contracture of the
lateral ligaments

B

Figure 2.39. (A) Adhesions of the extensor tendons at the metacarpal level. The position of the MP joint influences the degree of flexion possible for the PIP joint. (B) The contracture of the lateral ligaments of the PIP joint involves a restriction on mobility. The position of the MP joint does not influence the degree of flexion possible for the PIP joint when the lateral ligaments of the PIP joint are contracted.

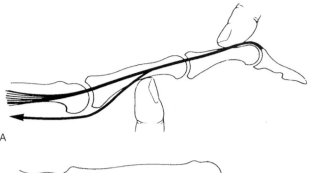

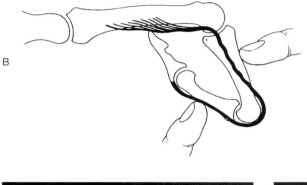

Figure 2.40. Finochietto–Bunnell test: swan-neck deformity. (A) and (C) When the proximal phalanx is maintained in extension, it is impossible to flex the middle phalanx. (B) and (D) Flexion of the proximal phalanx allows flexion of the middle phalanx. This maneuver indicates an interosseous muscle contracture.

A

B

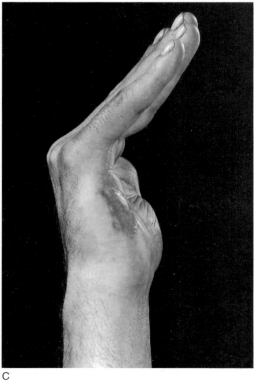

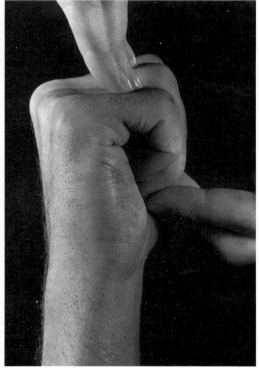

C

D

flexion is blocked during active thumb flexion, volar radial wrist pain is triggered (Linburg's sign).

Interosseous muscles contracture

The Finochietto-Bunnell test is the application of these phenomena to the interosseous muscles when they are contracted: when the metacarpophalangeal (MP) joint is in extension the contracted interosseous muscles impede flexion of the IP joint because they are extensors at this level. Flexion of the MP joint will relax them and flexion becomes possible at the IP joints (Figure 2.40).

Tenodesis effect
Flexion of the wrist will put the extensor tendons of the fingers under tension and will passively bring the MP joints into extension even without muscular contraction (see Figure 1.66). The result is that the extensor tendon function can not be correctly assessed with the wrist in flexion. The action of the flexor tendons in this position is limited by tension of the extensors.

Similarly, extension of the wrist will put the flexor apparatus under tension and relax the extensor apparatus.

Deformities due to tendon rupture or imbalance

Localized lesions of the tendon apparatus by division, rupture or elongation of traumatic or pathological origin will create an imbalance between the forces overlying each joint and will give rise to a characteristic deformity.

Tendon ruptures
Tendon ruptures in the hand are caused by a violent trauma or by attrition of the tendon against either a displaced bony structure or against a bone spur. Tendon ruptures are common in the rheumatoid hand caused by attrition or by direct invasion of the tendon by hypertrophic tenosynovitis. Tendon ruptures are far less common in the flexors than in the extensors:

Terminal avulsion of the flexor digitorum profundus after a violent effort or blow has been reported mostly in rugby and football players when, in grabbing an opponent's shirt, the distal phalanx of the finger is passively hyperextended while the phalanges of the other fingers remain flexed. These injuries are seen predominantly in the ring finger because of the anatomical arrangement of the extensor tendons. When the MP joints of the middle and little fingers are flexed 90 degrees, the ring finger cannot be fully extended because the extensor tendon of ring finger is pulled distally by the inter-tendinous connections (junctura tendinum) between the extensor communis tendons (Leddy and Packer, 1977). The index finger is less susceptible because the muscle body of the flexor profundus is independent. These avulsions can also cause a fracture at the base of the distal phalanx. The tendon may retract into the palm if the vincula are torn; it then loses a large part of its vascularization. If the tendon does not retract past the

217

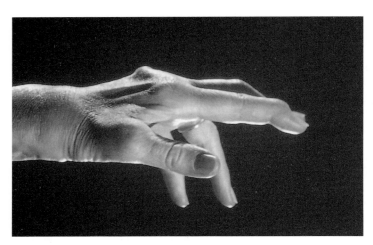

Figure 2.41. Rupture of the extensor tendons of the ring and little fingers.

proximal interphalangeal joint, leaving the vinculum longum intact, the prognosis is better.

Flexor tendon ruptures in rheumatoid arthritis: the diagnosis of flexor tendon rupture is easy as the patient will notice the inability to flex a digit. However, an isolated rupture of a flexor superficialis tendon may not be readily apparent. *Attrition ruptures* are caused by abrasion of the tendon on prominent bone spicules. The scaphoid bone is the most common site of this process. Additional sites include the trapezium, hook of the hamate and distal ulna. The flexor pollicis longus and the flexors superficialis and profundus to the index finger are the tendons most frequently involved because of their location. *Direct invasion* of the tendon by proliferative flexor synovitis involves all locations where the synovial sheath is present: within the carpal canal, palm or digital sheath. The prognosis of these flexor tendon ruptures is determined (1) by the etiology: attrition ruptures have a slightly better prognosis for the restoration of active flexion than ruptures by invasion; (2) by the location: ruptures within the digit have an unfavourable prognosis; (3) by the number of ruptured tendons and the degree of articular involvement.

Extensor tendon ruptures occur at the wrist level and in the digits: At the wrist level the extensor tendons, with their synovial sheaths, pass under the dorsal retinaculum on the back of the wrist before diverging toward the fingers. Tendon ruptures are frequent at this site in rheumatoid arthritis by attrition and direct invasion. Rupture of the extensor tendons of the little finger is most common, and is often the prelude to ruptures of the extensor tendons of the ring finger and then of the other finger extensor tendons (Figure 2.41). Tendon rupture of the little finger constitutes an indisputable indication for surgery, not only to repair the tendon but to prevent other ruptures. A synovectomy should be performed as soon as possible, with a careful removal of any body projection that might have been responsible for tendon attrition. The diagnosis of rupture of the finger extensor tendons relies on the defect of active extension of the proximal phalanx. The middle and distal phalanges can be extended by the interosseous muscles. The diagnosis of rupture of the extensor tendons in the little finger is not always made, for the defect in extension of the finger may be due

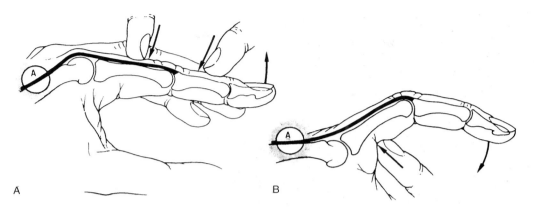

A   B

Figure 2.42. Extensor-plus test, showing the presence of a contracture or adherence of the extensor tendons. (A) Flexion of the proximal phalanx prevents flexion of the distal phalanx. (B) Release of the tension in the extensor tendon is obtained by hyperextension of the proximal phalanx. This permits flexion of the distal phalanges.

to subluxation of the tendon. To make this diagnosis, the finger is placed in passive extension, and the patient is asked to maintain this position. If the patient is unable to do this, there is probably a rupture. When possible, one can also flex the wrist, which, as a result of a tenodesis effect, will extend the finger if there is a luxation but not if there is a rupture.

Ruptures of the extensor pollicus longus tendon are also frequent, usually at the level of Lister's tubercle.

Elongations or ruptures of the extensor tendons are responsible for specific deformities: the boutonnière at the level of the PIP joint and the mallet finger at the distal joint.

Ulnar deviation of the fingers
This is physiological (see Figure 2.34) and is accentuated by active extension in the normal hand. This becomes pathological when the stabilizing capsuloligamentous structures lose their function. This is most commonly seen in rheumatoid arthritis, but it can occur in other diseases. It is accompanied by an ulnar deviation of the extensor communis tendons onto the ulnar side of the MP joints (*see* page 76).

Extensor-plus syndrome
The extensor-plus syndrome (Figure 2.42) (Kilgore et al, 1975) is caused either by shortening of the tendon or by adherence of the tendon proximal to the MP joint. It results in the inability to flex simultaneously the MP and PIP joints, although individually each joint can be flexed. The clinical test demonstrating this state is the opposite of Bunnell's intrinsic plus test.

Swan-neck deformity
In this deformity, the PIP joint is in hyperextension and the distal interphalangeal (DIP) joint in flexion (Figure 2.43). This is due to excessive traction by the extensor apparatus inserted on the base of the middle phalanx, whatever the origin of the force. This

219

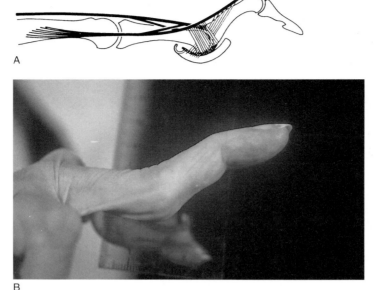

A

B

Figure 2.43. Swan-neck deformity. The PIP joint is in hypertension because of excessive traction of the central extensor tendon inserted on the base of the middle phalanx. The lateral extensor tendons are displaced toward the midline and their extensor effect on the distal phalanx consequently diminished.

deformity is at first reducible but the lesion gradually becomes fixed and will give considerable functional handicap. The deformity is favoured by a laxity of the PIP joint.

Swan-neck can be due to numerous factors which can be classified into:

- articular (lesion of the structures which prevent hyperextension of the PIP joint);
- intrinsic muscles factors (contracture of the interosseous muscles), palmar subluxation of the base of the proximal phalanx which brings the interosseous tendons into a position dorsal to the axis of the MP joints and so their force will act to increase the forces of extension of the extensor apparatus inserted on the base of the middle phalanx (Figure 2.44).
- factors acting on the extrinsic muscles to increase the power of extensor communis, i.e., chronic flexion of the wrist or destruction of the proximal insertion of the extensor communis at the MP level.

Boutonnière deformity

This involves flexion of the PIP joint and hyperextension of the DIP joint (Figure 2.45). It follows division, rupture or degeneration due to rheumatoid arthritis of the central tendon of the extensor apparatus on the dorsum of the PIP joint. This results in a lateral dislocation of the lateral extensor tendons in which the head of the proximal phalanx is "button holed" through the gap in the extensor apparatus. Without the insertion of the extensor apparatus on its base, the PIP joint is brought into flexion by the long flexor tendons. All the force of extension is transmitted to the distal phalanx, thus hyperextending the DIP joint.

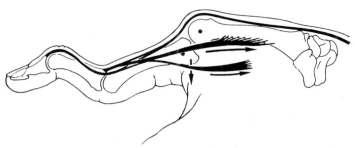

Figure 2.44 Contracture of the intrinsic muscles of the fingers causes excess traction on the base of the middle phalanx.

A

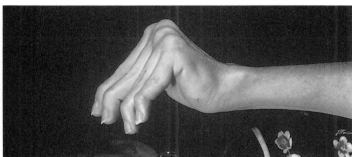

B

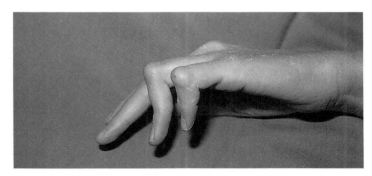

Figure 2.45 Boutonnière deformity. After rupture of the central extensor tendon, the lateral extensor tendons are subluxated volarly, creating a boutonnière.

A

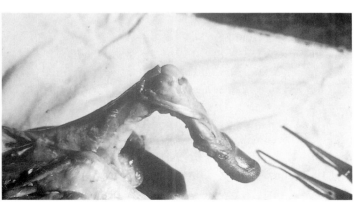

B

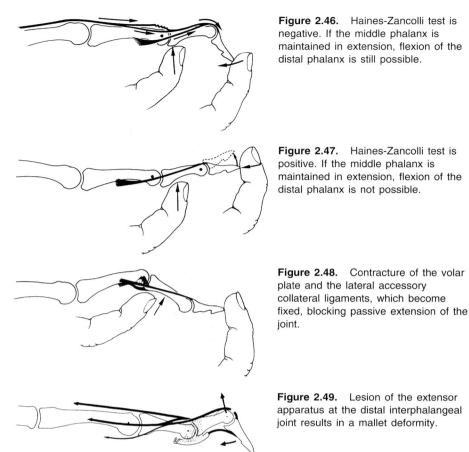

Figure 2.46. Haines-Zancolli test is negative. If the middle phalanx is maintained in extension, flexion of the distal phalanx is still possible.

Figure 2.47. Haines-Zancolli test is positive. If the middle phalanx is maintained in extension, flexion of the distal phalanx is not possible.

Figure 2.48. Contracture of the volar plate and the lateral accessory collateral ligaments, which become fixed, blocking passive extension of the joint.

Figure 2.49. Lesion of the extensor apparatus at the distal interphalangeal joint results in a mallet deformity.

At an early stage, the deformity is reducible. The Haines-Zancolli test is negative (Figure 2.46). Fixed contracture of the oblique fibers of the retinacular ligament prevents passive flexion of the distal joint, thus giving a positive Haines-Zancolli test (Figure 2.47). Fixed contracture of the transverse fibers of the retinacular ligament maintains the lateral tendons in the subluxed position but does not prevent passive correction of the flexion deformity at the PIP joint. Contracture of the volar plate and collateral ligaments leads to a fixed flexion contracture of the PIP joint (Figure 2.48). This lesion causes less functional impairment than a fixed swan-neck deformity.

Mallet finger
Because there is a loss of active extension of the DIP joint, the distal phalanx lies in a flexed position (Figure 2.49). This is due to the division or elongation of the terminal extensor tendon at the level of the DIP joint. This may be traumatic or inflammatory in origin.

222

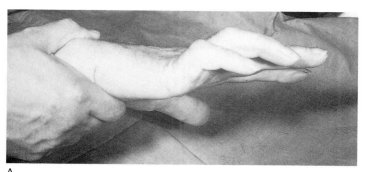

A

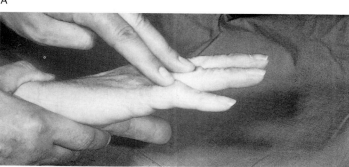

B

Figure 2.50. Claw hand deformity. In cases of interosseous muscle palsy (A), stabilization and prevention of hyperextension of the metacarpophalangeal joints (B) allow the extensor digitorum to extend the interphalangeal joints (Bouvier's sign).

Ulnar claw hand

This is seen in the ring and little fingers when attempting active extension (Figure 2.50). The MP joint is brought into hyperextension and the IP joints are kept in flexion. This is due to a loss of interosseous muscle function. The deformity does not occur in the index and middle fingers because these lumbrical muscles are innervated by the median nerve. If the median nerve is also injured, clawing extends to all four fingers.

Claw hand is one of the main symptoms of an ulnar nerve palsy (see Section 4) but it is important to know that not all ulnar palsies give rise to clawing. The clawing is worse in distal ulnar nerve lesions when the long flexors are still intact. If the examiner prevents hyperextension of the MP joints the intrinsic muscle force is moved distally to the IP joints and extension of the distal phalanges is re-established (Figure 2.50). This test, described by Bouvier (1851), is the principle of the reconstructive surgery for this condition.

For the classification of chronic finger deformities see Tubiana (1998b).

The thumb

Z deformity

This deformity shows a lack of extension of the MP joint and hyperextension of the IP joint (Figure 2.51). This is due to interruption or lateral dislocation of the extensor pollicis brevis tendon at the level of the MP joint, sometimes after trauma but more commonly in rheumatoid arthritis.

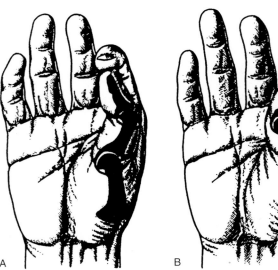

Figure 2.51. (A) Swan-neck deformity of the thumb. (B) Boutonnière deformity of the thumb.

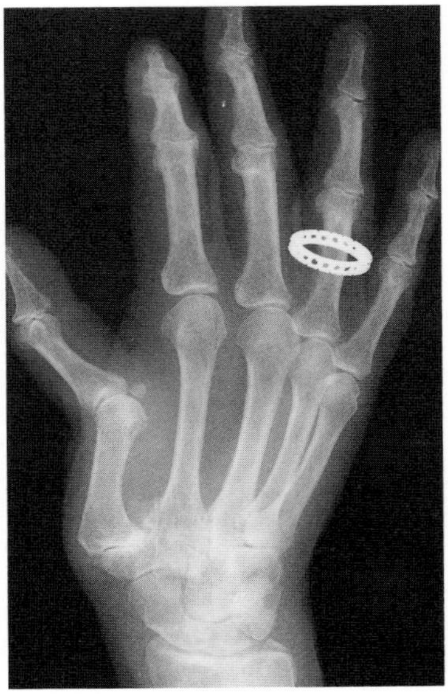

Figure 2.52. Radiograph of an adducted thumb.

The adducted thumb

This is a permanent adduction of the first metacarpal (Figure 2.52), i.e. contraction of the first web space with a compensatory hyperextension of the MP joint causing a boutonnière deformity of the thumb (see Figures 2.49 and 2.51). This is seen in lesions of the first carpometacarpal joint due to inflammatory or degenerative arthritis associated with a muscular contracture of the adductor pollicis and first dorsal interosseous.

Froment's sign

This is one of the best signs of ulnar nerve palsy and shows the weakness or paralysis of the adductor pollicis muscle. This is manifested by strong flexion of the IP joint when attempting to pinch a piece of paper being pulled by the examiner. The interpretation of this sign is discussed in Chapter 4.2.

Finkelstein's test

This test is the best sign of "De Quervain's disease" or tenosynovitis of the abductor pollicis longus tendon. De Quervain's disease is characterized by a triad of symptoms: swelling at the level of the radial styloid, tenderness just proximal to the tip of the radial styloid and a positive Finkelstein's test. The patient is asked to make a fist around the flexed thumb and the examiner passively deviates the wrist ulnarly, producing a sharp pain at the radial side of the wrist.

3 IMAGING

INTRODUCTION

Diagnostic imaging has progressed rapidly in recent years. In cases where diagnosis is difficult, consistent imaging can be invaluable—this requires an accurate clinical examination and good communication between the clinician and the radiologist.

Investigation of the skeleton and the circulation are described separately. Endoscopy is used in the upper limb at the level of the shoulder, elbow and wrist. Improved non-invasive techniques such as magnetic resonance imaging (MRI) will probably reduce the need for diagnostic imaging arthroscopy at the wrist level (Stanley and Saffar, 1994; Dautel and Merle, 1993; Legré et al, 1993).

3.1 RADIOLOGICAL EXAMINATION
by Ph Saffar

Radiological techniques without preparation

The hand

Posteroanterior (PA) and lateral views are the most common radiographic views taken. These usually allow visualization of the fingers and of the proximal interphalangeal (PIP) and distal interphalangeal (DIP) joints. They can be centered on the area of interest (Figure 3.1).

Oblique views are useful for the metacarpals and the metacarpophalangeal (MP) joints. The base of the metacarpals are easily seen with a few degrees of pronation and supination (Figure 3.2).

The thumb

The two phalanges of the first metacarpal and their adjacent joints can be seen on PA and lateral views of the thumb. Kapandji et al (1980) have described special views to obtain a true frontal and lateral projection of the base of the thumb.

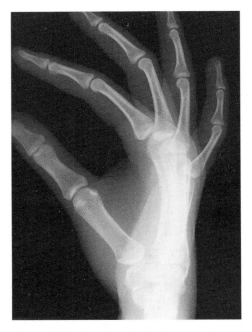

Figure 3.1. Lateral radiograph centered on the proximal interphalangeal joint.

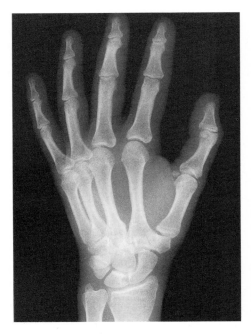

Figure 3.2. Oblique view showing the metacarpophalangeal joint.

For the lateral view, the wrist should be in 20 degrees of extension, 15–20 degrees of adduction, so that the lateral border of the forearm is in line with the thumb. The hand and the forearm are in pronation, the ulnar border is elevated so that the hand and the cassette will make an angle of 20–30 degrees. The beam is centered perpendicular to the MP (and not on the first carpometacarpal joint). The result is good if the two sesamoids are superimposed (Figure 3.3a).

For the anteroposterior (AP) view, the ulnar border of the forearm and of the hand are placed on the table. By pronation and extension of 15 degrees of the wrist, the plane of the nail is placed parallel to the table. The beam is centered on the TM, with an inclination of 30 degrees. The projection is good if the sesamoids have a symmetrical projection on the metacarpal head (Figure 3.3b).

These two views allow the exact visualization of the trapezio-metacarpal, the scaphotrapeziotrapezoidal and the trapeziotrapezoidal joints.

The wrist

PA view

The radius is in the same axis as the third metacarpal. The patient is seated with the arm and forearm on the table. The elbow is in 90 degrees of flexion and the shoulder abducted at 90 degrees (Figure 3.4a).

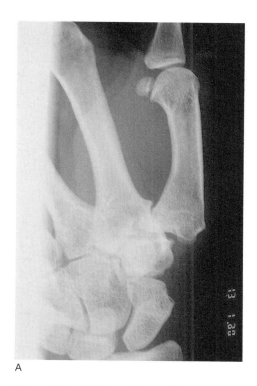 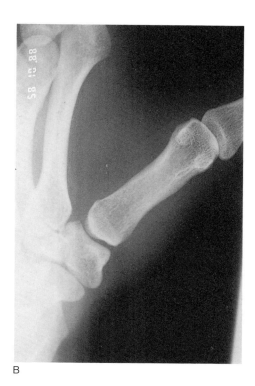

A

B

Figure 3.3. (A) Lateral view of the trapezio-metacarpal (TM) joint. (B) Frontal view of the TM joint.

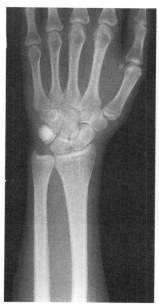 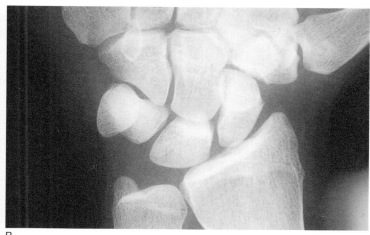

B

Figure 3.4. (A) Frontal view of the wrist in a posteroanterior (PA) view. (B) Frontal view of the wrist in an anteroposterior (AP) view.

A

227

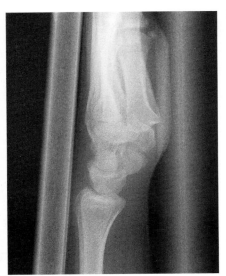

Figure 3.5. Lateral view of the wrist.

AP view

The AP view with the elbow extended shows the intercarpal joints better (Figure 3.4b).

Lateral view

The lateral view is very important: the axis of the distal radius and of the third metacarpal has to be in line. A special splint described by Meyrueis et al (1978) can be used to obtain this alignment (Figure 3.5).

When these PA and lateral projections include the head of the metacarpals, important radiographic measurements can be calculated:

- on the PA projections, carpal height and carpal translation (Youm et al, 1978);
- on the lateral projections, the scapholunate angle (Linscheid et al, 1972), the radiolunate angle (Meyrueis et al, 1978), and the radiocapitate angle (Sarrafian et al, 1977) (Figure 3.6).

Dorsal intercalated segment instability (DISI) and volar intercalated segment instability (VISI) can be assessed by these measurements (Linscheid et al, 1972) (Figure 3.7).

Scaphoid views

The scaphoid bone is the most frequently fractured bone of the wrist. As it cannot be seen fully on frontal and lateral projections of the wrist (Figure 3.8), many views have been described to improve visualization of this bone. Schnek (1933), Stecher (1937), Bridgman (1949), and many others have defined positions that give a more complete projection of the scaphoid. Radiographs taken with the hand in ulnar deviation are very useful to see a fresh fracture, which is often difficult to see on routine radiographs. It is sometimes possible to see a pseudoarthrosis on these views (Figure 3.9).

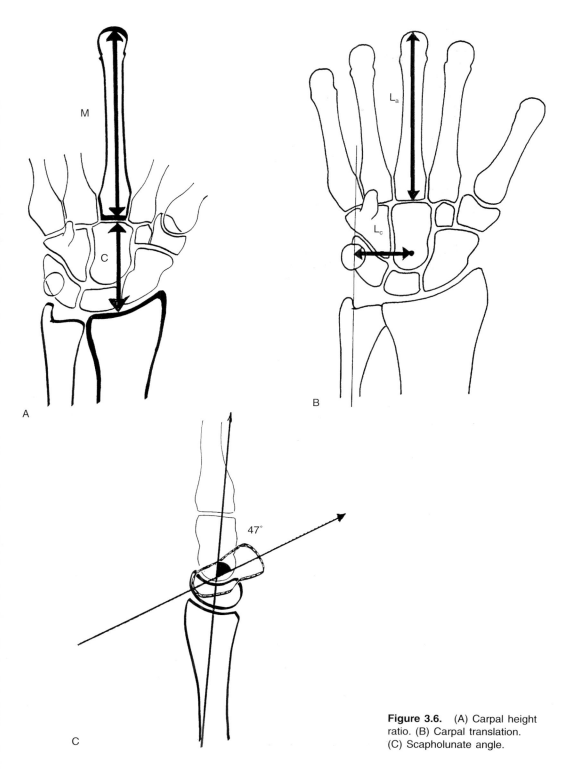

Figure 3.6. (A) Carpal height ratio. (B) Carpal translation. (C) Scapholunate angle.

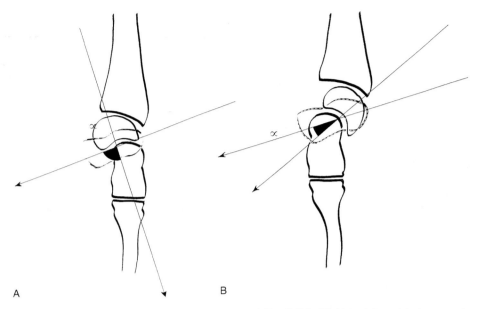

Figure 3.7. (A) Dorsal intercalated segment instability (DISI). (B) Volar intercalated segment instability (VISI).

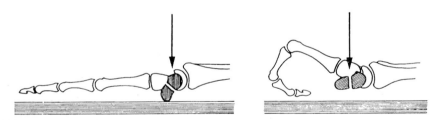

Figure 3.8. Diagram showing the slant of the scaphoid and the necessity of special views in order to see a fracture.

The instability series

The dynamics of the carpal bones are examined with dynamic x-ray imaging (Taleisnik, 1985).

PA views

PA views taken in radial and ulnar deviation show the dynamics of the scaphoid, foreshortened in radial deviation and elongated in ulnar deviation. The dynamics of the four medial ulnar carpal bones can also be checked (Figure 3.10).

With these static and dynamic radiographs, some abnormal features can be noted:

- existence of a gap between two carpal bones (most commonly a scapholunate gap; considered abnormal if over 2 mm) (Figure 3.11);

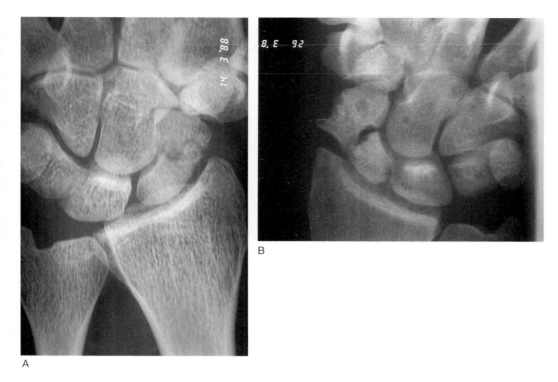

Figure 3.9. (A) Scaphoid fracture. (B) Scaphoid pseudoarthrosis.

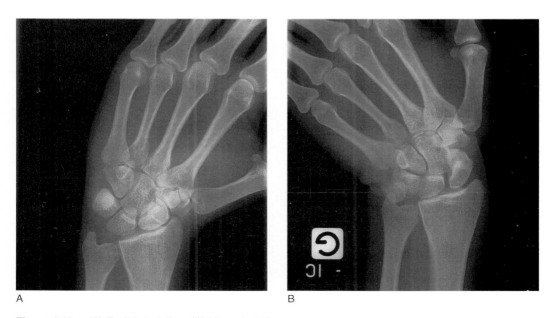

Figure 3.10. (A) Radial deviation. (B) Ulnar deviation.

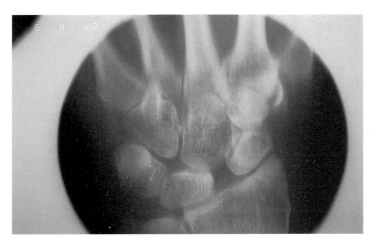

Figure 3.11. Scapholunate gap.

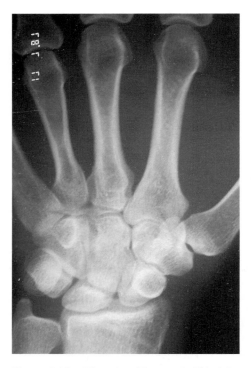

Figure 3.12. Ring sign. The scaphoid is fully flexed.

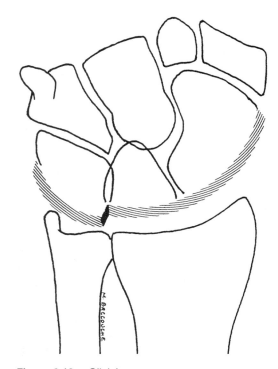

Figure 3.13. Gilula's arcs.

- ring sign is the cortical ring image of the distal pole of the scaphoid collapsed in volar flexion. The scaphoid appears shortest whatever the position of the wrist (Figure 3.12);
- rupture of the Gilula's arcs (Gilula et al, 1987) (Figure 3.13).

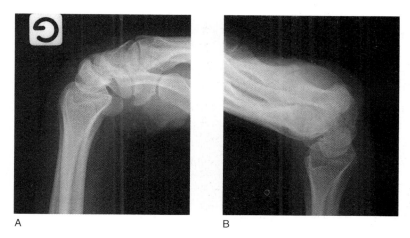

A   B

Figure 3.14. (A) Flexion on lateral view. (B) Extension on lateral view.

Lateral views

Lateral views with flexion and extension show the relative mobility of the radiocarpal and midcarpal joints (Figure 3.14).

Other views

Further stress views may be included:

- active – clenched fist position (Dobyns et al, 1975);
- passive – traction, compression, drawer's test (Schernberg and Gerard, 1983).

Distal radioulnar joint

The distal radioulnar joint (DRUJ) may be seen in these views. Early radiographic changes of rheumatoid arthritis are often seen there first (Figure 3.15).

Ulnar variance (the difference between the length of the radius and the ulna) can be estimated. In the ulna-minus variant, the ulna head lies proximal to the distal radial articular surface (Gelberman et al, 1975; Palmer et al, 1982; Kristensen et al, 1986; Steyers and Blai, 1989) (Figure 3.16).

Carpal tunnel views

The carpal tunnel projection (Hart and Gaynor, 1941) is useful for examining the carpal tunnel and its contents. The hook of the hamate, the triquetrum and the pisiform (Figure 3.17) are also shown in this view.

The hamate

The hook of the hamate can be seen also on various views described by Papilion et al (1988), but even so the bony anatomy is very difficult to demonstrate clearly on radiographs and CT scan may be indicated.

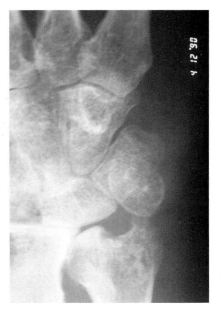

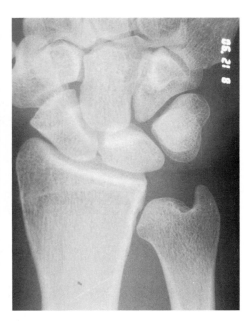

Figure 3.15. Early changes of rheumatoid arthritis at the distal radioulnar joint.

Figure 3.16. Short ulna (ulna-minus variant).

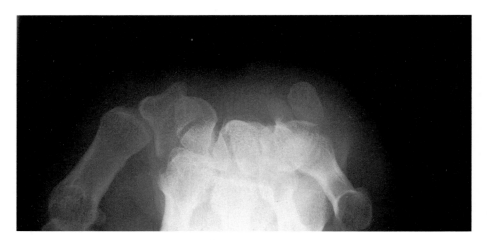

Figure 3.17. Carpal tunnel view.

The pisiform and the pisotriquetral joint
The pisiform and the pisotriquetral joint can be seen on a lateral view with 30 degrees of supination (Vasilas et al, 1960) (Figure 3.18).

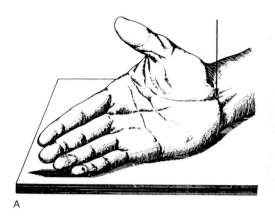

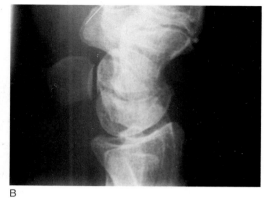

A   B

Figure 3.18.   Pisotriquetral joint.

Radiographic enlargements

> They are very useful to study the bony trabecular structure, especially in the case of bone tumors and fresh fractures, which can be difficult to see on plain radiographs.

Special techniques for imaging the hand and wrist

Tomography

> Tomography is not often requested because CT scan and MRI are useful to assess the staging of Kienböck's disease (Figure 3.19). Trispiral tomography has regained interest, specially for viewing the carpal bones, and it can be of great help in assessing scaphoid malunions, for example.

Bone scan

> Bone scan has a great sensitivity but a poor specificity. It reacts to activity around a lesion. The four principal indications are:

- following trauma, a fracture of the scaphoid may be suspected on clinical examination but not evident on radiograph views. A bone scan after 24 hours may demonstrate the fracture;
- diagnosis of first-stage algoneurodystrophy can be made by bone scan. This allows early treatment;
- osteomyelitis and inflammatory diseases may be localized by bone scan;
- some tumors, such as osteoma and osteoid or malignant tumors, give a high signal on isotope bone scan. It is, however, impossible to differentiate between benign and malignant tumors (Figure 3.20).

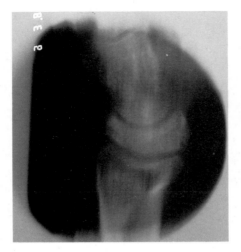

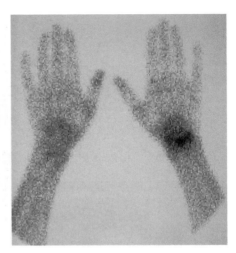

Figure 3.19. Lateral tomography revealing a Kienböck's disease stage III (avascular necrosis of the carpal lunate).

Figure 3.20. Bone scan of the wrist.

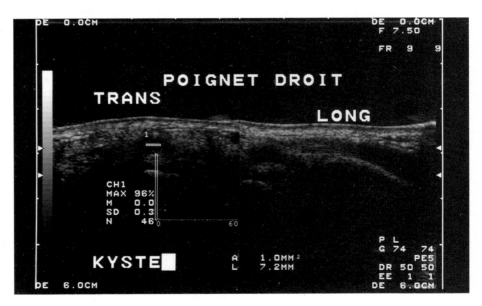

Figure 3.21. Sonography of a ganglion.

Sonography

Sonography has some applications in investigating disorders of the hand. It can allow dynamic study of tendons and show tenosynovitis. Some foreign bodies and tumors, such as occult ganglia, can be localized by this examination (Figure 3.21).

Nerve and arteries can also be seen and differentiated using sonography.

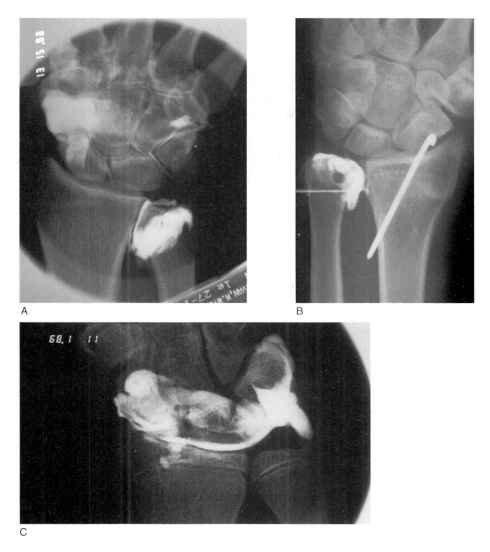

Figure 3.22. (A) Arthrography of the midcarpal joint. (B) Arthrography of the distal radioulnar joint. (C) Arthrography of radiocarpal joint.

Arthrography

Arthrography of the wrist has been described by many authors including Coleman (1956, 1960), Rieunau et al (1971), Martinek (1977a, 1977b), Gilula et al (1983), Palmer et al (1983), Braunstein et al (1985), Levisohn et al (1987), Wuttge et al (1988) (Figure 3.22). It has improved the diagnosis of carpal ligamentous injuries. The wrist joint is divided in three main compartments:

237

- radiocarpal
- mid-carpal
- distal radioulnar (DRUJ).

Radiocarpal joint arthrography was the first to be performed.

Arthrography is indicated when plain and dynamic radiographs do not show abnormal relationships in a painful wrist. It is mainly useful in dynamic scapholunate instabilities and in triquetrolunate instabilities.

Mainly used for the diagnosis of carpal instabilities, arthrography has now gained a great importance. The usual sequence of injections is first, the midcarpal and DRUJ compartments, and if this is not sufficient, injection of the radiocarpal joint two to three hours later. The patient often has to perform the movements of flexion–extension and radioulnar deviation to produce the leakage of the dye from one compartment to another. The extent of the ligamentous tear can be deduced from the amount of dye passing through the tear.

Midcarpal arthrography

Injection of the midcarpal joint is the most important: leakage of the dye between the scaphoid and lunate or between the triquetrum and lunate indicates a rupture of the interosseous scapholunate or triquetrolunate ligament where the dye enters the radiocarpal joint. Midcarpal arthrography is normal in midcarpal instability.

Arthrography of the DRUJ

Injection of the DRUJ gives increased pressure of this joint and when a TFCC tear is present, the radiocarpal joint is rapidly penetrated by the dye.

Radiocarpal arthrography

Arthrography of the radiocarpal joint shows the prestyloid recess and in 60 per cent of cases, the pisotriquetral joint; these are normal features.

Cineradiography

Cineradiography has been described by many authors, including Arkess (1966), Manaster (1986), and Imamura (1987). It is done when a midcarpal instability is suspected: the sudden jolt of the intact proximal carpal row on the second is clearly seen when the patient goes from radial to ulnar deviation with a clenched fist.

Cinearthrography

Cinearthrography, recorded on films and videotapes, combines the findings of arthrography and cineradiography (Resnick et al, 1984; White et al, 1984; Quinn et al, 1988) (Figure 3.23). The exact route of the contrast dye during the first 30 seconds after the injection is very important, and the surgeon can view this route as often as necessary. This examination is the most accurate available for sprains of the ulnocarpal interosseous ligaments. It is performed with the same machinery that is used for coronarography.

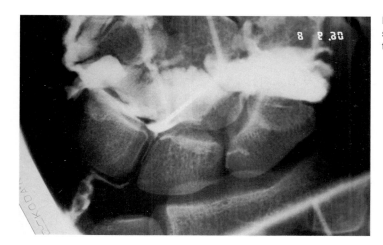

Figure 3.23. Cinearthrography showing a lunotriquetral ligament tear.

CT scans

CT scanning is not as useful in the wrist as that in other parts of the skeleton. However, it does have some specific indications (Cone et al, 1983; Bush et al, 1987; Schmitt and Lanz, 1992). Coronal and sagittal planes are not the only ones to be asked for and the surgeon must give precise information to the radiologist, explaining what is being looked for. Spatial resolution is limited but density resolution is better than in plain radiographs. CT slices can show a fracture of the base of the metacarpals or of the carpal bones that was not evident on plain radiographs.

CT scans of the scaphoid
CT slices of the scaphoid parallel to its long axis, and in the coronal and sagittal plane, are useful for:

- making an early diagnosis of a fracture (Figure 3.24);
- assessing a pseudoarthrosis and showing the extent of loss of substance, exact position of the fragments, and necrosis of the proximal pole; and
- following the healing of a fracture or a pseudoarthrosis after surgical treatment and ensuring that the length of the scaphoid has been restored.

Kienböck's disease
In Kienböck's disease, the vascularity of the lunate and any bony collapse can be assessed for staging and choice of surgical procedure. CT scanning can demonstrate a limited osteoarthritis and explain a localized tenderness.

Tumors
A tumor, particularly an osteoid osteoma, can be seen and precisely localized using a CT scan (Figure 3.25). The histological type of a tumor can be determined: density is measured in Hounsfield Units (HU):

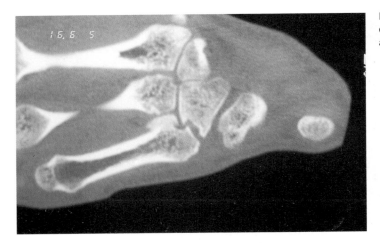

Figure 3.24. CT scan demonstrating a limited hamate and second metacarpal fracture.

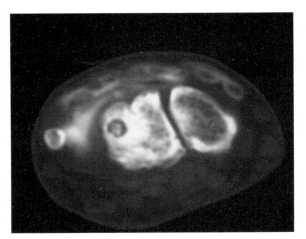

Figure 3.25. CT scan of an osteoid osteoma.

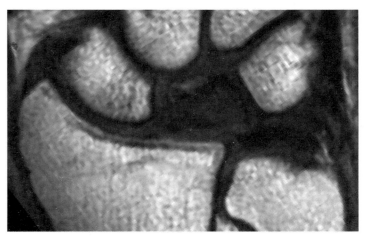

Figure 3.26. MRI scan of Kienböck's disease stage I.

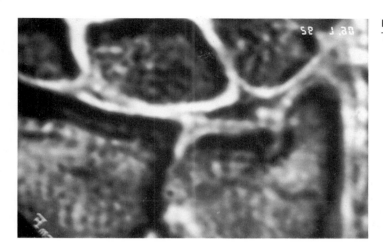

Figure 3.27. MRI scan of TFCC ligament.

bone = +1000 HU
air = 0 HU

A lipoma or a ganglion can be clearly differentiated from dense tumors, though it is difficult to be sure whether the tumor is benign or malignant. Peripheral infiltration can be estimated. Administration of contrast media can help in the diagnosis. Exploration of soft tissue is possible and the position of tendons and nerves can be estimated, specially inside the carpal tunnel.

Other uses of CT scans
Although not of clinical interest for the moment, 3-D reconstruction may be very useful in future (Weeks et al, 1985). Arthroscan is useful to assess the cartilage status or show ligament tears.

Magnetic resonance imaging
Magnetic resonance imaging (MRI) (Zlatkin et al, 1989; Pigeau et al, 1992) is the most sensitive technique currently in use. Its main application is in showing the soft tissues, the vascularity of both bones and soft tissues, and in assessing the extension of bony tumors into soft tissues (Figures 3.26, 3.27).

Using MRI, intrinsic and extrinsic ligaments of the wrist can now be seen, both in the coronal and sagittal planes. For the diagnosis of TFCC tears, it is a very important tool (Figure 3.28). Interosseous ligaments (the scapholunate (Figure 3.29) and luno-triquetral ligaments) and extrinsic ligaments (such as the radiocapitate and radiolunate ligaments) are elicited in special planes; these give significant information about carpal instability. T2-weighted sequences and spin echo and gradient-first and gradient-second echoes are used.

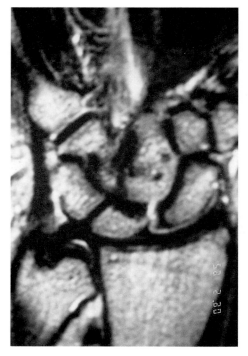

Figure 3.28. TFCC tear shown by MRI.

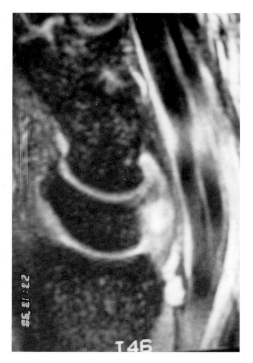

Figure 3.29. Scapholunate interosseous ligament tear shown by MRI.

Cartilage erosions and osseous avascular necrosis (eburnations) are evaluated mainly in T1-weighted sequences and are helpful for the surgical indications. Vascularization of the carpal bones can be assessed and enhancement by gadolinium injection can give information on the prognosis for revascularization.

Dynamic MRI will soon be available, and this will improve the results.

3.2 INVESTIGATION OF THE CIRCULATION

The circulation of the upper extremity is investigated in a variety of conditions. Diagnostic modalities have improved considerably in the past few decades. Physical examination remains the primary method of evaluating patients with vascular disease, but non-invasive techniques developed recently—such as radionuclide imaging, Doppler ultrasonography, capillaroscopy and pulse volume recording—have reduced the need for invasive methods such as arteriography. The introduction of digital angiography has made arteriography even less aggressive, using reduced doses of contrast media and finer puncture needles. Its adaptation to the venous circulation could also help in studying the vascular anatomy of the upper extremity.

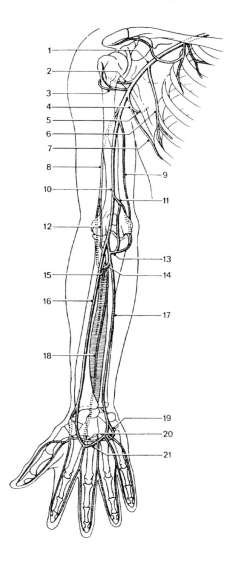

Figure 3.30. Arteries of the upper limb: (1) axillary artery; (2) posterior circumflex humeral artery; (3) anterior circumflex humeral artery; (4) subscapular artery; (5) circumflex scapular artery; (6) lateral thoracic artery; (7) subscapular artery; (8) arteria profunda brachii; (9) ulnar collateral artery; (10) brachial artery; (11) inferior ulnar collateral artery; (12) anterior branch of arteria profunda brachii; (13) ulnar recurrent artery; (14) interosseous artery; (15) dorsal interosseous artery; (16) radial artery; (17) ulnar artery; (18) volar interosseous artery; (19) deep ulnar artery; (20) deep palmar arch; (21) superficial palmar arch.

Radioanatomical studies

Accurate knowledge of the relationships and pathways of the major arterial structures in the upper extremity, as well as their patterns of variation, is of considerable importance for the investigation of normal or pathologic circulation (Figure 3.30).

Axillary artery

The axillary artery demonstrates a fairly consistent anatomical pathway. It begins as the continuation of the subclavian artery at the lateral aspect of the first rib and ends as the brachial artery at the inferior border of the pectoralis major. The vessel may be divided into three anatomical parts by its relationship to the pectoralis minor muscle (Figure 3.31). The numerous branches of the axillary artery include the superior thoracic artery arising from the first segment, the thoracoacromial and lateral thoracic arteries from the middle section, and the subscapular and anterior and posterior circumflex humeral arteries, which anastomose freely with each other and provide an abundant collateral blood supply in the thoracic–scapular–humeral region. The close relationship with the brachial plexus and axillary vein contributes to the frequent association of nerve injuries in addition to occasional post-traumatic arteriovenous fistulas following axillary arterial trauma.

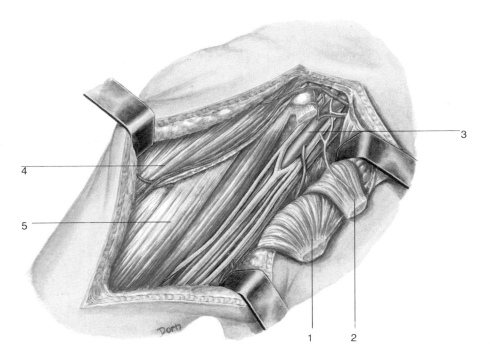

Figure 3.31.   (1) Pectoralis major; (2) pectoralis minor; (3) axillary artery; (4) deltoid; (5) biceps.

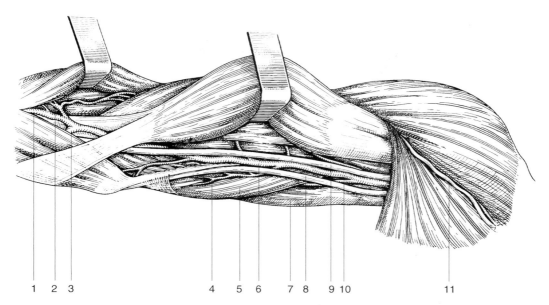

Figure 3.32. (1) Radial artery; (2) radial recurrent artery; (3) ulnar artery; (4) ulnar collateria artery; (5) medial head of triceps; (6) brachial artery; (7) long head of triceps; (8) ulnar nerve; (9) median nerve; (10) profunda brachii; (11) cephalic vein.

Brachial artery

Beyond the lower border of the teres major, the brachial artery leaves the axilla medially and deep to the median nerve, coursing distally and laterally (Figure 3.32) to terminate just beyond the antecubital fossa by dividing into the radial and ulnar arteries. The brachial artery has three major branches. The large profunda brachii passes downward between the medial and long heads of the triceps, branching to anastomose anteriorly with the radial recurrent artery and posteriorly with the posterior interosseous artery. A second branch, the superior ulnar collateral or inferior profunda artery, courses with the ulnar nerve, anastomosing distally with the posterior ulnar recurrent artery—all forming an extensive network of collateral vessels about the elbow.

Ulnar artery

In the forearm, the ulnar artery is usually the dominant artery (Figure 3.33). Proximally it gives rise to the large common interosseous artery, which bifurcates to either side of the interosseous membrane into the anterior and posterior interosseous arteries. These, combined with the radial artery, establish an excellent collateral network in the forearm consisting of four parallel arterial pathways with numerous intercommunications.

Radial artery

The radial artery lies more superficial in the forearm (Figure 3.34), running just under the anterior aspect of the brachioradialis and across the supinator to enter the anterior

245

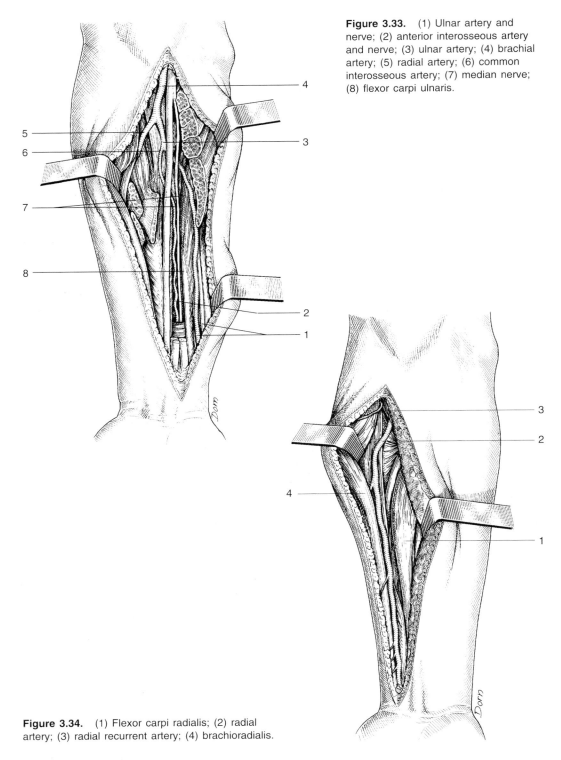

Figure 3.33. (1) Ulnar artery and nerve; (2) anterior interosseous artery and nerve; (3) ulnar artery; (4) brachial artery; (5) radial artery; (6) common interosseous artery; (7) median nerve; (8) flexor carpi ulnaris.

Figure 3.34. (1) Flexor carpi radialis; (2) radial artery; (3) radial recurrent artery; (4) brachioradialis.

and radial aspect of the forearm. At the proximal aspect of the wrist it generally is found between the flexor carpi radialis and the brachioradialis.

A persistent median artery, found in 10 per cent of limbs, contributes primarily to the superficial palmar arch, always passing deep to the transverse carpal ligament and often intimately associated with the median nerve.

Arterial supply of the hand

The hand is supplied through two main arteries—the radial and the ulnar. Under normal circumstances these two vessels are responsible for virtually the entire arterial supply. Other important channels are the interosseous arteries (especially the anterior interosseous artery), which arise from the common interosseous branch of the ulnar artery. These vessels, which are relatively unimportant under normal circumstances, may assume a vital role if either of the main forearm arteries is injured. In 8–9 per cent of cases the anterior interosseous artery gives off an artery that accompanies the median nerve; it is known as the median artery and usually anastomoses with the superficial palmar arch. These arteries, through their anastomoses, form the arterial arches. The main ones are the superficial and deep palmar arches; the accessory ones are the dorsal and palmar carpal arches.

The deep palmar arch

The deep palmar arch is formed by the terminal part of the radial artery and its anastomosis with the deep branch of the ulnar artery (Figures 3.35 and 2.7). It lies anterior to the upper extremity of the metacarpal shafts. It is seldom fully developed and the deep ulnar branch is often negligible. The dominance of the radial artery is readily demonstrable by the selective vascular compression test.

The deep palmar arch gives rise to the interosseous (or metacarpal) arteries. These are, from lateral to medial, the interosseous artery of the first interspace (which ramifies into the ulnar palmar collateral and the radial palmar collateral, also known as the princeps pollicis, and the radial collateral artery of the index finger) and the interosseous arteries of the second, third, and fourth interspaces.

The superficial palmar arch

The superficial palmar arch is formed from the anastomosis of the terminal branch of the ulnar artery with the superficial palmar branch of the radial artery (Figure 3.35). On an arteriogram it is seen to lie under the deep palmar arch and has a smaller caliber. It is fully developed in only 13–19 per cent of cases. In 60 per cent of cases it is formed from the ulnar artery alone and in 32 per cent from the superficial palmar branch of the radial artery. In 8 per cent of cases it results from the anastomosis of the median with the ulnar artery. Often one arch and its branches are obviously dominant.

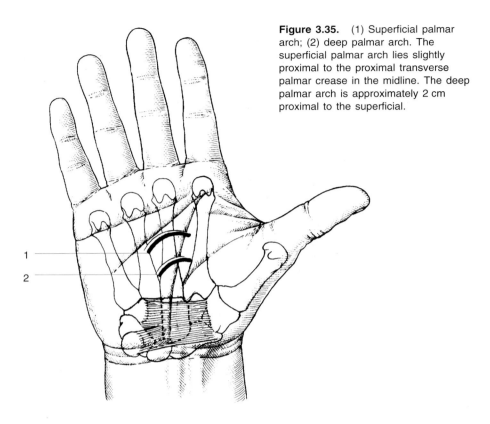

Figure 3.35. (1) Superficial palmar arch; (2) deep palmar arch. The superficial palmar arch lies slightly proximal to the proximal transverse palmar crease in the midline. The deep palmar arch is approximately 2 cm proximal to the superficial.

From its convex side the superficial palmar arch gives off four collaterals, known as the palmar digital arteries, which, from the ulnar to the radial side, are the first, second, third, and fourth digital arteries. There often is a fifth digital artery, which is of small caliber and anastomoses with the first palmar interosseous artery, itself a branch of the deep palmar arch.

The carpal arches

The dorsal carpal arch, when present, is formed by the union of homologous branches from the radial and ulnar arteries (Figure 3.36). The interosseous dorsal arteries of the second, third, and fourth interspaces, as well as the medial collateral of the little finger, are formed from this arch. Each dorsal interosseous artery splits into two dorsal collateral branches that terminate on the lateral aspects of adjacent fingers. The dorsal carpal arch can function as a collateral channel between the radial artery and the deep palmar arch; it often receives a significant contribution from the radial artery.

Much less commonly found is a palmar carpal arch; it seldom forms a recognizable arcade and frequently consists of a loose collateral nework known as the palmar carpal plexus. It usually connects the anterior interosseous artery with the radial and ulnar arteries.

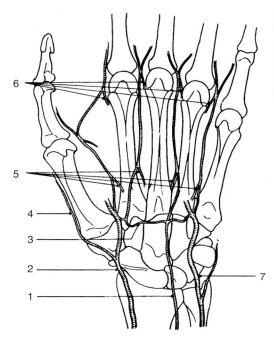

Figure 3.36. Dorsal arch of the carpus. (1) dorsal interosseous artery (of the forearm); (2) radial artery; (3) dorsal arch of the carpus; (4) radialis pollicis; (5) proximal perforating branches; (6) distal perforating branches; (7) ulnar artery.

The interosseous (or metacarpal) palmar and dorsal arteries anastomose with the palmar digital arteries and with one another through proximal and distal perforating channels to form the palmar collateral arteries of the fingers (Blonstein et al, 1977).

Vascularization of the digits
by F Brunelli

Vascularization of the fingers

The fingers are vascularized mainly by the palmar collateral arteries. The dorsal collateral arteries are narrow and generally taper out at the level of the PIP joint. The two palmar arteries for each digit run alongside the digital canal accompanied by the palmar collateral nerves.

At the level of the two proximal phalanges the neurovascular bundles are contained within a fibrous tunnel bounded by Grayson's ligament anteriorly, and Cleland's ligament posteriorly. The nerve is usually located medial to the artery with reference to the long axis of the finger. At the DIP joint the neurovascular bundles exit from this tunnel. The nerve continues distally to provide sensation to the pulp, and the artery runs medially to anastomose with the contralateral artery to form the pulpar arcade. This arcade is situated at approximately the mid-point between the distal flexion crease

249

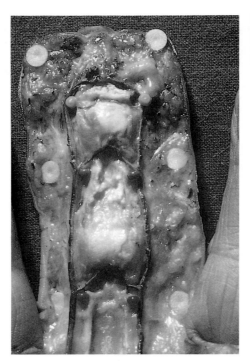

Figure 3.37. Anatomical dissection of a ring finger after colored latex injection. Following removal of the flexor apparatus the deep anastomoses are exposed.

and the fingertip and supplies the distal half of the pulp, the phalanx and the nailbed. There are in addition many palmar anastomoses between the two digital arteries, which are divided into superficial and deep:

- Superficial anastomoses (type 1) are tenuous, numerous and variable, lying in the immediate subcutaneous plane;
- Deep anastomoses (type 2) are more significant and more constant. They are formed from branches arising on the medial border of the collateral arteries which form the subtendinous arcades. The largest of these is situated deep to the fibrous flexor sheath over the distal metaphyses of the proximal and middle phalanges (Figure 3.37).

The collateral arteries are about 1 mm in diameter at the root of the finger, and taper progressively as they near the base of the finger. In general the two arteries are of equivalent diameter but there are occasional exceptions and it is necessary to be aware of potential vascular anomalies.

The two central fingers (ring and middle) show the most constant vascular pattern.

In approximately 10 per cent of index fingers the collateral radial artery vanishes at the middle phalanx (Figure 3.38). In 15 per cent of little fingers the ulnar collateral artery disappears at the same level. A basic guideline is that the dominant artery to a finger is that which faces the median axis of the hand (ulnar on the index finger and radial for the little finger) (Figure 3.39).

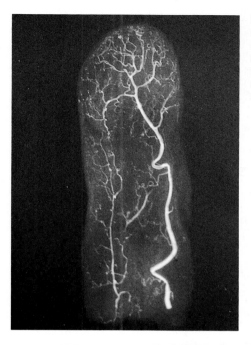

Figure 3.38. Angiogram of the palmar skin of the little finger. In this case, the ulnar collateral artery is very narrow and does not reach the DIP joint. In 15% of our series, the ulnar collateral artery of the little finger and radial collateral artery of the index finger showed this pattern.

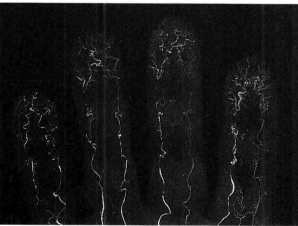

Figure 3.39. Angiogram of the palmar skin of the four long fingers. In general, the collateral arteries are of similar size. If there is a discrepancy, the dominant artery is the one facing the median axis of the hand.

Vascularization of the thumb

Palmar aspect

The arteries of the thumb vary in both size and number, thus making any surgical reconstruction quite delicate. Before starting any intervention, it is necessary to understand clearly the anatomical layout of the arteries, and this is even more important if an island flap or a microsurgical intervention is intended.

251

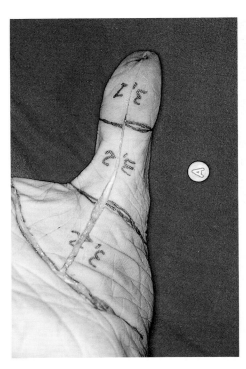

Figure 3.40. Division of the palmar aspect of the thumb in three segments: defined by the opposition, metacarpophalangeal and interphalangeal crease.

The most common variations of the palmar arteries can be schematized by dividing the thumb into three segments, defined by the metacarpophalangeal and interphalangeal flexion creases (Figure 3.40).

Although no constant arteries exist in anatomy, the above concepts can often make any gesture of research or dissection of the vessels easier and less traumatic.

The layout of the arteries is the result of innumerable variations regarding origin, transit, connections and size; some of these are sufficiently frequent to serve as a reasonable basis for surgical technique, but modification may become necessary during an intervention.

According to the classical layout, the "princeps pollicis" artery, the terminal branch of the radial artery, crosses the first intermetacarpal space, then runs along the ulnar side of the first metacarpal bone and along the volar surface of the adductor muscle, emerging onto the subcutaneous palmar tissue at the level of the cutaneous flexion crease of the metacarpophalangeal joint. Here it divides into two terminal rami, namely the collateral palmar arteries of the thumb, which run along the digital tunnel symmetrically and are of equal caliber, heading distally to finally unite in the pulp arcade (Figure 3.41). During their transit in the digital tunnel, they break off into numerous collateral branches, either cutaneous, articular or osseous.

An arcade located deep in the flexor tendon joins together the two arteries at the level of the distal metaphysis of the first phalanx, from where (and from another similar,

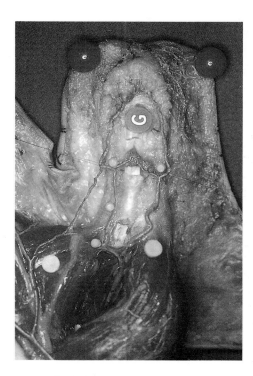

Figure 3.41. Classical layout of the palmar arteries of the thumb.

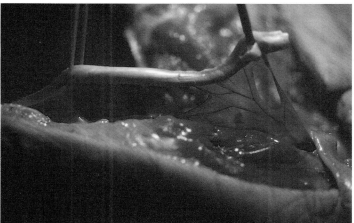

Figure 3.42. Arteries to the flexor tendon of the thumb including to the "vincula".

but more narrow and inconstant, arcade, situated at the level of the distal tendon insertion) the vessels originate which enter the "vincula" and irrigate the flexor tendon (Figure 3.42).

If the above is to be considered a reflection of the classical description of the palmar arteries of the thumb, it cannot be defined as "typical": in anatomical studies, only 15% of dissections fall into such a category.

Significant variations can modify the origin, the transit and the size of the two arteries. The arteries are located in three different segments:

- First segment: It is rare to find arteries of surgical interest on the volar surface of the thumb between the opposition crease and the metacarpophalangeal flexion crease. Although arteries of a significant size can sometimes be found emerging from the superficial arcade or the commissural artery, the artery of this region is located deeply and is more easily accessible from the dorsal surface. This is represented by the "princeps pollicis".

- Second segment: The two arteries run alongside the flexor tendon and behind the collateral nerves. In this area, the main artery is the ulnar collateral artery. Although sometimes absent (in which case it is replaced by the dorsal artery), it is more often easier to dissect than the latter, and its size enables the surgeon to achieve a more reliable microanastomosis. At this level the two collateral arteries are of a similar size, and the subtendinous anastomosis situated at the level of the neck of the first phalanx acts as "moderator" between the two arteries. In cases where the palmar ulnar collateral artery is absent, the dorsal artery takes its place by means of a branch through the subtendinous arcade from which the artery originates. The latter then joins up with the contralateral artery to form the pulp arcade.

- Third segment: In the pulp segment, as already stated, the two arteries are of similar size and run through the thick fatty subcutaneous padding, then cross over and convert into the ends of the digital nerves at the level of the median axis.

Dorsal aspect
The dorsal arteries of the thumb have not yet been the subject of an indepth anatomical study and are described in the classical anatomical literature as:

"stemming from the terminal branches of the radial artery at the level of the anatomical snuff-box and heading distally towards the dorsal surface of the thumb where they end up as periosteal and bony skin rami at first phalanx level" (Testut).

Such a description only partially corresponds to reality in that the quoted arteries are intended for the vascularization of the area corresponding to the posterior surface of the first metacarpal and metacarpophalangeal joint. Moreover, the posterior area of the thumb is vascularized by two arteries which originate from the palmar arteries (princeps, commissural or anastomoses of the superficial arcade) at the level of the first metacarpal. After having run laterally along the metacarpophalangeal joint, and continuing obliquely from volar to dorsal, these arteries then head in a distal direction remaining on the side of the two distal phalanges.

At the level of the neck of the first phalanx, an anastomosis can be found which originates from the palmar arteries. Similarly to the palmar arteries, they are joined by three arcades:

- one inconstant arcade located under the extensor tendon at the level of the neck of the first phalanx;

- the arcade of the nail matrix;
- the arcade of the nailbed.

The ulnar dorso-collateral artery generally stems from the "princeps pollicis" onto the medial border of the neck of the first metacarpal and heads distally remaining on the lateral surface of the first phalanx. It joins together at the level of the distal metaphysis of the first phalanx, receiving an anastomotic ramus coming from the palmar collateral artery or from the subtendinous anastomosis located deep to the flexor tendon. It then proceeds onto the ulnar side of the second phalanx and proximally to the base of the nail, continues laterally to meet up with the contralateral artery forming the arcade of the nail matrix. This artery can be large and dissected under the naked eye, or thin and necessitate the use of a microscope in order to identify it, but it is quite constant (Figure 3.43).

The radial dorso-collateral artery is slightly reminiscent of the internal collateral artery, as far as origin and connections are concerned. Its identification is more difficult despite the use of an optical microscope.

It should be emphasized that the layout of the arterial blood supply of the dorsal surface varies greatly from that of the other fingers.

Examination of an a radiograph of the dorsal skin of a thumb and a finger, having previously injected it with latex colouring mixed with lead, shows that a continuous longitudinal arterial vessel is present on the ulnar side (and in some cases also on the

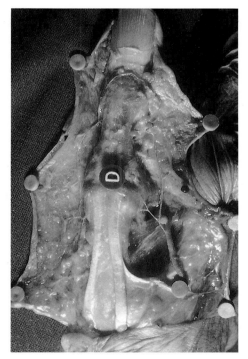

Figure 3.43. Anatomical dissection of the ulnar dorso-collateral artery of the thumb.

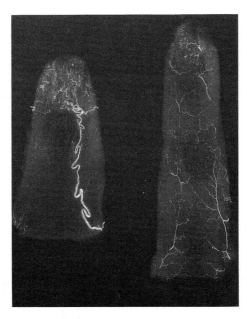

Figure 3.44. Angiogram of the dorsal skin of a finger and of a thumb. In the fingers vascularization is extremely segmental and dependent on the palmar anastomoses while in the thumb a longitudinal arterial vessel is present quite constantly on the ulnar side.

radial side) of the thumb. However, vascularization of the fingers is extremely segmented, dependent almost exclusively on numerous, variable and small vessels which stem from the palmar arteries at different levels (Figure 3.44).

The venous system

The palmar veins of the hand are few and small whilst the dorsal veins are large. The loose dorsal skin allows dilatation of the dorsal veins which are not compressed during gripping of the hand. The dorsal veins pass on either side of the digit, communicating at intervals via the dorsal venous arches (Figure 3.45).

The veins on the adjacent borders of the fingers form a network in the web space, before joining to form the dorsal metacarpal veins which drain into the dorsal venous arch. The dorsal veins of the thumb and index finger join the radial side of the arch, which continues proximally as the cephalic vein. The ulnar side of the arch receives the dorsal veins from the ulnar side of the little finger and becomes the basilic vein.

In the forearm, the three major superficial veins are on the anterior aspect: the cephalic vein, the median vein of the forearm and the basilic vein (Figure 3.46). The cephalic vein runs along the radial border of the forearm and continues on the lateral border of the belly of the biceps before entering the deltopectoral groove. The basilic veins runs along the ulnar border of the forearm and just below the elbow receives both the median vein of the forearm and the median cubital vein.

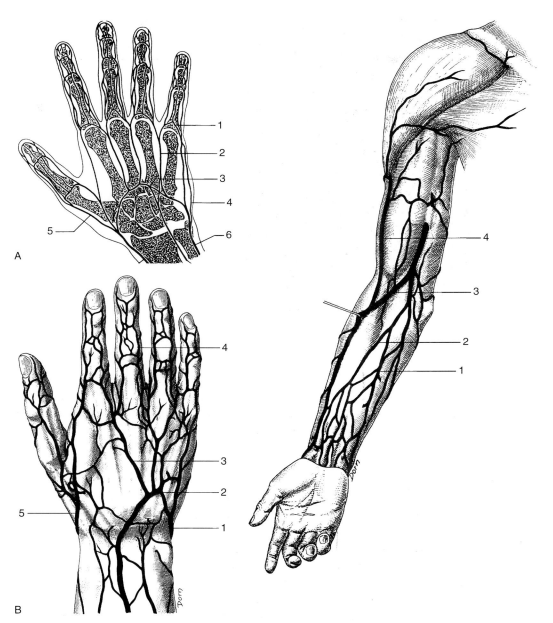

Figure 3.45. (A) Diagram of a normal phlebogram: (1) digital arcade; (2) metacarpal vein; (3) dorsal venous arcade; (4) dorsal vein; (5) dorsal vein of the thumb; (6) cubital vein; (7) radial vein; (8) accessory radial vein. (B) The dorsal veins of the hand: (1) basilic vein; (2) dorsal venous arch; (3) dorsal metacarpal veins; (4) dorsal digital veins; (5) cephalic vein.

Figure 3.46. The major superficial veins: (1) basilic vein; (2) median vein of the forearm; (3) median cubital vein; (4) cephalic vein.

257

Techniques of investigation of the arterial supply
by J P Melki

Non-invasive techniques

A logical sequence would start with non-invasive techniques before requesting the invasive ones.

Doppler ultrasonography

With Doppler ultrasonography it is possible to detect mobile structures and to measure their rate of movement.

The Doppler method can measure blood flow in different circumstances—at rest, during exertion, in different positions, and at different temperatures. Hence its relevance in functional studies of the circulation of the hand.

All the arteries of the upper limb can be studied by the Doppler method and echotomographic techniques, from the subclavian trunk down to the digital arteries.

Static tests: Static tests are used to detect changes in flow rate at a site or stenosis, occlusion, or an arteriovenous shunt. With the added help of echotomography, it is possible to measure the arterial output at rest and to determine the nature of a stenosis.

Dynamic tests: Dynamic tests reveal alterations in blood flow in different positions of the limb, in selective compression, and in induced hyperemia.

Capillaroscopy

Capillaroscopy is a method of observing the microcirculation of the skin *in vivo* (Vayssairat and Housset, 1980).

Capillaroscopy magnifies the cutaneous microcirculation by 50–300 times. This microcirculation is made physiologically opaque by transillumination of the epithelium, which is almost transparent. The alignment of the capillary bed of the skin is mostly perpendicular to the epithelium, except in a few areas such as the nail bed, the ocular conjunctiva where the capillaries can be examined as a horizontal network.

Pulse volume recording (PVR)

PVR (Zweifler et al, 1967), which measures changes in digital volume through an inflated cuff, is a reliable indicator of blood flow to the digits.

Invasive techniques

Advances in angiographic techniques and experience in interpretation have made angiographic study an invaluable means of investigating of circulation.

Computerized angiography (Figure 3.47) has now taken a large place in this type of exploration and it allows the examiner to assess the dimensions of the part to be explored. Opacification in a flow state (2 to 4 cm per second) is followed on the screen and covers all the vascular times until venous return.

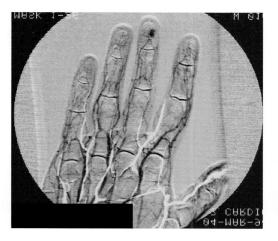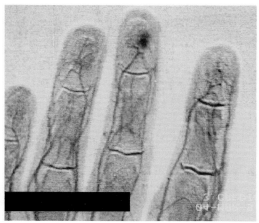

Figure 3.47. Computerized angiography showing a glomus tumor.

Digital subtraction angiography is used to depict the arteries of the hand using either the venous or the arterial route. The images obtained are the result of a digital analysis of the variations in luminosity per unit of surface area; these are projected on to a screen, on which visualization by direct subtraction is possible.

Selective angiography: The main advantage of selective angiography is its capacity to delineate a precise vascular territory, its arterial supply, and its venous channels.

Other techniques

Other techniques can also provide useful information regarding the vascularization of the hand and can be considered as complementary to those already described.

Phlebography

Phlebography is more useful in study of the venous return in the arm and forearm than in the hand (see Figure 3.47). By means of selective compression, more information can be gained, especially when investigating arteriovenous malformations. In addition, the late phases of an arteriogram can also help in studying the patterns of venous blood flow.

Lymphography

Lymphography is useful in the study of the lymphatic drainage of the upper limb but provides little information about the lymphatic network of the hand proper. The procedure can be difficult in the presence of lymphedema.

Phlebography and lymphography using radioisotopes

These potentially useful techniques have the same drawbacks as their radiological equivalents, in that they have limited application in the study of the venous and lymphatic circulations of the hand. Their main advantage is that they are non-invasive, a major asset in the study of a lymphedematous limb.

In practise, labeled colloids (usually with technetium) are injected subcutaneously for a lymphogram and intravenously for a phlebogram. The progress of the colloids is then followed using a gamma camera.

The scanner

The scanner is particularly helpful in the study of angiodysplasias. Indeed it may be useful in distinguishing between angiodysplasia and tissue hypertrophy, as well as in locating the exact site of the angiodysplasia (e.g. skin or muscle).

Thermography

Thermography is another complementary method of investigation that can be used in conjunction with the Doppler technique to follow the evolution of vascular lesions such as angiomas.

Plethysmography

Plethysmography remains useful in the study of acrosyndromes.

CONCLUSION

Plain radiographs are the best and most frequently used investigation. If the surgeon asks for radiographs after he has performed a thorough clinical examination and if he gives the radiologist sufficient information, the radiologist can choose the most appropriate views, which will give the diagnosis in the great majority of cases.

Bone scan localizes the site of pathology and can be the second examination of choice in some painful wrists where radiographs are normal.

All the other diagnostic tools should be used only with special reference to their specific indications and cost-effective results. These other investigations are useful in particular conditions, and algorithms are given by some radiologists to aid diagnosis by using special sequences of examinations.

4 EXAMINATION OF THE PERIPHERAL NERVE FUNCTION IN THE UPPER LIMB

INTRODUCTION

The nerves supplying the hand are in continuity with those of the rest of the limb and their function cannot be assessed separately. It is therefore necessary to describe in further detail the function of the peripheral nerves as a whole. This chapter will consider:

- innervation of the upper limb and clinical features of nerve paralysis
- assessment of motor function
- sensibility evaluation
- signs of neural regeneration.

4.1 INNERVATION OF THE UPPER LIMB AND CLINICAL FEATURES OF NERVE PARALYSIS

The brachial plexus

It is traditional to think of the brachial plexus (BP) (Figure 4.1) in the following manner:

- the fifth anterior cervical root (C5), after receiving the branch from the fourth root (C4), unites with the sixth root (C6) to form the superior trunk
- the first thoracic root, after receiving a branch from the second thoracic root, unites with the eighth cervical root (C8) to form the inferior trunk
- the seventh cervical root (C7) continues as the middle trunk.

Each of these trunks divides into two divisions, one anterior and one posterior. Then:

- the three posterior divisions unite to form the posterior cord from which the axillary nerve and radial nerve arise
- the anterior division of the superior trunk receives the anterior division of the middle trunk, and they unite to form the lateral cord from which the musculocutaneous nerve and the lateral root of the median nerve arise
- the anterior division of the inferior trunk remains independent and forms the medial cord from which the medial root of the median nerve, the ulnar nerve, and the medial brachial cutaneous nerve of the arm and forearm arise.

Thoracic outlet syndromes

The thoracic outlet syndromes (TOS) (Peet et al, 1956) comprise variations and combinations of neurologic and vascular symptoms affecting the upper limb, caused by abnormal compression and irritation of the brachial plexus. The condition can be congenital or acquired and can appear at one or several levels along the narrow channels that the nerves have to follow when descending from the intervertebral foramina toward the axilla. They are joined by the vessels leaving the upper thoracic aperture to irrigate and drain the upper limb (Figure 4.1c).

The commonly used Adson test (1927), which involves checking the radial pulse in various arm positions with the head turned and extended to the ipsilateral side has no

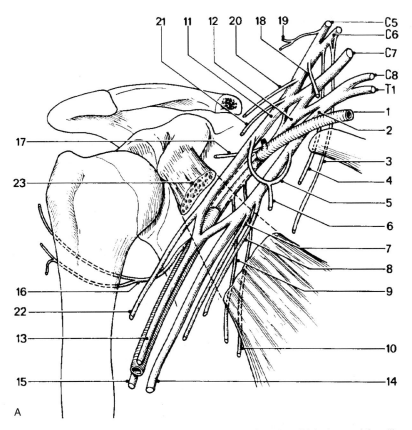

Figure 4.1. The brachial plexus. (A) Branches of the brachial plexus: (1) axillary artery; (2) medial cord; (3) nerve to serratus anterior; (4) upper subscapular nerve; (5) medial anterior thoracic nerve; (6) anterior thoracic nerve; (7) medial brachial cutaneous nerve; (8) medial antebrachial cutaneous nerve; (9) nerve to latissimus dorsi; (10) nerve to teres major; (11) lateral cord; (12) posterior cord; (13) median nerve; (14) ulnar nerve; (15) radial nerve; (16) axillary nerve; (17) inferior subscapular nerve; (18) dorsal scapular nerve; (19) nerve to subclavius; (20) suprascapular nerve; (21) lateral anterior thoracic nerve; (22) radial nerve; (23) pectoralis minor muscle. (*Continued*)

bearing on the compression of the brachial plexus and is obsolete (Ross, 1987). For Ross, the most effective and reliable test for evaluation of the three types of TOS (neurologic, venous and arterial) is the 3 minute elevated arm stress test (EAST) in the "surrender" position (Figure 4.1d). The position of this test tends to close the costoclavicular space and tense the neck and shoulder muscles to bring into play the abnormal compression mechanisms that may affect the brachial plexus nerves and subclavian vessels. With the arms in the frontal plane of the shoulders, the patient is asked to open and close the hands very slowly, about once every 2 seconds, and to describe any symptom that develops during the 3 minute test.

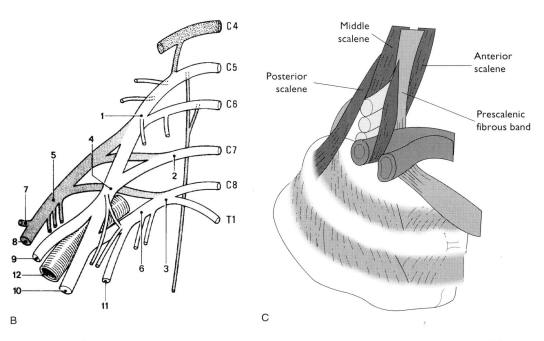

B

C

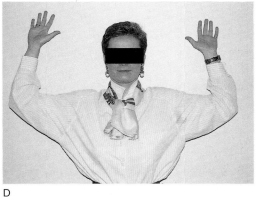

D

Figure 4.1 _contd_. The brachial plexus. (B) Structure: (1) superior trunk; (2) middle trunk; (3) inferior trunk; (4) lateral cord; (5) posterior cord; (6) medial cord; (7) axillary nerve; (8) radial nerve; (9) musculocutaneous nerve; (10) median nerve; (11) ulnar nerve; (12) axillary artery. (C) Brachial plexus, subclavian vessels and scalene muscles at the level of the first rib. (D) The Ross test.

A person who has a normal extremity can perform this test with no symptom other than mild fatigue. In the neurologic type of TOS, the patient will describe early tingling in the fingers that spreads through the hand and gradually through the forearm. The arm becomes unusually heavy and starts to ache and the patient has an urge to drop the arm.

In the venous type of TOS, the arm gradually becomes cyanotic from proximally to the extremity and the forearm and wrist veins become distended. In the arterial type, the pulse may be occluded, the arm and hand become ischemic, cadaverically white and the muscles quickly fail, forcing the arm to drop to the lap.

Peripheral nerves

We shall consider briefly the course, relations, and distribution of the main nerves of the upper limb and the clinical features of nerve paralyses of the upper limb.

Suprascapular nerve

The suprascapular nerve arises from the upper trunk of the BP and passes through the suprascapular notch deep to the suprascapular ligament (Figure 4.2). The suprascapular artery runs above the ligament. The nerve can be compressed in the suprascapular notch. It supplies both supra and infrasupinatus muscles.

Axillary nerve

Functional anatomy

The axillary or circumflex nerve (C5, C6) is the lateral terminal branch of the posterior cord. It runs alongside the posterior circumflex artery at the lower border of subscapularis. Together they form a neurovascular pedicle, which winds around the surgical neck of the humerus from medial to lateral and from posterior to anterior under cover of the deltoid muscle. It passes through the quadrilateral space, the boundaries of which are formed by the humerus and the long head of the triceps laterally, by teres minor above, teres major below, and the long head of the triceps medially (Figure 4.2).

The funicular pattern of the axillary nerve is quite variable, Sunderland (1968) noted that the number of funiculi ranged from 1 to 15. In the axilla there is usually a single large motor funiculus accompanied by fine satellites.

The axillary nerve supplies the teres minor and the deltoid. Paralysis of the nerve leads to loss of abduction of the arm. Its sensory fibers supply the skin on the posterolateral aspect of the shoulder.

Axillary nerve palsy

The axillary nerve can be injured by dislocation of the glenohumeral joint and by fractures of the surgical neck, and it can be compressed in the axilla, e.g. by crutches.

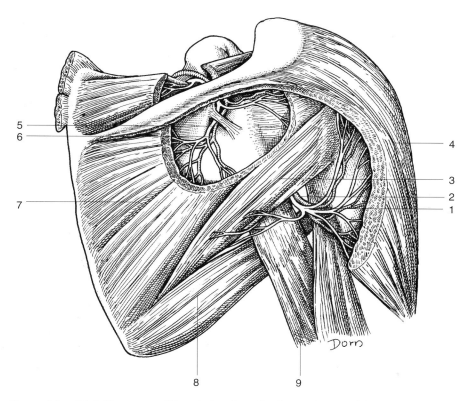

Figure 4.2. (1) Axillary nerve; (2) posterior circumflex humeral artery; (3) teres minor; (4) deltoid; (5) suprascapular artery; (6) suprascapular nerve; (7) infraspinatus (with a window); (8) teres major; (9) long head of triceps.

It is at risk during surgery when the shoulder joint or proximal humerus is approached from the posterior or lateral aspect.

Radial nerve

Functional anatomy (Figure 4.3)

The radial nerve is a continuation of the posterior cord. Its roots emerge at the C6, C7, C8, and T1 levels. Lying at first behind the axillary artery, it runs distally in the arm by winding around the posterior aspect of the humerus from medial to lateral (Figure 4.4). It continues in the lateral bicipital groove in the cubital fossa. As it reaches the humeroradial joint line, the radial nerve divides into two terminal branches (Figure 4.5)—the anterior sensory branch, which runs into the forearm under the brachioradialis lateral to the radial artery, and a posterior motor branch, the *posterior interosseous nerve*, which penetrates the supinator muscle by passing under the arcade of Frohse (Frohse and Frankel, 1908). This arcade is fibrous in about one-third of cases and may

265

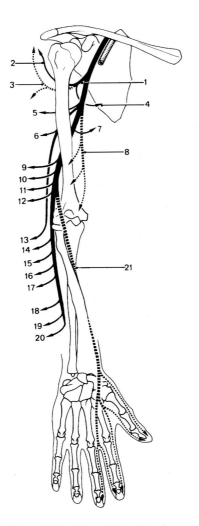

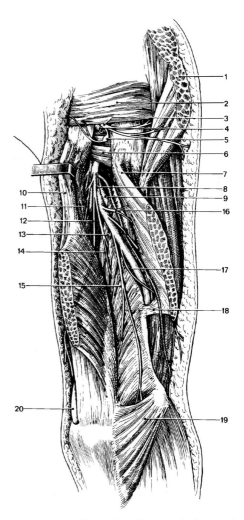

Figure 4.3. The radial and axillary nerves; muscles supplied and cutaneous distribution. The forearm is pronated. (1) Axillary nerve; (2) deltoid; (3) cutaneous branch to shoulder; (4) teres minor; (5) triceps (long); (6) triceps (lateral); (7) triceps (medial); (8) medial cutaneous branch; (9) brachioradialis; (10) extensor carpi radialis longus; (11) extensor carpi radialis brevis; (12) supinator; (13) anconeus; (14) extensor digitorum communis; (15) extensor digitorum to fifth digit; (16) extensor carpi ulnaris; (17) abductor pollicis longus; (18) extensor pollicis brevis; (19) extensor pollicis longus; (20) extensor indicis proprius; (21) anterior sensory branch. The sensory branches are shown as dotted lines.

Figure 4.4. Dissection of the posterior arm to show the axillary and radial nerves (right arm). (1) Deltoid muscle (posterior part reflected anteriorly); (2) teres minor; (3) axillary nerve emerging with posterior humeral circumflex artery (4) through the quadrilateral space; (5) branch to teres minor, showing a ganglion; (6) teres major; (7) lateral head of triceps; (8) radial nerve with the profunda brachii artery (9); (10) long head of triceps; (11) nerve to long head of triceps; (12) medial cutaneous nerve of arm; (13) short head of triceps; (14) superior nerve to short head of triceps; (15) inferior nerve to short head of triceps and anconeus; (16) superior nerve to lateral head of triceps; (17) inferior nerve to lateral head of triceps; (18) lateral intermuscular septum; (19) anconeus; (20) ulnar nerve.

266

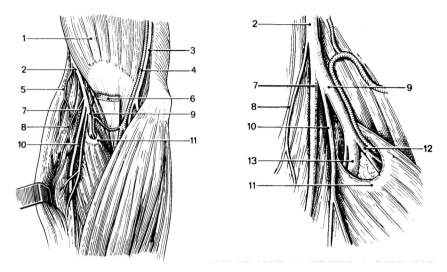

Figure 4.5. The radial nerve at the level of the elbow. (1) Brachialis; (2) radial nerve; (3) median nerve; (4) brachial artery; (5) branch to brachioradialis; (6) cut end of biceps tendon; (7) superficial branch of radial nerve; (8) branch to extensor carpi radialis longus; (9) posterior motor branch of radial nerve; (10) branch to extensor carpi radialis brevis; (11) arcade of Frohse; (12) branches to supinator; (13) posterior interosseous nerve.

compress the nerve. The nerve winds around the neck of the radius (between the two heads of the supinator). In 25 per cent of cases it lies flush against the periosteum for about 3 cm (bare area) when the forearm is supinated; it is more vulnerable at this level (Spinner, 1978). The nerve then emerges from the supinator in the posterior compartment of the forearm (Figure 4.6). After giving off branches to all the muscles in this compartment, it runs along the posterior aspect of the interosseous membrane and sends sensory branches to the wrist and carpometacarpal joint.

The radial nerve supplies all the extensors of the elbow, the wrist, and the fingers. By contrast, its sensory territory is relatively limited (the lateral half of the dorsum of the hand), but the autonomous zone is restricted to the dorsal aspect of the first interosseous space, so that sensory nerve palsy is functionally insignificant. However, sectioning of the small sensory branches of the radial nerve at the wrist can give rise to painful neuromas.

In the arm the anterior (superficial) and posterior (interosseous) divisions of the radial nerve can be traced as funiculi for 7.2–9.0 cm above their point of division. The single funiculus of the posterior interosseous nerve branches 35 mm distal to its origin, giving a branch to the supinator.

Radial nerve palsy
On the motor side, radial palsy results in paralysis of the triceps (rare after injury because the fibers supplying this muscle arise high in the axilla) and paralysis of the

267

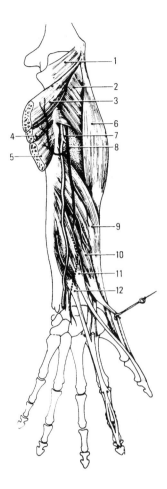

Figure 4.6. The posterior compartments of the forearm showing the posterior interosseous nerve and its branches (deep planes only). (1) Anconeus; (2) supinator; (3) extensor digitorum; (4) extensor digiti minimi; (5) extensor carpi ulnaris; (6) brachioradialis; (7) posterior interosseous artery; (8) motor branch of radial nerve (posterior interosseous); (9) abductor pollicis longus; (10) extensor pollicis brevis; (11) extensor pollicis longus; (12) extensor indicis.

supinator (partially compensated for functionally by the biceps and by shoulder movements). By contrast, three movements that are essential to hand function are lost and cannot be compensated for—extension of the wrist (all three wrist extensors are supplied by the radial nerve), extension and retroposition of the thumb (brought about by the extensor pollicis longus, abductor pollicis longus, and extensor pollicis brevis), and extension of the metacarpophalangeal joints of the fingers (Figure 4.7).

The close anatomical relationship of the radial nerve with the humeral shaft accounts for the high incidence of radial nerve injuries in fractures of the humerus.

As it crosses the spiral groove on the posterior aspect of the humerus, the nerve is not in contact with the bone. They are kept apart by thin sheets of muscle. They come into direct contact only at the lateral supracondylar border of the bone. At this level the nerve crosses the inextensible posterior intermuscular septum to enter the lateral bicipital groove; it is somewhat stretched at this point, and lack of mobility accounts for its vulnerability in humeral fractures (Holstein and Lewis, 1963).

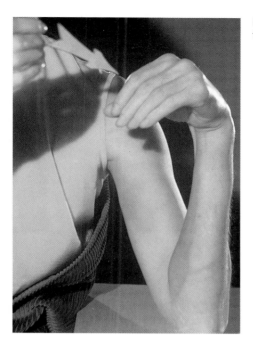

Figure 4.7. The characteristic wrist and finger drop in radial nerve palsy.

Treatment of radial nerve palsy

Primary radial nerve palsies are commonly associated with fractures of the middle and distal thirds of the humeral shaft. These fractures are usually characterized by lateral angulation and overriding of the distal fragment. Seddon (1943) demonstrated that actual division of the nerve is rare. Thus, emergency treatment should be directed at proper closed management of the fracture with frequent evaluation of the status of the nerve injury before any operative intervention is undertaken.

This conservative approach is now being reconsidered. Vichard (1982) found that in more than 25 per cent of his cases of radial nerve palsy associated with a humeral fracture there was either complete disruption or significant entrapment of the nerve. The advantage of early operative intervention in these cases is obvious. It is possible that this increase in the severity of the radial nerve lesions is a result of the frequent association today of severe multisystem trauma with this injury.

Iatrogenic radial nerve palsy is a separate problem. It results from the technique of closed reduction or surgical exposure and is unrelated to the type of fracture.

Musculocutaneous nerve

Functional anatomy

The musculocutaneous nerve arises from the lateral cord of the brachial plexus lateral to the axillary artery. It enters the arm by piercing the coracobrachialis from medial to

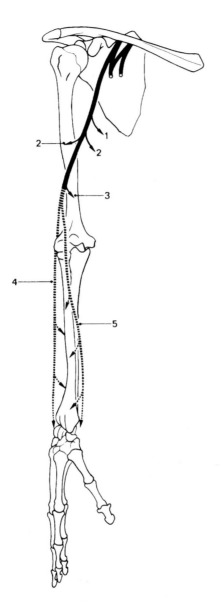

Figure 4.8. The musculocutaneous nerve; muscles supplied and cutaneous distribution. (1) Coracobrachial branch; (2) biceps brachii; (3) anterior brachial branch; (4) posterior branch (sensory); (5) anterior branch (sensory). The sensory branches are shown as dotted lines.

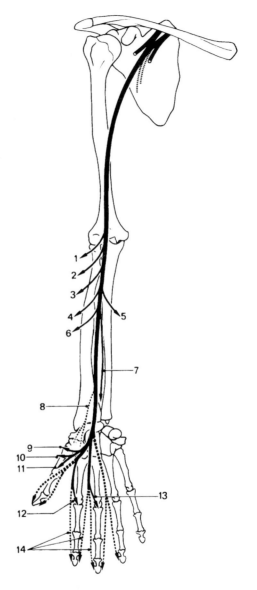

Figure 4.9. The median nerve; muscles supplied and cutaneous distribution. (1) Pronator teres; (2) palmaris longus; (3) palmaris brevis; (4) flexor digitorum superficialis; (5) flexor digitorum profundus to second and third digits; (6) flexor pollicis longus; (7) pronator quadratus; (8) palmar cutaneous branch; (9) abductor pollicis brevis; (10) superficial branch to flexor pollicis brevis; (11) opponene pollicis; (12) first lumbrical; (13) second lumbrical; (14) digital nerves (sensory). The sensory branches are shown as dotted lines.

lateral and runs between the biceps anteriorly and the brachialis posteriorly to the lateral bicipital groove of the cubital fossa (Figure 4.8). It then becomes superficial on the lateral side of the biceps tendon and medial cephalic vein, and as the lateral cutaneous nerve of the forearm divided into its two terminal branches—an anterior branch for the antero-lateral aspect of the forearm and a posterior branch that supplies the posterolateral skin.

Musculocutaneous nerve palsy

The collateral motor branches supply the coracobrachialis, biceps, and brachialis. Lesions of these branches result in considerable impairment of elbow flexion. Loss of the adductor action of the coracobrachialis can be compensated for by the pectoralis major.

The segment of the nerve traversing the coracobrachialis muscle is impossible to dissect. The terminal branch, the lateral cutaneous nerve of the forearm, has a similar pattern.

Median nerve

The median nerve arises by two roots—one from the lateral cord of the brachial plexus (C6, C7) and the other from the medial cord (C8, T1). The two roots arch around the axillary artery and join anterior to it (Figure 4.9). Thus formed, the median nerve runs distally in the anteromedial compartment of the arm. In the cubital fossa the nerve lies medial to the artery, covered by the bicipital aponeurosis, and passes between the two heads of the pronator teres and under the fibrous arch, joining the two heads of the flexor digitorum superficialis. It crosses anterior to the ulnar artery and enters the anterior compartment of the forearm, closely bound to the deep surface of the flexor digitorum superficialis within the muscle sheath (Figure 4.10). As the muscle changes to tendon in the lower half of the forearm, the median nerve runs at first lateral to the index tendon and then anterior to it and lateral to the tendon of the middle finger. It runs under the flexor retinaculum, and as it emerges from the carpal tunnel, it divides into its terminal branches to the lateral thenar muscles, the radial two lumbrical muscles, the skin of the radial half of the palm and palmar skin of three and one-half digits, and the skin covering the dorsum of the distal and medial phalanges of the radial three and one-half digits. The median nerve is the most important sensory nerve.

The median nerve gives off numerous motor branches to all the superficial volar muscles of the forearm except flexor carpi ulnaris. The medial epicondylar branch to the pronator teres arises just above the elbow. Distal to the elbow, the anterior interosseous nerve accompanies the anterior interosseous artery and lies on the interosseous membrane. It supplies the flexor pollicis longus, the flexor profundus to the index finger and the pronator quadratus.

The *fascicular anatomy* of the median nerve is relatively constant in the forearm, presenting clearly defined bundles. The recurrent thenar branch is composed of two fascicles. It joins the nerve on its volar–radial side and can be traced proximally for about 70 mm.

The palmar cutaneous branch also presents two separate bundles; they can be traced proximally for about 190 mm.

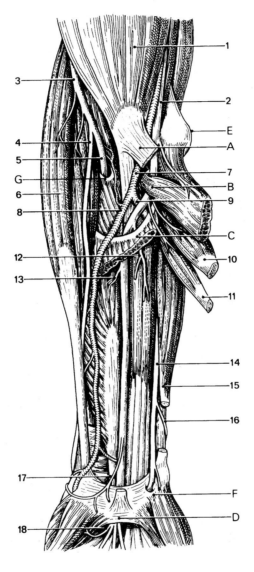

Figure 4.10. Dissection of the anterior aspect of the forearm to show the median nerve, radial nerve, and ulnar nerve. The common sites of compression of the three nerves are shown. (1) Biceps brachi; (2) median nerve; (3) radial nerve; (4) sensory branch of radial nerve; (5) motor branch of radial nerve; (6) brachioradialis; (7) brachial artery; (8) radial artery; (9) ulnar artery; (10) flexor carpi radialis; (11) palmaris longus; (12) branch of anterior interosseous nerve to flexor digitorum profundus to index and middle fingers; (13) branch of anterior interosseous nerve to flexor pollicis longus; (14) ulnar nerve; (15) flexor carpi ulnaris; (16) dorsal cutaneous branch of ulnar nerve; (17) palmar cutaneous branch of the median nerve; (18) thenar branch of the median nerve.

Common sites of nerve compression in the forearm. Median nerve: (A) expansion of biceps; (B) two heads of pronator teres; (C) flexor digitorum sublimis; (D) carpal tunnel. Ulnar nerve: (E) medial epicondylar groove; (F) Guyon's canal. Radial nerve: (G) arcade of Frohse.

The anterior interosseous nerve can be traced for about 150 mm. In its intraneural course it gives off the motor branch to the flexor carpi radialis.

The pronator teres branch dissects within the nerve for 100 mm without any interfascicular connections.

Median nerve compression

The median nerve can be compressed at several points along its course: between the heads of pronator teres, in the fibrous bridge between the heads of the flexor digitorum superficialis, and of course within the carpal tunnel.

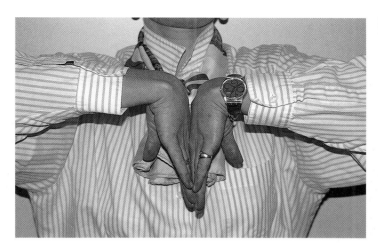

Figure 4.11. The Phalen test.

Carpal tunnel syndrome (CTS)

The diagnosis of CTS, essentially based on interrogation of the patient, is easy when the typical history of nighttime numbness and tingling, limited to the distribution of the median nerve is elicited. These paresthees are reproduced by clinical tests that cause an increase in pressure in the carpal tunnel.

Phalen's test is probably the most reliable, holding the wrist in maximum flexion (Figure 4.11 and see Section 1.1, Figure 1.13c). It becomes significant when symptoms follow within 60 seconds. Nevertheless, 34% of patients with electrical signs of compression have negative results of Phalen's test, and 20 per cent of subjects without any clinical signs have positive results on Phalen's test (Seror, 1988).

Median nerve palsy

During its superficial course across the wrist, the median nerve is particularly exposed to trauma; hence the high incidence of low median nerve palsies. These result in the loss of the most essential function of the nerve, sensibility of the prehensile zone, which includes the all important pulp skin of the thumb and index and middle fingers.

Section of the median nerve causes paralysis of the lateral thenar muscles, resulting in loss of the anteposition of the thumb. The median and ulnar nerves jointly ensure the movement of opposition and the interdependence of their actions is mirrored in the frequent overlapping of their respective territories. The flexor pollicis brevis is partly or wholly supplied by the ulnar nerve and is therefore frequently spared (Figure 4.12).

Section of the median nerve above the elbow produces, in addition to the intrinsic lesions of the hand, paralysis of the flexor pollicis longus, flexor digitorum superficialis, and the lateral half of the flexor profundus, resulting in loss of flexion of the distal phalanges of the thumb, the index finger, and sometimes the middle finger. Pronation of the forearm is usually preserved because the high branches to the pronator teres are

273

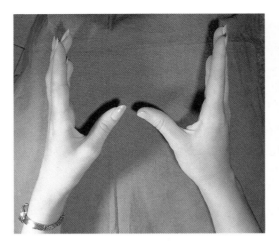
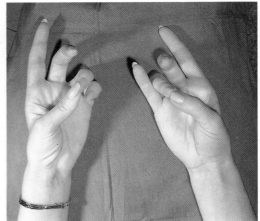

Figure 4.12. Paralysis of the median nerve on the left side. The flexor pollicis brevis is partly or wholly supplied by the ulnar nerve and is therefore frequently spared.

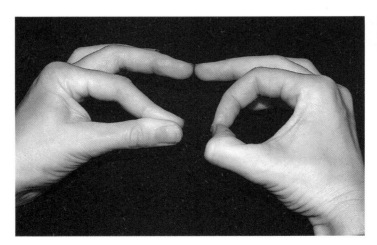

Figure 4.13. Typical pinch attitude in anterior interosseous nerve palsy (left hand).

given off above the elbow. More proximal lesions of the median nerve severely impair pronation.

Dissociated median nerve forearm palsy resulting from compression or sectioning of the anterior interosseous nerve supplying the flexor pollicis longus, the radial half of the flexor digitorum profundus, and the pronator quadratus also produces a characteristic deformity known as the "anterior interosseous nerve syndrome" (Kiloh and Nevin, 1952; Tinel, 1915; Figure 4.13). During pinch the distal phalanges of the thumb and index finger cannot flex and stay in extension (the Benediction sign). Pronation of the forearm is usually preserved because the high branches to the pronator teres are given off above the elbow. More proximal lesions of the median nerve severely impair pronation.

Ulnar nerve

Functional anatomy

The ulnar nerve arises from the medial cord of the brachial plexus and lies at this point medial to the medial cord contribution to the median nerve. Its fibers come from the C7, C8, and T1 roots. It runs medial to the humeral artery, goes through the medial intermuscular septum, and passes between the medial epicondyle of the humerus and the olecranon (Figure 4.14). It enters the forearm between the humeral and ulnar origins of the flexor carpi ulnaris and descends within the anteromedial compartment of the forearm under cover of the flexor carpi ulnaris. At the wrist, lying on the medial side of the ulnar artery, it runs with the latter, in the so-called Guyon

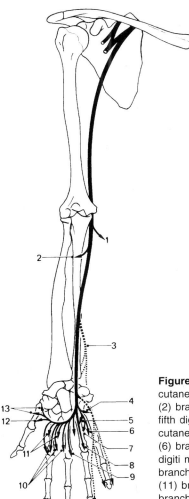

Figure 4.14. The ulnar nerve; muscles supplied and cutaneous distribution. (1) Branch to flexor carpi ulnaris; (2) branch to flexor digitorum profundus supplying fourth and fifth digits; (3) dorsal cutaneous branch; (4) palmar cutaneous branch; (5) branch to abductor digiti minimi; (6) branch to opponens digiti minimi; (7) branch to flexor digiti minimi; (8) fourth lumbrical branch; (9) third lumbrical branch; (10) branch to palmar interosseous muscles; (11) branch to dorsal interosseous muscles; (12) deep branch to flexor pollicis brevis; (13) branch to adductor pollicis. The sensory branches are shown as dotted lines.

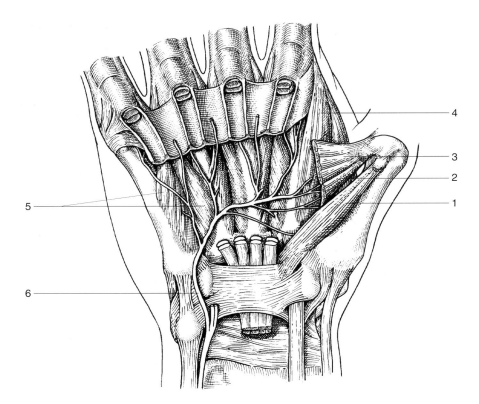

Figure 4.15. Dissection of the palm to show the deep branch of the ulnar nerve. (1) Deep head of flexor pollicis brevis; (2) adductor pollicis, oblique head; (3) adductor pollicis, transverse head; (4) first dorsal interosseous muscles; (5) interossei; (6) deep motor branch of ulnar nerve.

osseofibrous canal (distinct from the carpal tunnel). Just distal to the pisiform it divides into its two terminal branches, the superficial sensory branch, which supplies the medial skin of the hand, and the deep motor branch, which winds around the hook of the hamate, crosses the sharp lower border of the opponens digiti minimi muscle, and, under cover of the deep flexor tendons, reaches the adductor pollicis and flexor pollicis brevis muscles on the lateral side of the hand (Figure 4.15).

The ulnar nerve supplies the flexor carpi ulnaris and the two ulnar heads of the flexor digitorum profundus. In the lower third of the forearm it gives off the dorsal cutaneous branch, which supplies the skin of the ulnar half of the dorsum of the hand. Between them the median and the ulnar nerves supply all the intrinsic muscles of the hand; the deep terminal branch of the ulnar nerve sends fibers to all the intrinsic muscles (except the two lateral lumbricals), to the adductor pollicis, and to the deep head of the flexor

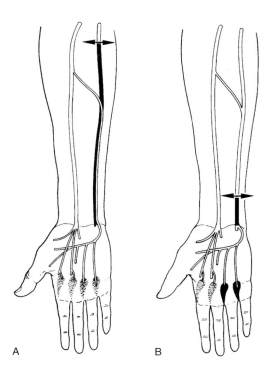

Figure 4.16. Diagram to show the Martin–Gruber anastomosis between the median and ulnar nerves in the forearm. In high lesions of the ulnar nerve (A), the anastomosis from the median nerve can result in prevention of paralysis of the ulnar innervated intrinsic muscles. In lesions of the ulnar nerve distal to the anastomosis (B), this will not occur.

A

B

pollicis brevis. In fact the respective territories of the median and ulnar nerves are poorly defined. Anastomoses occur in the forearm (Martin–Gruber anastomosis) in 15 per cent of the cases according to Mannerfelt (1966) and in the palm (anastomoses of Riche and Cannieu; Riche, 1897), which explain the frequent anomalies of distribution (Figure 4.16).

Ulnar nerve compression
The ulnar nerve can be compressed at several points:

1 In the lower third of the arm, the nerve enters the posterior compartment by passing through an osseofibrous foramen (Figure 4.17a). This is formed laterally by the medial intermuscular septum (which is attached to the humerus), above by a fibrous expansion of the coracobrachialis, and medially by the medial head of the triceps. Distally the foramen may be narrowed by inconstant insertions of the triceps, which form "Struthers' arcade" (Struthers, 1854).

2 At the elbow the nerve passes through a narrow channel between the epicondyle and the olecranon where it may be compressed by the bone or joint (Figure 4.17b). Next the nerve runs between the humeral and ulnar heads of the flexor carpi ulnaris under a fibrous arcade, which must be divided to relieve compression at that level (Osborne, 1970).

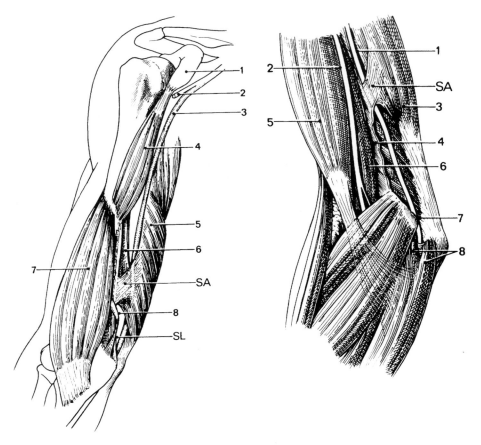

Figure 4.17. (A) Dissection to show the ulnar nerve in the arm and its common sites of compression: (1) coracoid process; (2) musculocutaneous nerve; (3) ulnar nerve; (4) coracobrachialis; (5) medial head of triceps; (6) medial intermuscular septum; (7) brachialis; (8) supracondylar spur; (SA) Struther's arcade; (SL) Struther's ligament. (B) The ulnar nerve at the elbow: (1) ulnar nerve; (2) median nerve; (3) triceps; (4) medial intermuscular septum; (5) biceps; (6) brachialis; (7) medial epicondylar groove; (8) two heads of flexor carpi ulnaris; (SA) Struther's arcade.

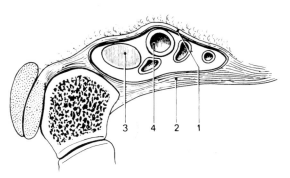

Figure 4.18. The space of Guyon (transverse section). (1) Volar ligament of wrist; (2) flexor retinaculum; (3) ulnar nerve; (4) ulnar artery.

3 The nerve also can be compressed in the wrist as it courses through Guyon's canal whose floor is formed by the flexor retinaculum (inserted on the pisiform) and its roof by an expansion of the flexor carpi ulnaris (Figure 4.18).

The deep terminal branch dives under the fibrous band that stretches from the pisiform to the hook of the hamate, from which arise the abductor and flexor digiti minimi brevis. The ulnar nerve is most vulnerable at the elbow and at the wrist.

Funicular anatomy

The distal part of the ulnar nerve can be easily microdissected. The dorsal cutaneous branch forms an independent fascicle that can be traced proximally well above the epicondyle. Jabaley et al (1980) suggested the use of this branch as a graft in cases in which it is considered expendable.

Sensory ulnar palsy affects both the palmar and the dorsal aspects of the ulnar half of the hand. The autonomous zone of the ulnar nerve is limited to the skin of the distal two phalanges of the little finger.

Motor ulnar palsy

Motor ulnar palsy, by contrast, has far more functional consequences (Table 4.1). Distal ulnar nerve lesions produce the classic claw deformity. The claw hand consists of hyper-extension of the proximal phalanx while the two distal phalanges are in flexion. It is important to be aware that every ulnar paralysis does not result in a claw hand. This deformity is caused by the paralysis of the intrinsic muscles, when the extrinsic muscles, i.e., the long flexors and the long extensors of the fingers are active.

This deformity is present in varying degrees, depending on the extent of the paralysis and the suppleness of the digits. It involves the four fingers in cases of associated paralysis of the ulnar and median nerves (see Figure 4.18). It involves only the ring and small fingers in cases of isolated ulnar paralysis, because the two radial lumbricals, innervated by the median nerve, prevent deformity of the index and long fingers when the hand is at rest. The third lumbrical may be innervated by both the median and ulnar nerves, and clawing is more severe in the little finger than in the ring finger (Kaplan and Spinner, 1980). The deformity is more marked when the nerve lesion is distal and the long flexors are intact (Figure 4.19).

To explain these deformities, one must recall the action of the intrinsic and extrinsic muscles of the fingers (*see* page 42).

Dynamic problems producing troubles of prehension are far more bothersome than the claw hand itself. All the pinch grip modalities are disturbed by intrinsic muscle paralysis.

Precision pinch

Precision pinch between the thumb and fingers becomes extremely difficult, because the patient is unable to adapt the position of the distal phalanges, which are deprived of active extension. The thumb also presents with flexion of its distal phalanx during pinch: this is Froment's sign.

Original description by	Year	Symptoms and signs
Duchenne	1867	Clawing of the ring and little fingers The little finger cannot be adducted to the ring finger; inability to play high notes on the violin because the flexor carpi ulnaris and opponens digiti quinti are paralyzed and there is loss of sensibility of the little finger
Jeanne	1915	Hyperextension of the metacarpophalangeal joint of the thumb in pinch grip (Jeanne's sign)
Froment	1915	Pronounced flexion of the interphalangeal joint of the thumb during adduction toward the index finger (Froment's sign)
Masse	1916	Flattening of the metacarpal arch
André-Thomas	1917	The wrist tends to fall into volar flexion during action of the extensors of the middle finger
Pollock	1919	Inability to flex the distal phalanx of the fifth finger
Pitres-Testut	1925	The transverse diameter of the hand is decreased Radial–ulnar abduction of the metacarpophalangeal joint of the middle finger is impossible Inability to shape the hand to a cone
Wartenberg	1939	Inability to adduct the extended little finger to the extended ring finger (Wartenberg's sign)
Sunderland	1944	Inability to rotate, oppose, or supinate the little finger toward the thumb (Sunderland's sign)
Fay	1954	Inability of the thumb to reach the little finger in true opposition (probably a misinterpretation of the author because the little finger cannot always reach the thumb in cases of paralysis of the opponens of the little finger)
Bunnell	1956	The thumb no longer pinches against the index finger to make a full circle
Egawa	1959	Inability of the flexed middle finger to abduct radially and ulnarly and to rotate at the metacarpophalangeal joint
Mumenthaler	1961	On abduction of the little finger against resistance, no normal dimple appears in the hypothenar region because of paresis of the palmaris brevis musculature
Mannerfelt	1966	Hyperflexion sign Thumb: Interphalangeal joint flexed; metacarpophalangeal joint slightly hyperextended; the thumb is markedly supinated Index finger: With increasing force in the collapsed pinching grip, a flexion position (often more than 90°) of the proximal interphalangeal joint is seen; the distal interphalangeal joint is hyperextended, and the radial part of the pulp slides in a proximal direction along the ulnar part of the thumb

Table 4.1. Symptoms and signs in ulnar nerve paralysis (adapted from Mannerfelt, 1966)

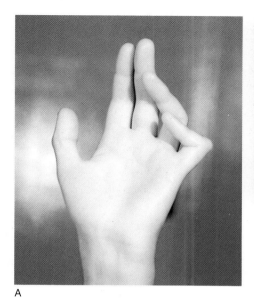

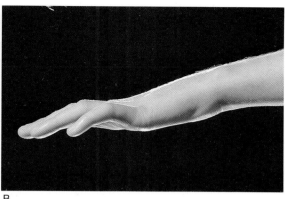

Figure 4.19. (A) Distal ulnar palsy. (B) Proximal ulnar palsy. Note the relative lack of deformity secondary to paralysis of the long flexors.

The interpretation of this sign has been the subject of numerous commentaries (McFarlane, 1962). Thus for Froment (1920), lack of extension of the distal phalanx is caused by the paralyzed adductor. At the level of the interphalangeal IP joint, extension depends partly on the thenar muscles, which, as shown by Duchenne (1867), have attachments through their dorsal expansions into the extensor apparatus like those of the intrinsic muscles at the level of the fingers

Although these expansions to the extensor pollicis longus (EPL) arise from both the abductor pollicis brevis (APB) and the adductor (i.e. the medial and lateral muscles) an extension lag of the distal phalanx is not found after an isolated paralysis of the median nerve. On the contrary, after an isolated ulnar nerve paralysis, a flexion deformity of the distal phalanx occurs when an object is grasped. This deformity is not fixed (at least not initially); it is dynamic, and the degree of flexion augments with increasing effort.

This difference in position of the distal phalanx between median and ulnar nerve paralysis is explained by the predominance of muscles innervated by the ulnar nerve. For Bunnell (1938), flexion of the distal phalanx is due to the collapse of the thumb column and is secondary to the hyperextension of the metacarpophalangeal (MP) joint (Jeanne's sign) that causes tension of the flexor pollicis longus (FPL). It is, in effect, sometimes possible to diminish the flexion of the distal joint by stabilizing the MP joint in slight flexion. One can, however, observe effort-induced flexion of the distal phalanx of the thumb unaccompanied by hyperextension of the proximal phalanx when the flexor pollicis brevis (FPB) is not paralyzed.

The flexion deformity of the distal phalanx of the thumb is functionally disabling because it hinders the most useful type of pinch. Furthermore, during finger–thumb

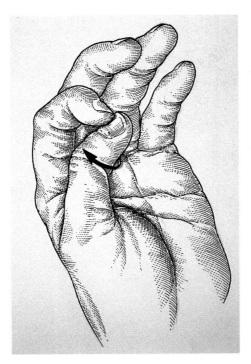

Figure 4.20. The "crank-handle" effect.

pinch pressure from the index is exerted on the dorso-ulnar aspect of the distal phalanx of the thumb, forcing the thumb into supination when there is a paralysis of all the intrinsic muscles of the thumb (the "crank-handle" effect; Brand, 1985; Figure 4.20).

Grasp
Grasp is also disturbed for several reasons:

1 Lack of extension of the distal phalanges, which prevents the grasping of large objects.
2 Inversion of the sequence of phalangeal flexion. Normally, finger flexion begins at the level of the proximal interphalangeal (PIP) and MP joints and is followed by distal interphalangeal (DIP) joint flexion. In cases of interosseous paralysis, the sequence of flexion is altered. Finger flexion is accomplished by the long flexors alone, which act first on the distal phalanges. The MP joint flexes last. With flexion, the pulps of the fingers shave the palm, and the hand cannot grasp large objects (Figure 4.21). This "dyskinetic finger flexion" is one of the most awkward functional consequences of these paralyses.
3 For a long time, intrinsic muscle strength has been underestimated. This strength is far from negligible, especially in the peripheral digits (*see* Chapter 1). The more proximal the ulnar paralysis, the more marked is the deficit of the strength of finger flexion, because the flexor profundus paralysis of the ring and little finger is added to the intrinsic paralysis. When there is concomitant proximal median nerve paralysis, all the digital flexors, intrinsics and extrinsics, are paralyzed.

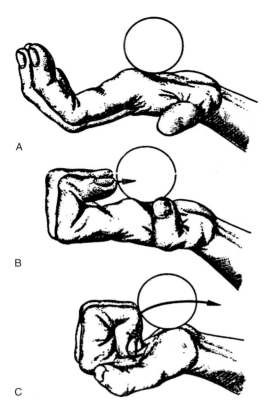

Figure 4.21a, b and c. Alteration of grasp with intrinsic paralysis. Flexion begins with the distal phalanges.

A

B

C

4 The disturbance in finger flexion causes a modification of the location of pressure zones during grasp. Normally during grasp the pressure over the zone of contact is widely distributed on the palmar aspect of the fingers, on the metacarpal heads, and on the thenar and hypothenar eminences. When an ulnar-paralyzed hand grasps an object, it is the extremities of the flexed fingers that do the grasping, and the pressure on these limited zones of contact is considerable (Figure 4.22). This can cause ulceration of the fingertips, especially when troubles of pressure distribution are associated with a sensory disturbance.

5 Flattening of the palmar arch and absence of fifth MP flexion considerably weaken the power to grasp large objects and may need to be corrected for certain manual laborers.

6 A considerable lack of thumb strength is always added to the lack of finger strength, because the adductor pollicis (AP), and often the FBP, are paralyzed. Measurements performed by Mannerfelt (1966) showed that residual strength of thumb adduction in ulnar palsy is only 17–20 per cent of normal. This deficit is far greater than the estimations of Björkesten (1946) and Bunnell (1956), who evaluated the residual force at about one-half or one-third of normal. A lack of hand strength is a major complaint of patients with ulnar palsy.

283

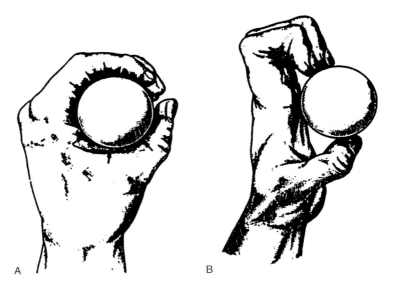

Figure 4.22. Comparison of pressure zones in (A) normal grasp and (B) grasp in a hand with intrinsic paralysis.

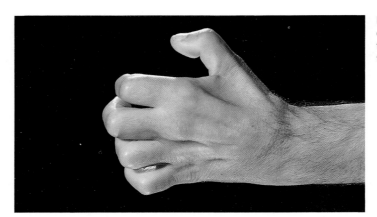

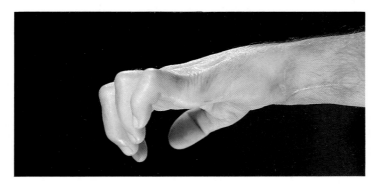

Figure 4.23. Claw hand deformity involving the four fingers (associated paralysis of the ulnar and median nerves).

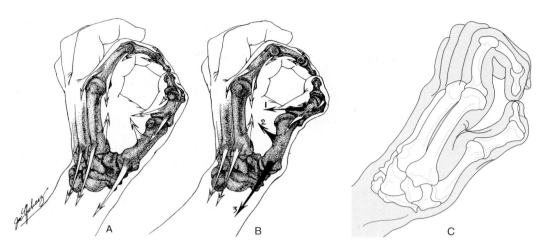

Figure 4.24. (A) Normal; (B) dysequilibrium of thumb column; (C) dysequilibrium of both index and thumb columns secondary to intrinsic paralysis produces terminal pinch.

Added to these thumb deformities caused by ulnar paralyses are those of the other digits, which further aggravate thumb–finger pinch disturbances (Figure 4.23). With palsy of the first dorsal interosseous, the index finger loses its abduction power and cannot resist pressure from the thumb. Also, in all the fingers, palsy of the interosseous muscles produces an extension deficit in the distal phalanges when the flexor digitorum profundus muscles produce increased IP flexion in an effort to flex the MP joints. Instead of the usual pulp-to-pulp pinch, these patients substitute with a terminal pinch between the flexed extremities of the phalanges of the thumb and fingers, which is infinitely less useful.

In the terminal thumb–index pinch (Figure 4.24), the patient cannot make an "O" with the two digits (Bunnell, 1956); the metacarpophalangeal joints have a tendency to hyperextend and the proximal interphalangeal joint of the index finger tends to hyperflex (Mannerfelt, 1966).

4.2 ASSESSMENT OF MOTOR FUNCTION

This section deals with tests that are used to demonstrate clinically the motor activity of each of the muscles of the upper limb. These tests do not necessarily make use of the normal activity of each individual muscle but aim at dissociating the muscle from its synergists. Most of the maneuvers described are used to produce active mobilization of a more distal segment; it is not so much the actual contraction of a muscle as its efficiency that is tested.

Weakening or disappearance of voluntary movement may be due to one of several causes: paralysis of the afferent nerve, destruction of muscle tissue (often as a result of ischemia of the fleshy part of the muscle), rupture of the tendon, and tendon block because of adhesions are the more obvious causes. However, it should be remembered that alteration at its point of angulation will reduce or annul the efficiency of a muscle. This is the case when the pulleys of the flexors are damaged or when the extensor tendons are dislocated into the intermetacarpal spaces. It is also obvious that these tests are valid only if the joint has a normal range of movement.

An abnormal hand posture may be characteristic and establish the diagnosis, as with a typical ulnar claw (see Figure 4.18) or as with wrist drop and flexion of the wrist and metacarpophalangeal joints, pathognomonic of radial nerve palsy (see Figure 4.7).

Somewhat less typical is the dissociated radial palsy simulating an ulnar claw in which extension of the thumb and index and middle fingers is preserved (Marie et al, 1917).

Analytical examination of the muscles

The main features of a motor palsy are muscle atrophy and the absence of voluntary contraction.

Demonstration of voluntary contraction is not always easy. Not all muscles are palpable. The nerve supply can be anomalous, and a contraction of a normally innervated muscle can be transmitted to the fibers of an adjacent paralyzed muscle. The reflexes must be tested and compared with those on the healthy contralateral side.

The key of this part of the examination is the study of voluntary movements. Accurate assessment of the individual muscles is essential. Muscle power is graded by using the Highet scale adopted by the British Medical Research Council (1941) or one of its variations. We use the version devised by Merle d'Aubigné et al (1956):

M0: no contraction
M1: flicker (no joint motion)
M2: contraction with mobility with gravity eliminated
M3: contraction against gravity
M4: contraction with active movement of normal amplitude against gravity and some resistance
M5: normal power.

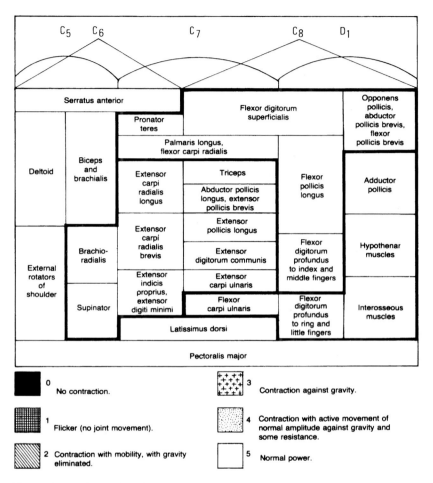

Figure 4.25. A standard form used to record motor function in the upper limb (after Merle d'Aubigné). The areas outlined in heavy black lines enclose those muscles usually supplied by the median, radial, and ulnar nerves. The area on the form for each muscle should be cross hatched or stippled according to its power (scale 0–5): (M0) no contraction; (M1) flicker of activity (no joint motion); (M2) contraction + joint motion (gravity eliminated); (M3) contraction + joint motion (against gravity); (M4) contraction against gravity + some resistance; (M5) normal power.

Examinations are repeated periodically and the results are noted on an appropriate form, such as that shown in Figure 4.25.

We will stress here the importance of testing for movements originating in the arm, forearm, and shoulder. These examinations are mandatory in high trunk lesions and injuries of the brachial plexus (see Figure 4.1).

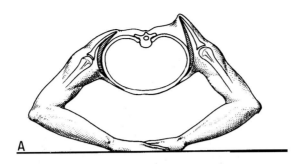

Figure 4.26. Serratus anterior palsy. (A) Winging of scapula on the left side as seen in this cross section of the trunk. (B) Clinical test to demonstrate winging of the left scapula.

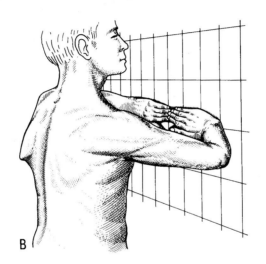

Testing the voluntary movements of the scapular muscles

Serratus anterior
Nerve supply. Long thoracic nerve ("respiratory" nerve of Bell; C5, C6, C7).
Action. Pulls the scapula forward against the ribs.
Test of muscle function. Using the upper limbs, the patient pushes his body away from a fixed plane. The medial border of the scapula is held against the thoracic plane by the serratus anterior unless the latter is paralyzed (Figure 4.26).

Rhomboid
Nerve supply. Nerve to the rhomboid (C4, C5).
Action. Pulls the lower half of the scapula medially.
Test of muscle function. The patient attempts to push his shoulder backward against resistance. Contraction of the muscle can be felt and sometimes seen (Figure 4.27).

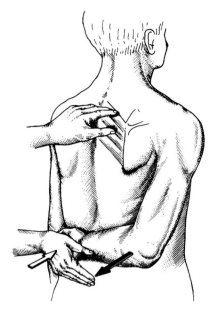

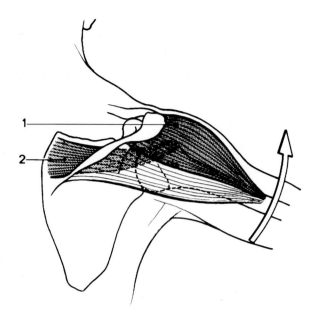

Figure 4.27. Paralysis of the rhomboids. With his arm behind his back, the patient presses his hand backward against resistance. The rhomboid muscle can be seen to contract.

Figure 4.28. The abductors of the shoulder: (1) middle part of deltoid; (2) supraspinatus.

Analysis of arm and shoulder movements

Abduction

Abduction of the arm at the shoulder joint is brought about by the middle part of the deltoid and the supraspinatus (Figure 4.28).

Flexion

Flexion is produced by the anterior part of the deltoid, the clavicular head of the pectoralis major, the coracobrachialis, and the short head of the biceps (Figure 4.29).

Extension

Extension results from the action of the posterior part of the deltoid, the latissimus dorsi, the teres major, and the long head of the triceps (Figure 4.30).

Adduction

Adduction is due to the combined action of anterior and posterior muscles—anteriorly, the pectoralis major and coracobrachialis and posteriorly, the posterior part of the deltoid, the long head of the triceps, the teres major, and the latissimus dorsi (Figures 4.31 and 4.32).

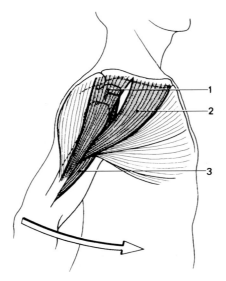

Figure 4.29. The flexors of the shoulder: (1) anterior part of deltoid; (2) clavicular head of pectoralis major; (3) coracobrachialis.

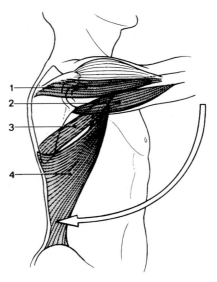

Figure 4.30. The extensors of the shoulder: (1) posterior part of deltoid; (2) long head of triceps; (3) teres major; (4) latissimus dorsi.

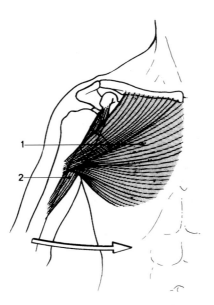

Figure 4.31. The adductors of the shoulder, anterior muscles: (1) pectoralis major; (2) coracobrachialis.

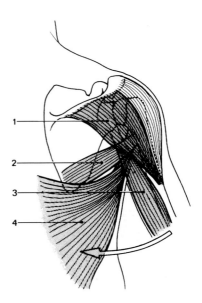

Figure 4.32. The adductors of the shoulder, posterior muscles: (1) posterior part of deltoid; (2) teres major; (3) long head of triceps; (4) latissimus dorsi.

290

Medial rotation

Medial rotation of the arm is brought about by the subscapularis, the teres major, the pectoralis major, and the latissimus dorsi (Figure 4.33).

Lateral rotation

Lateral rotation is achieved by the infraspinatus, the teres minor, and the posterior part of the deltoid.

Pectoralis major

Nerve supply. Lateral (C8, C7, C8) and medial (T1) pectoral nerves.

Action. Adducts, lowers, and medially rotates the arm.

Test of muscle function. The patient pulls his arm toward his chest against resistance (Figure 4.34).

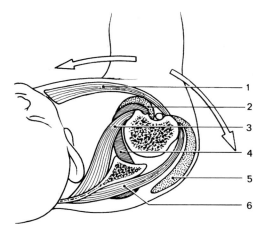

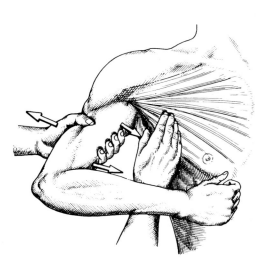

Figure 4.33. Medial and lateral rotators of the shoulder. Medial rotators: (1) pectoralis major; (2) latissimus dorsi; (3) subscapularis; (4) teres major. Lateral rotators: (5) posterior part of deltoid; (6) infraspinatus.

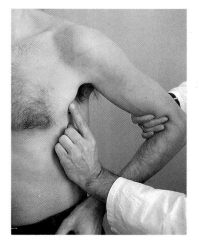

Figure 4.34. Pectoralis major. When the patient adducts his arm against resistance, the muscle belly can be seen and felt.

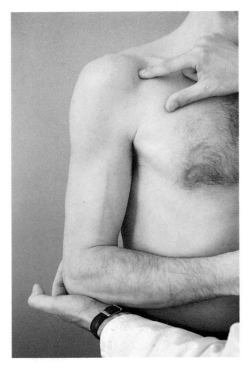

Figure 4.35. Pectoralis minor. The patient depresses his shoulder against resistance. The tendon can be felt at the coracoid process.

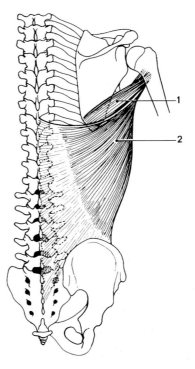

Figure 4.36. Anatomy of the teres major (1) and latissimus dorsi (2).

Pectoralis minor
Nerve supply. Branches to the pectoralis minor (C8).
Action. Lowers the shoulder.
Test of muscle function. Lowering the shoulder against resistance; the tendon can be felt on the coracoid process (Figure 4.35).

Latissimus dorsi
Nerve supply. Thoracodorsal nerve from the posterior cord of C6, C7, and C8.
Action. Adductor, extensor, and medial rotator of the arm.
Test of muscle function. Adduction of the arm against resistance demonstrates the lateral border of the latissimus dorsi. The teres major contracts at the same time (Figures 4.36 and 4.37). Active adduction can be tested with the limb raised or lowered. Moberg (1978a), remembering the name given to the muscle by ancient anatomists (musculus scapultor ani: "muscle used to scratch one's bottom"), asks the patient to carry his hand to his buttock against resistance applied by the examiner.

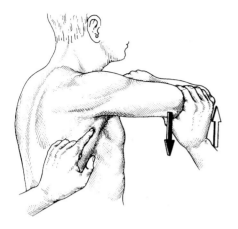

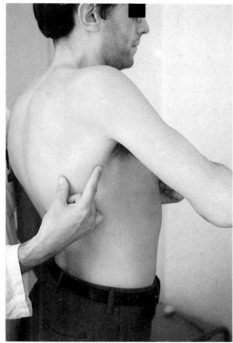

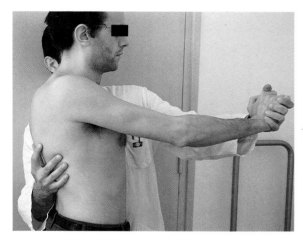

Figure 4.37. Clinical demonstration of the latissimus dorsi. The muscle can be seen when the patient adducts his arm against resistance.

Deltoid

Nerve supply. Axillary nerve (C5, C6).

Action. Abductor of the arm. In addition the anterior fibers carry the arm forward and the posterior fibers carry it backward (Figure 4.38).

Test of muscle function:

1 Middle fibers: The patient is asked to abduct his arm against resistance, in the range of 15 to 90 degrees of abduction (Figure 4.38a,b).
2 Anterior fibers: Elevation of the arm anteriorly against resistance (Figure 4.38c).
3 Posterior fibers: Elevation of the arm posteriorly against resistance (Figure 4.38d).

Supraspinatus

Nerve supply. Suprascapular nerve (C5).

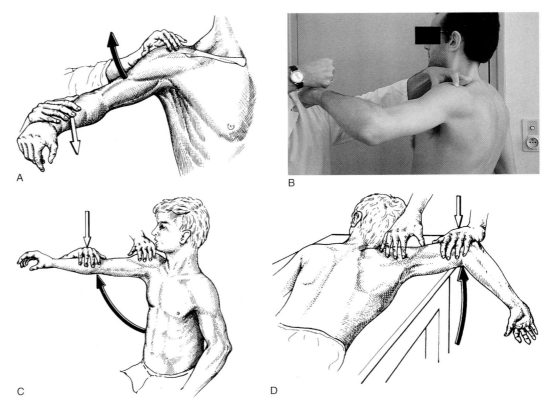

Figure 4.38. Clinical demonstration of the deltoid. (A and B) The middle part of the deltoid is palpated between the thumb and index finger of the examiner when the arm is abducted against resistance and flexed anteriorly 15 to 90 degrees. (C) Clinical demonstration of the anterior part of the deltoid. The patient is asked to elevate his arm anteriorly against resistance. (D) Clinical demonstration of the posterior part of the deltoid. The patient is asked to extend the arm posteriorly at the shoulder against resistance.

Action: Initiates abduction.

Test of muscle function: With the arm resting alongside the body, the patient attempts to abduct it against resistance. The muscle contraction normally can be felt under the upper part of the trapezius (Figure 4.39).

Infraspinatus

Nerve supply: Suprascapular nerve (C5).

Action: Rotates the arm laterally (Figure 4.40).

Test of muscle function: Standing up with his arm against his chest and the elbow in 90 degrees of flexion, the patient tries to carry his forearm laterally against resistance (Figure 4.41a). Or, lying prone with his arm in 90 degrees of abduction and his forearm hanging down from the couch, the patient tries to externally rotate his arm against resistance (Figure 4.41b).

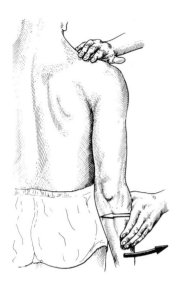

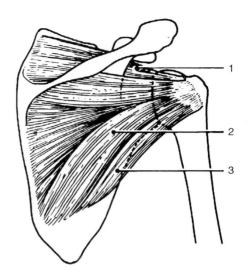

Figure 4.39. Clinical demonstration of the supraspinatus. As the patient abducts his arm against resistance, the muscle contraction can be felt.

Figure 4.40. Anatomy of the supraspinatus (1), infraspinatus (2) and teres minor (3).

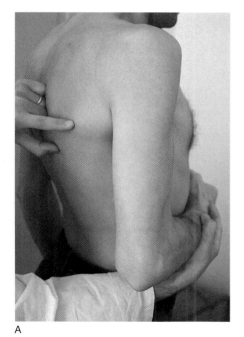

A

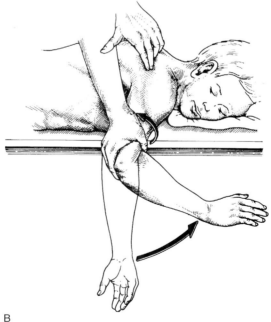

B

Figure 4.41. Clinical demonstration of the infraspinatus. (A) The muscle can be palpated when the patient attempts to rotate the arm externally from the position of internal rotation. (B) The patient lies prone with his shoulder abducted to 90 degrees, the elbow flexed to 90 degrees, and the forearm hanging down. The muscle can be palpated when he externally rotates the arm against resistance.

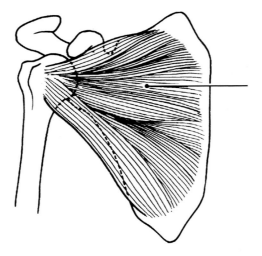

Figure 4.42. Anatomy of the subscapularis.

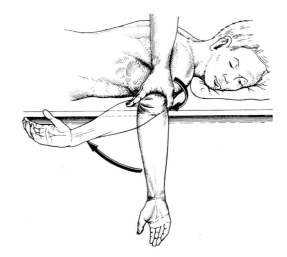

Figure 4.43. Clinical demonstration of the subscapularis. With the patient prone, the reverse procedure for testing the infraspinatus is performed.

Subscapularis

Nerve supply. Upper and lower branches of the scapular trunk, arising from the posterior division (C6, C7, C8; Figure 4.42).

Action. Medial rotation of the arm, adduction.

Test of muscle function. The patient in the prone position (as for infraspinatus testing) tries to internally rotate his arm against resistance (Figure 4.43).

Analysis of movements of the elbow and forearm

Elbow flexion

Elbow flexion is brought about by biceps, the brachialis, the brachioradialis, and the pronator teres (Figure 4.44).

Elbow extension

Elbow extension is effected by the triceps and the anconeus (Figure 4.45).

Forearm pronation

Forearm pronation is effected by the pronator teres and the pronator quadratus (Figure 4.46).

Forearm supination

Forearm supination is effected by the biceps and the supinator (Figure 4.47).

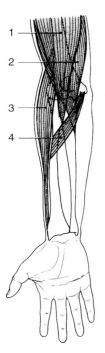

Figure 4.44. Flexors of the elbow: (1) biceps; (2) brachialis; (3) brachioradialis; (4) pronator teres.

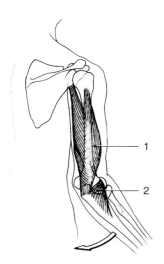

Figure 4.45. Extensors of the elbow: (1) triceps; (2) anconeus.

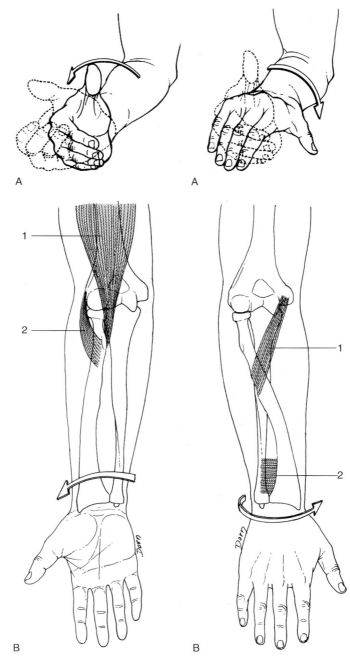

Figure 4.46. Supination of the forearm. (A) Movement of supination. (B) Muscles of supination: (1) biceps; (2) supinator.

Figure 4.47. Pronation of the forearm. (A) Movement of pronation. (B) Muscles of pronation: (1) pronator teres; (2) pronator quadratus.

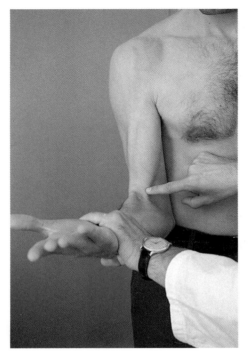

Figure 4.48. Clinical demonstration of the biceps brachii by flexion of the elbow against resistance.

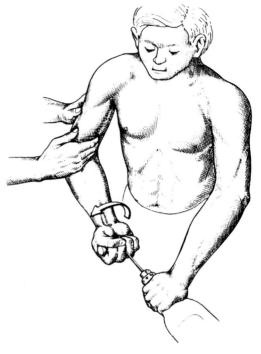

Figure 4.49. Clinical demonstration of the biceps brachii. Flexion of the elbow and supination, as in using a corkscrew, demonstrate the muscle.

Biceps brachii
Nerve supply: Musculocutaneous nerve (C5, C6).
Action: Flexes the elbow and supinates the forearm.
Test of muscle function: Flexion of the elbow against resistance with the forearm supinated (Figures 4.48 and 4.49).

Triceps
Nerve supply: Radial nerve (C5, C6, C7, C8).
Action: Extends the elbow; the long head also adducts the arm.
Test of muscle function: With the arm in 90 degrees of abduction, to eliminate the action of gravity, and the forearm hanging down, the patient tries to extend the elbow (Figures 4.50 and 4.51).

Brachioradialis
Nerve supply: Radial nerve (C5, C6, C7).
Action: Flexes the elbow; also acts as a pronator in full supination and as a supinator in full pronation.

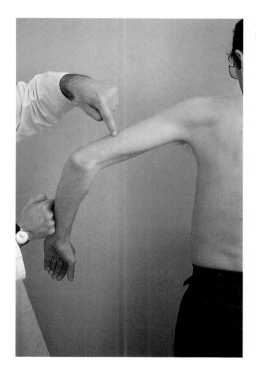

Figure 4.50. Clinical demonstration of the triceps by use of resisted elbow extension.

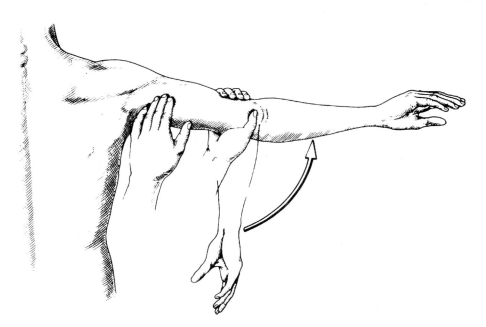

Figure 4.51. Clinical demonstration of the triceps. When testing the triceps, it is important to prevent trick movements that can extend the elbow by using gravity. The arm therefore should be placed horizontally to eliminate the effect of gravity.

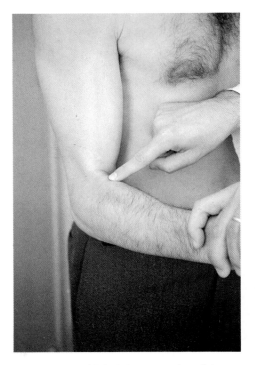

Figure 4.52. Clinical demonstration of the brachioradialis. Resisted elbow flexion is effected with the forearm in 90 degrees of flexion and neutral pronation and supination.

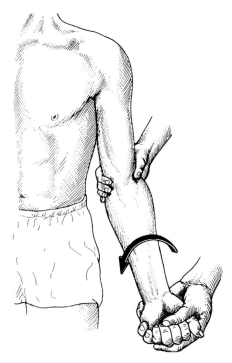

Figure 4.53. Clinical demonstration of the supinator. With the arm hanging by the side and the elbow extended to eliminate the action of biceps, the patient attempts to supinate the forearm against resistance.

Test of muscle function: Flexion against resistance with the elbow in 90 degrees of flexion and the forearm halfway between pronation and supination (Figure 4.52).

Supinator
Nerve supply: Radial nerve (C5, C6).
Action: Supinates the forearm.
Test of muscle function: With the arm hanging and the elbow extended, the patient attempts to supinate the forearm against resistance (Figure 4.53). With the elbow flexed, contraction of the muscle can be felt when the patient attempts to supinate the forearm against resistance (Figure 4.54).

Pronator teres
Nerve supply: Median nerve (C6, C7).
Action: Pronates the forearm, flexes the elbow.
Test of muscle function: With the elbow flexed, the patient pronates the forearm against resistance. Contraction of the muscle usually can be felt and seen (Figure 4.55).

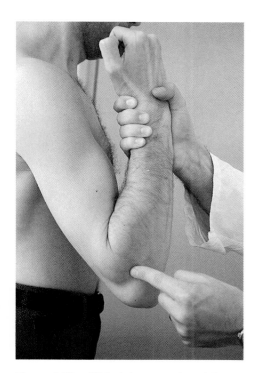

Figure 4.54. Clinical demonstration of the supinator. Supination of the forearm against resistance.

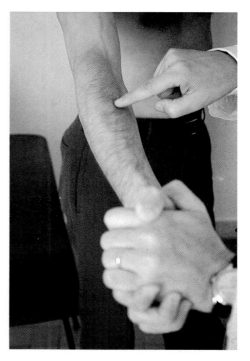

Figure 4.55. Clinical demonstration of the pronator teres. With the elbow and fingers flexed, the patient attempts to pronate the forearm against resistance.

Analysis of movements of the wrist

Wrist flexion

Wrist flexion is brought about by the flexor carpi radialis, palmaris longus, and flexor carpi ulnaris.

Wrist extension

Wrist extension is brought about by the extensor carpi radialis longus, extensor carpi radialis brevis, and extensor carpi ulnaris.

Radial deviation

Radial deviation is brought about by the abductor pollicis longus, extensor carpi radialis longus and brevis, and flexor carpi radialis.

Ulnar deviation

Ulnar deviation is brought about by the flexor carpi ulnaris and extensor carpi ulnaris.

301

Flexor carpi radialis
Nerve supply: Median nerve (C6).
Action: Flexes the wrist.
Test of muscle function: Flexion of the wrist against resistance (Figure 4.56).

Palmaris longus
Nerve supply: Median nerve (C6).
Action: Flexes the wrist.
Test of muscle function: Flexion of the wrist against resistance (Figure 4.56).

Flexor carpi ulnaris
Nerve supply: Ulnar nerve (C8, T1).
Action: Flexes the wrist with ulnar deviation.
Test of muscle function: Flexion and ulnar deviation of the wrist against resistance (Figure 4.57).

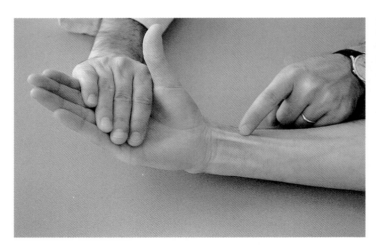

Figure 4.56. Counterflexion of the wrist allows one to test the flexor carpi radialis and palmaris longus; the tendons are accessible to direct examination.

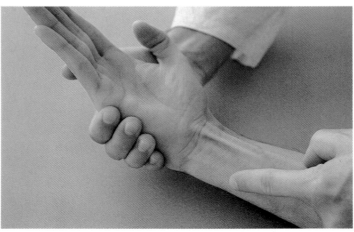

Figure 4.57. The flexor carpi ulnaris is evaluated by a movement counter to ulnar deviation and wrist flexion. Its tendon can be palpated at its insertion into the pisiform.

Extensor carpi radialis longus
Nerve supply. Radial nerve (C6, C7).
Action: Radial deviation and extension of the wrist.
Test of muscle function: Extends and deviates radially the wrist against resistance. The tendon is palpable over the base of the second metacarpal (Figure 4.58).

Extensor carpi radialis brevis
Nerve supply. Radial nerve (C6, C7).
Action: Extension of the wrist.
Test of muscle function: Extends the wrist against resistance. The tendon is palpable over the base of the third metacarpal (Figure 4.59).

On an anatomical preparation, traction on the ECRL causes marked radial deviation of the wrist (Figure 4.60). Traction on the ECRB also causes radial deviation, though less pronounced (Figure 4.61). In reestablishment of wrist extension by tendon transfer after paralysis, the motor tendon should be inserted in the ERCB and ECRL

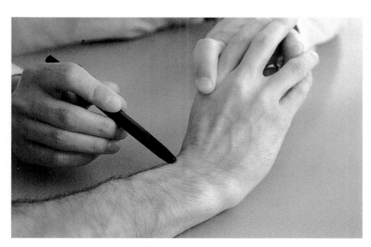

Figure 4.58. Isolated contraction of the extensor carpi radialis longus effects radial deviation of the hand when the wrist is extended. Its tendon is palpable over the base of the second metacarpal.

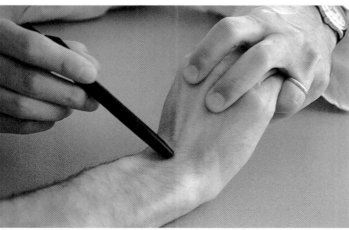

Figure 4.59. Only the extensor carpi radialis brevis is able by itself to effect direct extension of the wrist. Its tendon is palpable over the base of the third metacarpal.

303

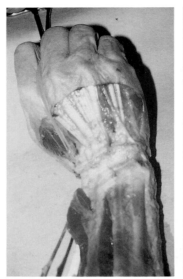 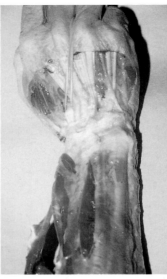 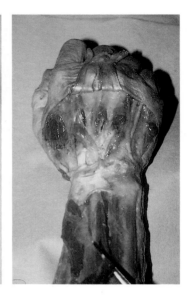

Figure 4.60. Traction of the extensor carpi radialis longus causes marked radial deviation.

Figure 4.61. Traction on the extensor carpi radialis brevis causes less marked radial deviation.

Figure 4.62. Correction of wrist extension by traction or by tendon transfer on ECRB and L after centralization of the ECRL tendon.

tendons after centralization of the ECRL tendon on the ulnar side of the base of the third metacarpal (Tubiana et al, 1989; Figure 4.62).

Extensor carpi ulnaris
Nerve supply. Radial nerve (C7).
Action. Extensor of the wrist in supination, ulnar deviation in pronation.
Test of muscle function. Ulnar deviation of the wrist against resistance in pronation. The tendon is palpable over the base of the fifth metacarpal (Figure 4.63).

Analysis of the movements of the fingers

Finger flexion
Finger flexion is brought about by the flexor digitorum superficialis, flexor digitorum profundus, and the interosseous muscles.

Finger extension
Finger extension is brought about by the extensor digitorum communis, extensor indicis proprius, extensor digiti quinti proprius, and the interosseous and lumbrical muscles.

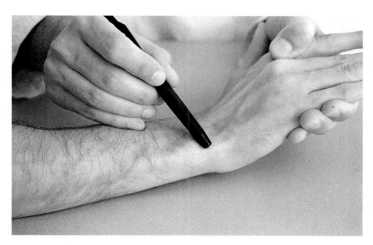

Figure 4.63. The extensor carpi ulnaris is evaluated by counterextension and ulnar deviation of the wrist. Its tendon can be felt at its insertion on the fifth metacarpal.

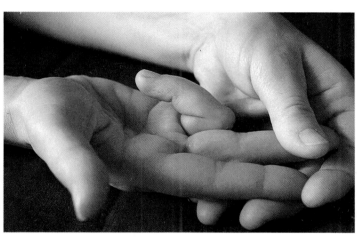

Figure 4.64. Testing the flexor digitorum superficialis.

Finger abduction
Finger abduction is brought about by the dorsal interosseous muscles and the abductor digiti quinti.

Finger adduction
Finger adduction is brought about by the palmar interosseous muscles.

Flexor digitorum superficialis
Nerve supply. Median nerve (C7, C8, T1).
Action. Flexion of the proximal interphalangeal joint.
Test of muscle function. Active flexion of the proximal interphalangeal joint of one finger while all the other fingers are held in full extension (Figure 4.64) to eliminate the action of the flexor profundus.

305

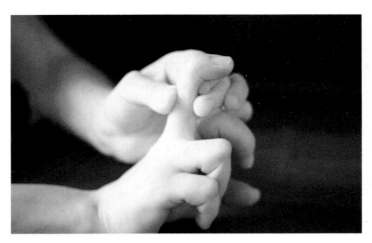

Figure 4.65. The flexor profundus flexes the distal phalanx. If the wrist and the two proximal joints of a finger are put into extension, and the muscle body is kept on tension, contractions can be detected.

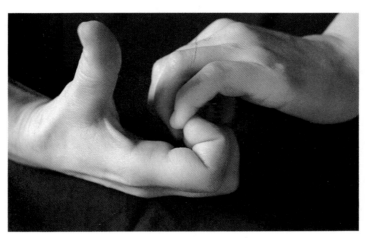

Figure 4.66. The strength of the flexor profundus is evaluated by applying counterpressure to the pulp on the flexed fingers.

Flexor digitorum profundus

Nerve supply. Median nerve (volar interosseous branch; C8, T1) for the index and long fingers; ulnar nerve (C8, T1) for the ring and little fingers.

Action. Flexion of the distal interphalangeal joint.

Test of muscle function. Flexion of the distal phalanx; the two proximal phalanges are held in extension (Figures 4.65 and 4.66).

Extensor digitorum communis

Nerve supply. Radial nerve (C7).

Action. Active extension of the metacarpophalangeal joints of the fingers.

Test of muscle function. Extension of the proximal phalanx against resistance (Figure 4.67).

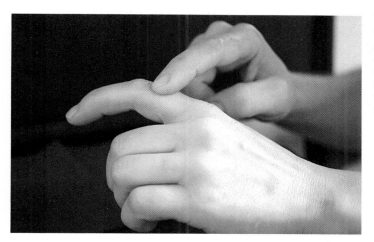

Figure 4.67. Evaluation of the extensor muscle. Passive dorsiflexion of the wrist excludes automatic metacarpophalangeal extension by a tenodesis effect; resistance is applied to the dorsal aspect of the proximal phalanx.

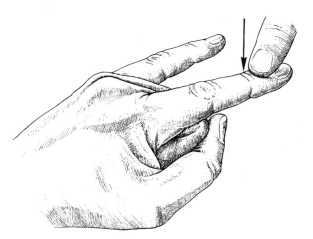

Figure 4.68. Testing extensor indicis proprius and extensor digiti quinti proprius.

Extensor indicis proprius
Nerve supply. Radial nerve (C7).
Action. Extension of the metacarpophalangeal joint of the index finger.
Test of muscle function. With the metacarpophalangeal joints of the long and ring fingers completely flexed to eliminate the action of the extensor communis, the proximal phalanx of the index finger is extended against resistance (Figure 4.68).

Extensor digiti quinti proprius
Nerve supply. Radial nerve (C7).
Action. Extension of the metacarpophalangeal joint of the little finger.
Test of muscle function. With the metacarpophalangeal joints of the long and ring fingers completely flexed, the proximal phalanx of the little finger is extended against resistance (Figure 4.68).

307

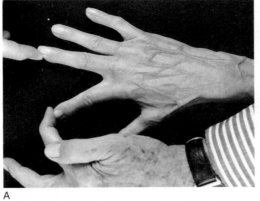

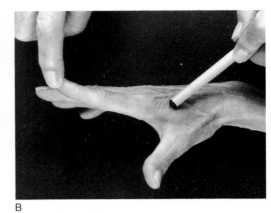

A

B

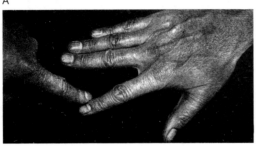

C

Figure 4.69. (A) The first dorsal interosseous muscle effects active strong radial deviation of the index finger. (B) The muscle belly is palpable; its strength is evaluated by applying counterpressure to the radial side of the finger. (C) The first palmar interosseus is evaluated by applying counterpressure to the ulnar side of the index finger.

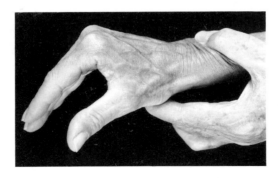

Figure 4.70. The interosseous muscles alone are capable of flexing the metacarpophalangeal joints simultaneously, with extension of the interphalangeal joints. This is the intrinsic-plus position.

Interosseous muscles

Nerve supply. Ulnar nerve (C8).

Action. The interosseous muscles as a group flex the metacarpophalangeal joints and extend the proximal and distal interphalangeal joints. The dorsal interosseous muscles abduct the index, ring, and little fingers away from the long finger. The palmar interosseous muscles are adductors.

Test of muscle function. Side to side movements of the fingers are partly dependent on the action of the extrinsic muscles. Each finger is tested separately with the metacarpophalangeal joint extended (Figures 4.69–4.71).

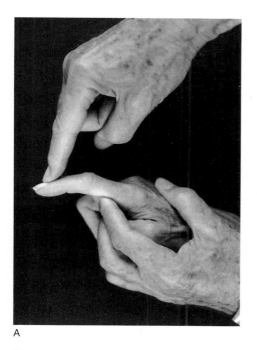
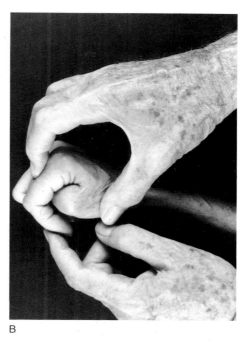

A   B

Figure 4.71. (A) By putting the metacarpophalangeal joints into extension first, one can demonstrate a contracture of the interosseous muscles of the corresponding finger, which keeps the interphalangeal joints extended. (B) When the proximal phalanx is flexed, the distal phalanges can be flexed.

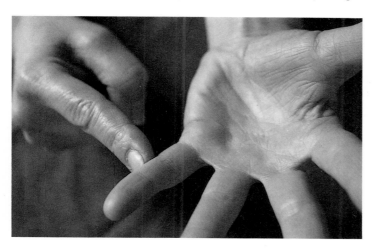

Figure 4.72. The abductor digiti minimi effects strong ulnar deviation of the finger. The contraction of its muscle belly is visible, and its strength can be evaluated by applying counterpressure on the ulnar border of the proximal phalanx.

Abductor digiti minimi
Nerve supply. Ulnar nerve (C8).
Action. Abducts the little finger and flexes the metacarpophalangeal joint.
Test of muscle function. Abduction of the little finger against resistance (Figure 4.72).

309

Opponens digiti minimi
Nerve supply. Ulnar nerve (C8).
Action. Flexion of the fifth metacarpal.
Test of muscle function. Flexion of the fifth metacarpal against resistance (Figure 4.73).

Flexor digiti minimi
Nerve supply. Ulnar nerve (C8).
Action. Abduction of the little finger. Cannot be tested specifically.

Analysis of the movements of the thumb

Flexion
Flexion is produced by the flexor pollicis longus and the flexor pollicis brevis.

Extension
Extension is produced by the extensor pollicis longus and extensor pollicis brevis.

Pronation
Pronation is produced by the abductor pollicis brevis and flexor pollicis brevis.

Supination
Supination is produced by the adductor pollicis and extensor pollicis longus.

Analysis of the movements of the first metacarpal

Anteposition
Anteposition is produced by the abductor pollicis brevis and opponens pollicis.

Retroposition
Retroposition is produced by the extensor pollicis longus.

Flexion–adduction
Flexion–adduction is produced by the adductor pollicis and flexor pollicis brevis.

Extension–abduction
Extension–abduction is produced by the abductor pollicis longus.

Opposition
Opposition is a combined movement involving all three segments of the thumb column: the first metacarpal moves in anteposition and then in flexion–adduction. This movement is accompanied by an "automatic" longitudinal rotation into pronation. The proximal phalanx flexes, pronates, and radially deviates (Figure 4.74). The distal phalanx flexes and slightly pronates (see Chapter 3).

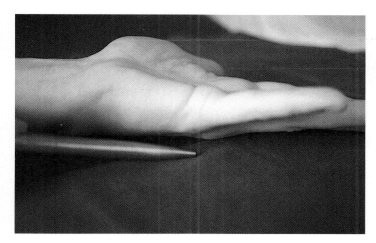

Figure 4.73. The opponens digiti minimi performs active flexion of the fifth metacarpal. Palmar counterpressure on its head can be used to evaluate its strength.

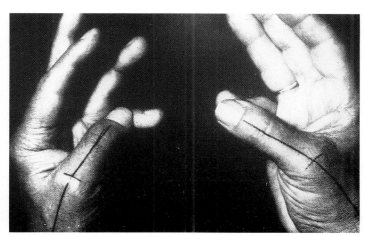

Figure 4.74. Opposition of the thumb. The proximal phalanx flexes, pronates and radially deviates.

Flexor pollicis longus
Nerve supply. Median nerve (C8, T1).
Action. Flexion of the interphalangeal joint of the thumb.
Test of muscle function. Flexion of the distal phalanx of the thumb against resistance (Figure 4.75).

Extensor pollicis longus
Nerve supply. Radial nerve (C7).
Action. Extension of the interphalangeal joint and of the metacarpophalangeal joint of the thumb as well as retroposition, adduction, and supination of the thumb column.
Test of muscle function. Retroposition of the thumb column (Figure 4.76).

311

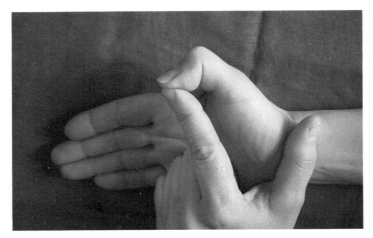

Figure 4.75. Flexion of the interphalangeal joint of the thumb against resistance applied to the pulp makes it possible to evaluate the strength of the flexor pollicis longus.

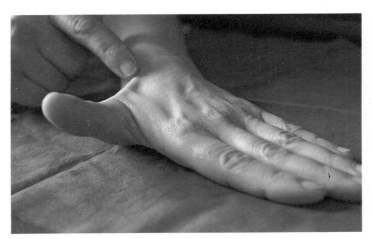

Figure 4.76. Only the extensor pollicis longus is capable of effecting active retropulsion of the column of the thumb and active interphalangeal hyperextension of the thumb.

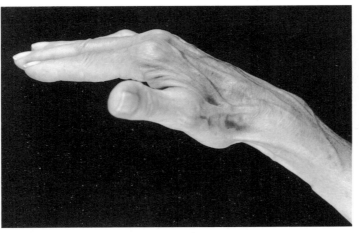

Figure 4.77. Extension of the metacarpophalangeal joint of the thumb simultaneously brings into play the short and long extensors. Evaluation of the short extensor by counter-pressure on the dorsal aspect of the proximal phalanx is not as reliable as when the interphalangeal joint is semiflexed.

Extensor pollicis brevis
Nerve supply. Radial nerve (C7).
Action: Extension of the metacarpophalangeal joint of the thumb.
Test of muscle function: Extension of the proximal phalanx with the distal phalanx semiflexed (Figure 4.77).

Abductor pollicis longus
Nerve supply. Radial nerve (C7).
Action: Radial abduction of the thumb column.
Test of muscle function: The patient is asked to move his thumb in radial abduction; the tension of the tendon is felt on the extensor border of the anatomical snuffbox (Figure 4.78).

A

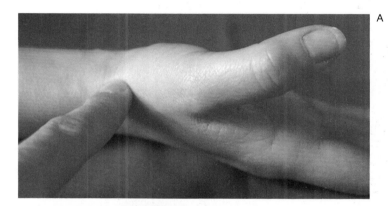

B

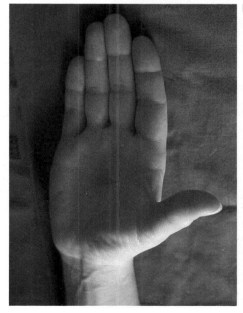

Figure 4.78. (A) Tension in the abductor pollicis longus palpable at the anterior border of the snuffbox is perceptible at the beginning of antepulsion, before the short abductor comes into play. (B) Separation of the thumb in the plane of the palm is effected by the abductor pollicis longus and extensor pollicis brevis.

313

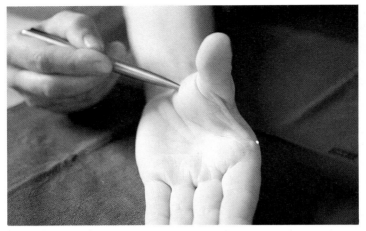

Figure 4.79. The abductor pollicis brevis performs antepulsion of the column of the thumb accompanied by pronation and radial deviation. Its strength can be evaluated by applying resistance to the radial aspect of the proximal phalanx.

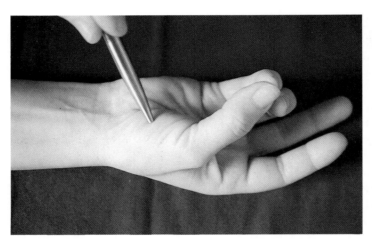

Figure 4.80. The contraction of the muscle belly of the opponens is perceptible in the pulp-to-pulp opposition of the thumb against the little finger.

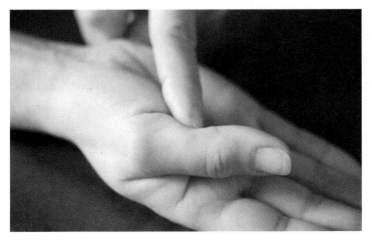

Figure 4.81. Testing muscle function of the flexor pollicis brevis.

Abductor pollicis brevis
Nerve supply: Median nerve (C6, C7).
Action: Anteposition of the thumb column in the plane perpendicular to the palm as well as lateral deviation and pronation of the proximal phalanx.
Test of muscle function: Anteposition of the thumb against resistance (Figure 4.79).

Opponens pollicis
Nerve supply: Median nerve (C6, C7).
Action: Anteposition of the first metacarpal.
Test of muscle function: Direct palpation of the muscle during anteposition of the thumb against resistance (Figure 4.80).

Flexor pollicis brevis
Nerve supply: Median nerve (C6, C7) for the superficial portion; ulnar nerve (C8) for the deep portion.
Action: Flexion of the metacarpophalangeal joint of the thumb as well as flexion–adduction and pronation of the thumb column.
Test of muscle function: Difficult to demonstrate unless the other thenar muscles are paralyzed (Figure 4.81).

Adductor pollicis
Nerve supply: Ulnar nerve (C8).
Action: Approximation of the first to the second metacarpal, flexion–adduction and supination of the thumb column, and extension of the distal phalanx.
Test of muscle function: Approximation of the first and second metacarpals, without flexing the thumb (to eliminate the flexor pollicis longus action) and the wrist extended (to relax the extensor pollicis longus; Figure 4.82).

Difficulties in testing voluntary movements

Errors of interpretation can have serious consequences. They are due to associated lesions, compensatory movements, and trick movements.

Associated lesions

Associated traumatic or post-traumatic lesions not involving nerves, such as tendon divisions, bone and joint injuries, adhesions, and stiffness, can interfere with muscle movements.

Compensatory movements

One must always remember that no muscle functions in isolation and that the simplest movements require the participation of several muscles (which may well be supplied by different nerve roots). The prime movers, which initiate the movement, are assisted by synergists and checked by antagonists and stabilizers. The final movement results from the modulation of these various forces.

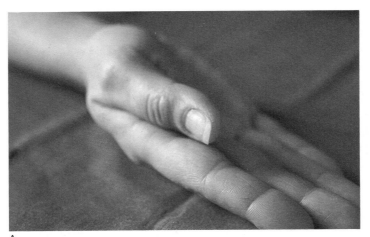

A

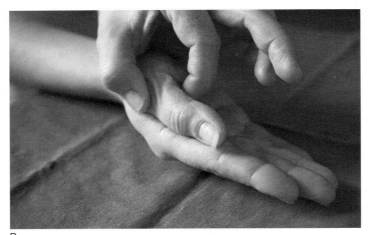

B

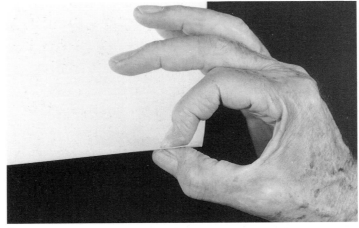

C

Figure 4.82. The strength of active closure of the first commissure (A) is evaluated by trying to separate the first and second metacarpals, held voluntarily closed. However, the long muscles of the thumb participate in this adduction. (B) Participation of the adductor pollicis in closure of the commissure can be verified by direct palpation of the transverse fibers during thumb–index finger pinch. (C) When the thumb is forced against the index finger, compensatory flexion of the interphalangeal joint is a sign of weakness of the adductor muscle of the thumb (Froment's sign).

The examiner should always take into account possible muscle "compensation." A muscle may have a secondary action, which is usually masked and becomes evident only when the adjacent muscles are paralyzed. Thus, the brachioradialis by itself can flex the elbow when the biceps and brachialis are paralyzed; the extensor digitorum communis can extend the interphalangeal joints if the interosseous muscles are paralyzed, provided the metacarpophalangeal joints are stabilized and hyperextension is prevented (see Figure 2.32). The dorsal expansions of the thenar muscles can extend the distal phalanx of the thumb in paralysis of the extensor pollicis longus, and the abductor pollicis longus can flex the wrist when the flexors are paralyzed.

Deceptive or trick movements

Trick movements have a number of causes, one of which is the effect of gravity (Jones, 1919). For example, when one is testing the function of the triceps muscle, the shoulder should be abducted to 90 degrees and internally rotated; thus the muscle can be tested with gravity eliminated. Gravity itself will cause extension of the elbow, even when the triceps is paralyzed, in certain positions of the arm.

Moreover, sudden relaxation of a contracting muscle whose antagonist is paralyzed can simulate movement in the latter; this is seen in paralysis of the long flexors of the fingers when sudden relaxation of the extensors triggers passive flexion of the metacarpophalangeal joint. In a multiarticular kinetic chain, such as the hand, the extrinsic tendons of the fingers cross several joints. Movements of the proximal joint, e.g. the wrist, can have a tenodesis effect and produce movements of the phalanges. Conversely, in radial palsy, flexion of the fingers can extend the wrist (Figure 4.83).

The commonest sources of error, however, are anomalous innervation and variations in the territories of nerve supply. Such variations are seen most often with the flexor digitorum profundus communis and with the thenar muscles. The territories can be differentiated only by means of selective trunk anesthesia (Highet, 1942).

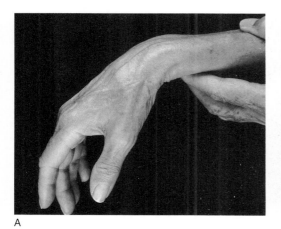
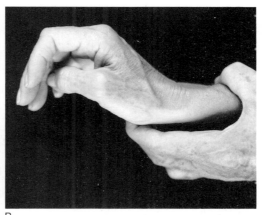

A B

Figure 4.83. (A) In radial palsy, flexion of the fingers (B) can extend the wrist.

Testing sensory function

Testing sensation is an essential part of the examination of the hand (see Section 4.3 on sensibility evaluation). The normal cutaneous sensory distribution of the nerve roots and the individual peripheral nerves are shown in Figures 4.84 and 4.85. Sensory skin territories have ill-defined boundaries, and adjacent territories overlap extensively. Thus, sectioning of the radial nerve may produce little to no clinically detectable anesthesia on the dorsum of the hand. The so-called "autonomous" zone of skin supply is much smaller than its potential sensory territory.

Scales for the assessment of sensibility, more or less similar to the motor scales, are based mainly on the British Medical Research Council scale (Seddon, 1975).

Sensory recovery

S0: Absence of sensibility in the autonomous area

S1: Recovery of deep cutaneous pain sensibility within autonomous area of nerve

S2: Return of some degree of superficial cutaneous pain and tactile sensibility within the autonomous area of the nerve

S3: Return of superficial cutaneous pain and tactile sensibility throughout the autonomous area, with disappearance of any previous over-response

S3+: Return of sensibility as in stage 3, with some recovery of two point discrimination within the autonomous area

S4: Complete recovery

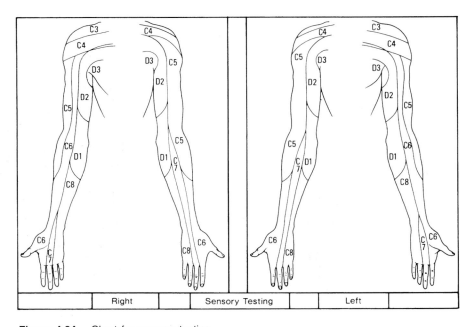

Figure 4.84. Chart for sensory testing.

318

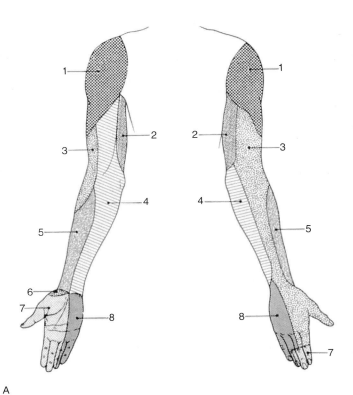

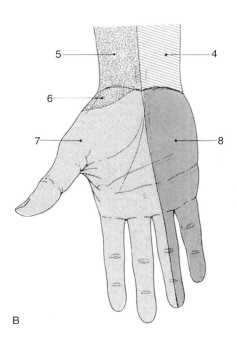

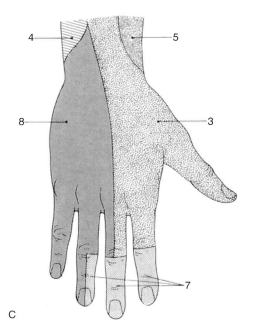

Figure 4.85. (A) Cutaneous sensory distribution of the peripheral nerves of the upper limb. (B) Volar aspect of the hand. (C) Dorsal aspect of the hand: (1) axillary nerve; (2) intercostobrachial nerve; (3) radial nerve; (4) medial cutaneous nerve of forearm and arm; (5) lateral cutaneous nerve of forearm (musculocutaneous nerve); (6) palmar cutaneous branch of radial nerve; (7) median nerve; (8) ulnar nerve. There is a considerable variation in the cutaneous areas supplied by each nerve.

A

B

C

319

Pain assessment

Pain can interfere with all these functional tests, because it affects the normal activity of the patient. As with the Ritchie system, the most objective way of measuring pain is probably the centimeter scale (from 1 to 10) on which the patients themselves place a mark indicating the intensity of pain (10 = no pain, 0 = intolerable pain).

Deep sensibility

Study of deep sensibility is not in current use in surgical disorders of the hand, because problems of deep sensation of the hand are less important than those of superficial sensation in lesions of nerve trunks.

Occasionally one must evaluate deep sensibility with precision when palliative surgery is contemplated in cases of central paralysis and in pure lesions of the motor cortex, as, for instance, in infantile hemiplegia. In such cases one must evaluate the state of basic deep sensation while looking at the same time for disruption of the position sense of the fingers.

Joint-position sense

In order to test joint-position sense, the examiner holds each side of the digit and flexes or extends the interphalangeal joints. The patient, who has his eyes closed, reports the position of the joints and can be asked to mimic this position by moving the normal contralateral digits. Sensibility to pressure is tested by asking the patient to weigh in his hand objects of different weights. Sensation to vibration is determined by using a tuning fork placed on the metacarpal heads and on the radial and ulnar styloid processes.

Stereognosis

The study of recognition of the shapes of objects, or stereognosis, is an important part of this examination, because this ability is necessary for the hand to keep its functional value, no matter what partial substitution may be provided by vision when deep sensation is lacking. One can evaluate only the extent to which this sensibility is preserved.

Stereognosis can be lost by two mechanisms. Sometimes objects are not recognized because their shape, size, texture, and weight are poorly identified. In other cases these different characteristics are correctly analyzed but the patient is unable to correlate them or to recognize in them the significant characteristics for identification of the object. These purely tactile asymbolisms are rare.

Assessing sympathetic function

It is customary to group arbitrarily under the heading "sympathetic" the various trophic disorders that follow peripheral nerve lesions. Lesions of the sympathetic fibers have a direct action on sweating and circulation. Other so-called "trophic disorders" depend on both sensory and sympathetic fibers.

After sectioning of a peripheral nerve, one often sees changes in the texture of the skin, which becomes dry, loses its elasticity, and develops a thinner epithelium. The nails become striated and brittle; their growth is slowed. The hairs may be longer and bushier, and elsewhere they atrophy and disappear, especially in patients with causalgia. In such patients the skin is often cyanosed, an indication of reduced blood flow. As a rule, the temperature of the skin is lower in the paralyzed zone, and even after re-innervation the part remains sensitive to cold. The consistency of the subcutaneous tissues also changes: the fat pads of the pulps and palm atrophy; this is most evident in the index finger after median nerve palsy. Atrophy of the skin, changes in blood flow, loss of sensation, and impairment of protective reflexes all increase the risk of injury and predispose to ulceration. These appear readily as a result of repeated minor trauma, pressure, or burns. Healing is slow to occur. The exposed anesthetic zones must be protected by wearing gloves, and the patient should be warned against injuries, which may lead to mutilation.

Electrical tests in lesions of the peripheral nerves

Electrodiagnosis tests are particularly useful for the detection, localization, and prognosis of lesions of the peripheral nerves (see Section 4.4 on electrodiagnosis). They include electromyography, nerve conduction speed measurements distal to the lesion, and the study of action potentials.

Global movements in the hand

In the course of a routine clinical examination it is impossible to test the whole motor system of the hand. In this section, therefore, we shall consider movements that contribute to everyday manual activities and study overall function rather than individual muscle action. Such function is the result of a number of factors affecting the joints (stiffness), the muscles (power), the tendons (adhesions or deviation), and the skin (scars). A test of function therefore is not used to diagnose or localize a specific lesion, as this has been dealt with already. We shall study the movements involved in opening and closing the hand, in opposition, and in the common grips.

Opening the hand

The movements involved in opening the hand determine the maximal size of the object that can be grasped. Such movements can thus be studied by asking the patient to grasp cylindrical objects of increasing sizes up to 11 cm in diameter, which usually represents the limb of cylindrical grasp.

In the fingers, the quality of the movements depends on the efficiency of the extensor muscles (radial palsy) and the mobility of the joints (hyperextension of one joint may sometimes compensate for fixed flexion in another). One flexed finger is sufficient to prevent the hand from grasping a sizeable object.

321

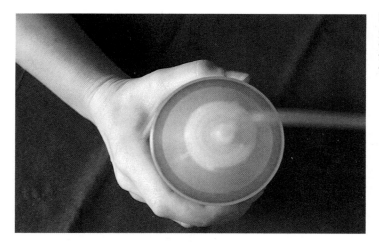

Figure 4.86. The size of objects that can be gripped by opening the hand depends on the ability of the first web space to open up.

In the thumb the movements depend on the ability of the first web space to open up (Figure 4.86). This is achieved by the action of the extensors and abductors of the thumb, but passive opening of the web depends on the absence of contracture of the skin and of the thumb adductor muscle and on the mobility of the carpometacarpal and metacarpophalangeal joints. Hyperextension of the latter may compensate to a certain extent for stiffness of the former.

Closing the fingers

As we have seen earlier, closing of the fingers involves a sequence wherein the metacarpophalangeal joint, proximal interphalangeal joint, and distal interphalangeal joint are flexed in turn. If this normal sequence is disturbed and the interphalangeal joints are the first to flex, grasping of a large object will become impossible.

The amplitude of the flexion, however, determines the size of the smallest object that the closed fingers can hold safely. It also determines the strength with which objects of a slightly larger size can be held. This amplitude depends on the range of mobility of the flexors, the suppleness of the joints, the overall flexor power, and the pliability of the soft tissues. It is usually best appreciated in terms of the distal palmar crease.

Normal morphological variations and the usual presence of two distinct creases define this landmark as a transverse line joining the ulnar end of the distal palmar crease to the radial end of the proximal palmar crease (Figure 4.87). In the normal hand the terminal part of the four digital pulps can be actively brought into contact with the palm along this line (Figure 4.88). When the fingers come into contact with the palm on the proximal side of this landmark, this usually implies a flexion deficit in the interphalangeal joints, which is more or less compensated for by increased metacarpophalangeal flexion (Figure 4.89). If the flexion deficit is more severe, the pulps will fail to reach the palm. The overall flexion deficit is then measured in terms of the distance in centimeters between the pulps and the palm (Figure 4.90).

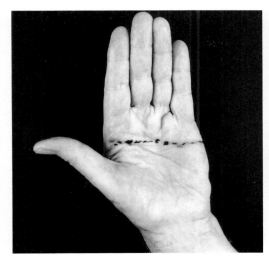

Figure 4.87. The transverse palmar crease for reference is a line joining the ulnar extremity of the distal palmar crease to the radial extremity of the proximal palmar crease.

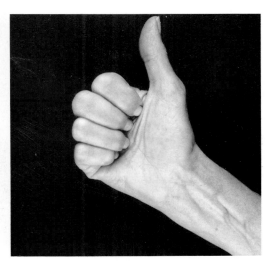

Figure 4.88. Complete flexion brings the distal extremities of the pulps to the palmar crease.

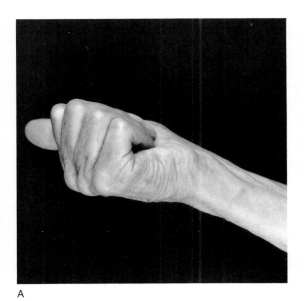

A

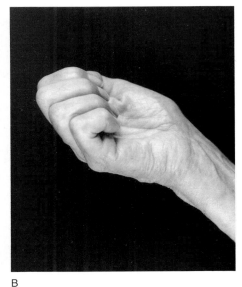

B

Figure 4.89. (A) Isolated interphalangeal stiffness can be compensated for by hyperflexion at the metacarpophalangeal joint. However, the pulps then touch "proximal" to the palmar crease. (B) Isolated metacarpophalangeal stiffness can be compensated for by interphalangeal hyperflexion, but the pulps then touch the palm distal to the palmar crease.

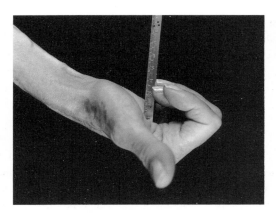

Figure 4.90. When the fingers cannot reach the palm, the palm-pulp distance in centimeters measures the lack of flexion.

Opposition

From the point of view of the mechanics and of the motor muscles involved, the movement of opposition is particularly complex (see pp. 193–99). We shall consider it under three headings.

1 The ability of the thumb successively to oppose the four fingers during the "long range" of the first metacarpal, that is, staying wide of the palm and keeping the first web space open. As long as this ability is retained, opposition will be virtually normal.
2 The ability of the thumb to oppose successively the four fingers during the short range of the first metacarpal, that is, with the first commissure closed. Preservation of only this type of opposition constitutes a major functional handicap.
3 Rotation of the pulp of the thumb, which determines the efficiency of a pulp grip. Between the position of full extension and abduction of the thumb in the plane of the palm and that of opposition with the little finger, pulp rotation may reach 90 to 120 degrees. It is normally possible to place the pulps of the thumb and little finger in the same plane at the end of the movement of opposition.

A simple method of assessing opposition of the thumb has been proposed by Kapandji (1986) using the patient's own hand as a reference point and allowing for comparison with a normal hand. It requires no special apparatus and gives an unequivocal numerical score for the functional range of movement of the hand. The degree of opposition of the thumb ranges from merely touching the lateral aspect of the index finger gradually reaching across the hand to touch the tip of each of the individual fingers and finally working its way down the palmar aspect of the little finger towards the ulnar end of the transverse palmar crease (see Figure 2.17).

Functional assessment

In addition to range of movement it is often necessary to have some assessment of global hand function, particularly to evaluate the hand with multiple pathologies such as the rheumatoid hand.

324

Assessment of function is useful to assess the patient's condition and to detect whether it is deteriorating. Preoperative and postoperative assessment of function will allow an objective assessment of hand surgery performed. If repeated at intervals postoperatively it will also give some indication of the durability of that surgical procedure allowing comparison of varying surgical procedures and a choice of the best based on objective measurements.

Traditionally, hand function has been assessed by hand therapists using an assessment of activities of daily living and, although these relate directly to the patient's activities and handicaps, they are very time consuming and highly subjective. Often the test is too insensitive to measure quality of function rather than the patient's ability to perform a specific task. For instance, it may be that the patient is unable to turn a key in a lock, and if they fall just short of the mark, this would be recorded as a complete inability to turn a key. Clearly what is required is some way of quantitatively and objectively assessing how much key-turning force the patient is capable of producing and only when this is known can it later be assessed whether the patient is deteriorating or whether they have improved as a result of a surgical procedure.

With a quantitative objective measurement the threshold of force required to perform a particular task can also be measured. It may also be possible to predict how far away the patient is from that crucial threshold. The importance of this is that patients who are particularly close to the threshold but deteriorating could be given priority for the reconstructive surgery that has been shown to improve that particular function.

Function of the hand is highly intricate and as such involves many factors, anatomical and psychological. The best way to minimize the influence of all these factors to allow an objective assessment is to use the patient's opposite hand as a control, if it is normal. Although there is an approximately 5–10 per cent difference between dominant and non-dominant hands, this is a smaller difference than the vast variations between patients.

Grip strength is one aspect of function which is amenable to objective and repeatable measurement. However it is often done with unfamiliar equipment and measures only a single static reading, which may bear little relationship to the patient's actual function. The Jamar grip strength meter (see Figure 4.100) shown is an example of this, it is not possible for patients with rheumatoid arthritis of the wrist to use this effectively. A fair degree of understanding is often necessary from the patient before they can comply with the test correctly. A simple compromise would be to measure the force available for performing simple everyday tasks. These tasks have been chosen because they illustrate the standard grip positions of the hand.

lateral pinch	turning a key
terminal pinch grip	gripping a pen-shaped object
tripod grip	” ”
diagonal grip	turning a door knob
span grip	opening the lid of a coffee jar
extended grip	lifting a plate

Each of these common functional maneuvers can be assessed by a simple strain gauge to which a series of different tests are attached in turn. Each test takes a few seconds to perform and with a connection to a microcomputer with analogue input, a graphic display of force and time can be given on the screen and printed on paper for the patient's notes.

Not only peak forces can be assessed but also decay with time. This helps to eliminate the effect of stoical patients who will hurt themselves to achieve high initial force but are unable to maintain this. It is also possible to know the threshold value below which, for example, a key cannot be turned in a lock. This threshold can be drawn automatically on the graph and the patient's position in relation to it noted. The most important use of these objective repeatable measurements is for surgeons and therapist to assess the success of their own activities and so allow them to plan further efficacitions treatment for their patients.

Nature and power of the common grips

(*See* "Grip and prehension" pages 161–8 and "Grasp and prehension" pages 343–4.)

"Spherical" grip

The "spherical" grip is used to catch hold of rounded objects. The four fingers and the thumb are extended and play an equal part in the grip. Grip is tested by asking the patient to lift a rounded object (e.g. an ashtray).

"Cylindrical" grip, or grasp

Grasp is the commonest form of power grip; it is used for handling tools and machinery controls. It is produced by wrapping the flexed thumb and fingers around the object. The size of the object that can be grasped depends, as we have seen, on the ability of the fingers to close. This grip is tested by using objects of decreasing size.

Prehensile force usually means the power grip. It is measured with a metal blade dynamometer of standard caliber (see Figure 4.100). The readings are interpreted by comparison with the contralateral limb because there are wide individual differences.

According to a study by Swanson (1960), the dominant hand is only 5–10 per cent more powerful than its counterpart. However, these figures are probably valid only in a population whose left-handed members are not taught to alter their dominance.

Age and sex also have an influence on the force of prehension, the average for women being one-third to one-half that for men. In men prehensile force decreases after the age of 50 (in women after 40) by about 10–20 per cent.

Thumb–finger pinch

Measurement of thumb–finger pinch requires a special dynamometer because the forces generated are smaller (see Figure 4.101).

The thumb–unidigital pulp-to-pulp pinch is not frequently used. Its clinical study is the basis for Froment's sign. The patient holds a sheet of paper between the pulp of the thumb and that of the index finger, and the examiner tries to pull it away. If the adductor pollicis is paralyzed, the patient, in an effort to hold on to the sheet, will flex the distal phalanx of the thumb (positive Froment's sign). It is worth noting, however, that the strongest thumb–unidigital pinch is that involving the middle finger.

The only common thumb–unidigital pinch is the terminoterminal hold between the thumb and index finger, which is used for picking up very small objects. The important factor here is not so much the force as the sensitivity of the pulps, which is responsible for its precision.

The most common thumb–digital pinch is that between the pulps of the thumb, index, and middle fingers. This hold is most powerful when the interphalangeal joint of the thumb is extended. It is studied by asking the patient to unscrew a bottle top or to hold a small cylindrical object (pen or pencil), which the examiner tries to pull away. The power of this grip, measured with an adapted dynamometer, varies between one-fifth and one-sixth of the so-called force of prehension.

In the subterminal lateral pinch (or key pinch), the proximal part of the pulp of the thumb is opposed to the lateral aspect of the middle phalanx of the index finger. It must be examined because of its practical importance (Figure 4.91). It is usually slightly weaker than the tridigital pinch already described. In major multiple palsies, it is often the only type of pinch that can be restored by palliative surgery.

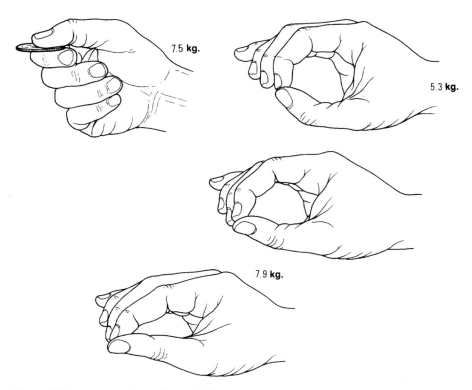

Figure 4.91. Average force of pollicidigital pinch.

4.3 SENSIBILITY EVALUATION

Introduction

Although sensibility evaluation of the hands has been studied for centuries, it is still by no means completely understood. Much of the literature and widely practiced techniques of sensibility evaluation remain in need of further scientific investigation.

Sensory receptors in the skin

The many techniques for testing sensibility confirm that we have much to learn about the tactile cutaneous system innervated by the peripheral nerves. Although it is accepted that there are differentiated sensory receptors in the skin which respond to mechanical and thermal stimuli, a complete understanding of these receptors remains elusive. Each receptor has a unique transfer function, which converts the stimulus to encoded information in a stream of action potentials. These are in turn transferred to the cerebral cortex where they are interpreted.

There are two types of receptors, based on their speed of response:

- pacinian corpuscles, which respond quickly to a stimulus but then begin to fade; and
- merkel discs, which respond more slowly but continue to give a sustained response.

These two types of receptors play an important part in the differentiation of touch. Experiments show, however, that the response of some receptors falls in between that of the usual slowly or quickly adapting receptors. The role of these "in-between" responses and how they work together with others in sensibility has yet to be determined (Bell-Krotoski, 1991; Jarvilehto, 1977; Vallbo and Johansson, 1978).

Quality of sensory function

Moberg (1960) long emphasized that the important factor in sensory function is one of quality and not merely the presence or absence of sensibility. He observed, "Why should the mere perception of touch or pain by the hand be accepted as a sign of normal sensation, when the perception of light is never identified with the normal capacity to see?"

We must therefore question whether hand sensibility as it pertains to function can be discussed merely on the basis of known modalities for touch, pain, cold, and warmth. Testing the skin with a safety pin for pain, with cotton wool for touch, and with test tube contact for warmth or cold has its limitations. Tests that apply a stimulus that is too variable cannot approach the sensitivity of the cutaneous sensory system. In addition, variation in application on repeated applications and from examiner to examiner makes it difficult to duplicate these tests periodically and obtain comparable quantitative results (Omer and Spinner, 1975).

Reliability and reproducibility of tests

The goal of evaluating the end result of a nerve repair has increased the need for clinicians to insist on reliability and validity (Fess, 1986) in the testing instruments they use before they can have confidence in the data. We need to know whether one type of surgical technique is better than another. Postoperative results must be compared with the preoperative status to indicate whether the repaired nerve is recovering and how well the patient can use his hand with the limited nerve supply he may have. What can he expect? The goal of sensibility testing is to evaluate this recovery on a quantitative anatomical basis and on a functional basis.

Moberg (1978) defined the problem by stating that only the pooled results from many centers can provide us with answers, but to be meaningful these data must result from measurements taken on an identical scale with identical devices. Most current clinical instruments used for testing sensibility lack the necessary sensitivity and are too variable. As a result, even if these instruments have been used in controlled clinical studies, or are in common use, their results cannot be replicated with repeated testing. As a consequence, changes in sensibility may go unrecognized, and may only be detected in the later stages of peripheral nerve abnormality, when treatment is likely to be less effective. Furthermore, early detection of reduced sensation is vital to prevent the patient from unintentional self-inflicted damage, which can occur with reduced protective sensation.

Sensibility tests

Sensibility tests are divided into three main categories:

- threshold tests
- functional tests
- objective tests.

Threshold tests

Threshold tests assess cutaneous function and include:

- pinprick perception
- temperature perception
- light touch–deep pressure
- vibration.

Pinprick perception

Protective sensation is the ability to perceive painful or potentially harmful stimuli on the skin and in the subcutaneous tissue. The most commonly used test of protective sensation is the safety pin. Testing for protective sensation with a pin requires that the patient be able to differentiate between the sharp and dull sides of the pin. It is not

329

enough to require the patient to say "touch" when touched with the sharp end of the pin because he may be respondingly simply to the pressure of the stimulus and not to the sharpness.

The tester must keep in mind that during nerve regeneration there can be a period of hypersensitivity to pinprick. In such an area, the response to pinprick will be hyperacute and extremely unpleasant for the patient. Therefore, the number of applications in one zone of the hand should be minimized. The uninvolved hand is tested first in order to determine the amount of pressure necessary to evoke correct responses: this is used as a guide for the pressure to be used on the involved hand (Callahan 1990).

Sunderland (1978) noted that the perception of pinprick ranges along a hierarchy that includes:

- absence of awareness
- pressure sensation without distinguishing between sharp and dull
- hyperanalgesia with radiation
- sharp sensation with some radiation and gross localization
- sensation of sharpness with or without slight stinging or radiation and fair localization
- normal perception.

Seddon (1975) likewise grades the response to pinprick along several parameters.

Temperature perception

Test tubes filled with hot and cold fluids are useful for determining protection from thermal or cold injury. However, the limitation of these instruments is gross if the temperatures are not carefully controlled. The tester can determine if the patient can distinguish between hot and cold, but not if the patient can distinguish between temperatures of, say, 1° C and 5° C, as the normal hand can. The tester also cannot determine if the patient can distinguish between +/– degrees of sensitivity along the entire range of very hot to very cold. The tester must be cautious in reporting that the patient has normal temperature sensation, if he has only tested hot and cold at one level in the range.

Because of this difficulty in controlling the variability of the temperature of the applied stimulus, test-tube testing within a test and between tests and its lack of correlation with functional sensation, many clinicians do not test for temperature, preferring to allow the presence of pinprick perception to be sufficient evidence of protective sensation. Others satisfy themselves with testing for determining the perception of cold and hot on a gross level (Callahan, 1990; Dellon, 1981; Moberg, 1962).

Light touch–deep pressure

Von Frey first described the use of graded stimuli to evaluate cutaneous sensibility in the late 1800s. In an attempt to standardize the technique, he found that horsehairs of varying thicknesses bend at specific milligrams of axial loading pressure. By pressing on the skin with a thorn glued to the end of a hair until the hair started to bow, von Frey obtained a measure of the pressure sensibility of nerve fibers in the skin. He calibrated the hairs on a balance, varying stiffness by changing length and by using hairs of different densities. He recorded pressure sensibility by noting whether a given hair touched to the skin produced any sensation.

In 1960, Semmes et al made the testing procedure more exact when they re-introduced von Frey's method, using nylon monofilaments mounted in Lucite rods. The monofilaments, known as the Semmes–Weinstein pressure aesthesiometer, are calibrated to exert specific pressures. Twenty filaments, graded in thickness, are included in the testing kit. The filaments are marked with numbers ranging from 1.65 to 6.65 (Figure 4.92). The filament number represents the logarithm of 10 multiplied by the force in milligrams required to bow the filament. Except for the very largest, all filaments buckle as the examiner presses them against the skin (Figure 4.93). As long as first-order

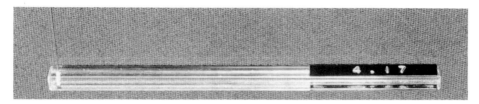

Figure 4.92. Twenty calibrated filaments, varying in pressure, are included in the testing kit. Close-up view of a filament.

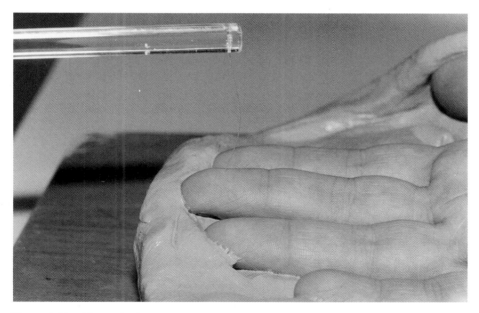

Figure 4.93. First-order buckling. The monofilament is applied perpendicular to the surface of the hand or digit surface. Pressure is increased until the monofilament bends. The patient's hand is supported in putty because motion of the hand misleadingly improves test results.

331

buckling is maintained, the pressure exerted on the skin varies only with the length and diameter of the calibrated filament, not with the force applied by the examiner. First-order buckling is the bowing produced in a properly applied Semmes–Weinstein filament when the examiner applies only those lateral forces necessary to keep the top end directly over the lower end when the filament is in contact with the skin (Levin et al, 1978). The filaments control the application force, because when they bend they reach a peak force, and maintain a constant force, within a very small deviation, until removed (Bell-Krotoski, 1992).

In 1967, von Prince and Butler used the Semmes–Weinstein monofilaments in a clinical setting to test light touch–deep pressure in patients with nerve injuries from war wounds. They required perception of touch by a given filament and localization of the area of touch for an accurate response. They correlated two-point discrimination and perception of light touch as measured by the monofilaments, and so were able to develop an interpretive scale that divides the patient's performance into graduated levels of sensibility. These levels are designated as:

- normal
- diminished light touch
- diminished protective sensation
- loss of protective sensation.

The stimulus is activated by the mechanical deformation of the skin. The filament bends the skin and skin deformation causes the firing of nerve endings. Despite variables, such as callousing of the hand and the age of the patient, the Semmes–Weinstein monofilaments are recognized as the best hand-held instrument to monitor sensory change or recovery, especially when the patient is repeatedly tested with the same instrument by the same tester (Bell and Buford, 1988). The monofilaments provide controlled, objective, reproducible force stimuli for testing peripheral nerve function. Implicit in this statement is the assumption that the monofilaments are of correct length and diameter. If these two measurements have been calibrated and are correct, the application forces of the filaments are repeatable within a predictable range (Bell-Krotoski and Tomancik, 1987).

Testing of the monofilament application forces has shown that the 20 monofilaments in the traditional filament kit may not all be necessary. Bell-Krotoski (1990a,b) reported that the variation in force range of one filament may overlap with its neighbor. Brand (1985) suggested that no more than five forces need to be used ordinarily in diagnostic tests, and perhaps only one or two for monitoring progress or recovery.

Therefore, the monofilaments used can be reduced in number with no significant loss in sensitivity of the test. Bell-Krotoski (1990a,b) reported that the "mini-kit" (Figure 4.94a) of five specially selected forces of the 20 available in the full Semmes–Weinstein kit is considered adequate for most testing. It is more cost effective and less time consuming than the full kit. The increments between the filaments in the mini-kit are spaced sufficiently far apart so that they do not overlap; thus, they can reliably show progressive return or diminution in peripheral nerve function. The five

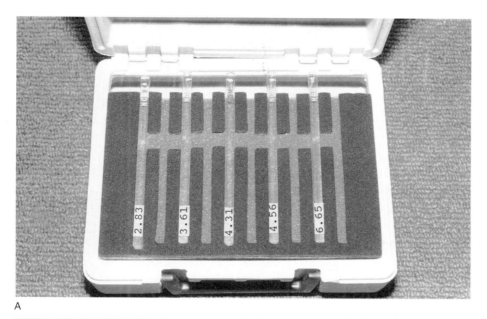

A

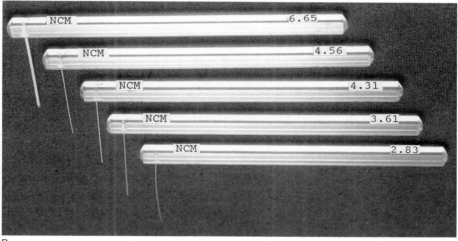

B

Figure 4.94. (A) Mini-kit. (B) The five filaments represent the cut-off forces for each functional level of sensibility.

filaments represent the cut-off forces for each functional level of sensibility (normal, diminished light touch, diminished protective, and loss of protective sensation); two filaments are included for loss of protective sensation (Figure 4.94b). Examiners should be able to expect a set of monofilaments in which each individual filament has been carefully calibrated for force (Bell-Krotoski et al, 1993) (Figure 4.95).

333

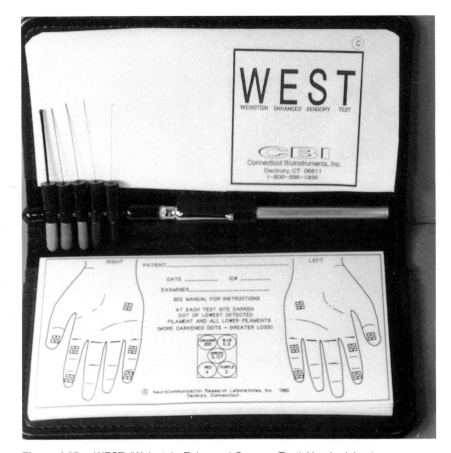

Figure 4.95. WEST (Weinstein Enhanced Sensory Test) Hand mini set.

In an effort to eliminate the need for separate test filaments and to place the mini-kit filaments in one instrument, Bell-Krotoski (1990b) developed Pocket Filaments (Figure 4.96a). The five colored filaments, which correspond to the colors used for mapping peripheral nerve involvement, are arranged in increasing sizes and can be separated and reassembled easily. Telescoping rods allow the filaments to be stored in a small case and extended for use (Figure 4.96b).

Vibration

Tuning fork
Tuning forks of 30 Hz and 256 Hz have been advocated for vibration testing but come under the same concerns as for light touch–deep pressure testing regarding uncontrolled stimuli. Tuning forks are dependent upon the method of application (for example, whether the side or the tip is applied) and force of application (Bell-Krotoski and Buford, 1988).

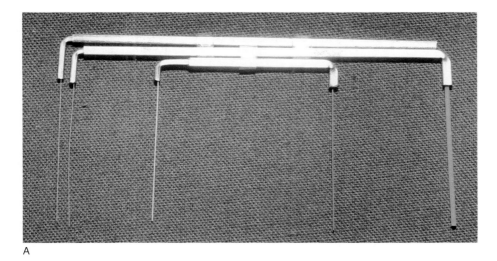

A

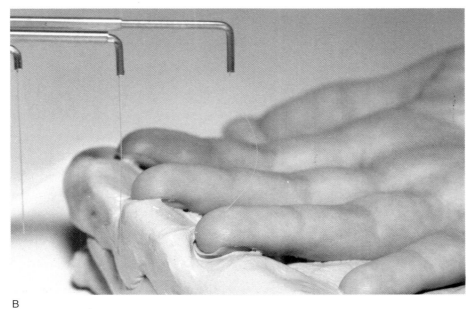

B

Figure 4.96. (A) Filaments. (B) Telescoping rods allow the filaments to be stored in a small case and extended for use.

Dellon (1981) reported that the 30 Hz tuning fork is best to evaluate the quickly adapting fiber/receptor system of the superficial dermis and that the 256 Hz tuning fork is best to evaluate the quickly adapting fiber/receptor system of the deep dermis and subcutis. However, tuning forks do not just produce the specified vibration of 30 Hz or 256 Hz, but also produce other high and low frequency signals throughout a broad

335

spectrum (Bell-Krotoski, 1991). Dellon recommends that, for convenience, the 256 Hz tuning fork be used to assess nerve compression and nerve division.

Dellon's technique of evaluating vibration sensibility in the hand is as follows.

1 The tuning fork is struck against a surface and then one of the ends of the prong is held tangentially to the fingertip. Tuning forks are highly subject to variation in application forces; therefore the examiner should try to control the intensity of amplitude by attempting to maintain the same striking force with each application of the tuning fork. The patient's vision must be occluded and the finger being tested should be supported. The area to be tested is always compared to the contralateral side. In addition, the area involved is compared to an ipsilateral fingertip.

2 The tuning fork is applied to the test site and the control site and the patient is asked, "Did the two applications feel different?" If the answer is "yes", it is followed with the question "How did they feel different?" Responses judged "positive" for abnormal perception are: "didn't feel anything", "softer", "louder" etc. Dellon also requires that the patient localize the perception.

Vibrometer

The vibrometer (Bio-Thesiometer) consists of a hand-held, variable-amplitude, fixed-frequency vibrator and a voltage meter (which measures increasing voltage as vibration amplitude is increased). Although the vibrometer has the same limitations as other hand-held instruments, it provides a more quantitative assessment of vibration than the tuning fork, thus allowing for a more reliable comparison of preoperative and postoperative thresholds (Callahan, 1990).

Functional tests

Functional tests assess the quality of sensibility. Is sensibility present on a gross level or on a fine discriminative level? Is it useful for fine prehension tasks? Is it adequate for the patient's activities of daily living in which the patient must recognize and manipulate objects with vision occluded?

Functional tests include:

• two-point discrimination
• localization
• the Moberg pick-up test.

Constant two-point discrimination

The two-point discrimination test introduced by Ernst Heinrick Weber, Professor of Anatomy in Leipzig, in 1953 measures the quality of sensation that has returned and, therefore, assesses the digit's ability to function as a sensory organ. Weber described the use of calipers whose points were held against the skin at different distances apart. The test determines the minimum distance at which the patient can distinguish whether he is being touched with one or two points in contact with the skin.

Although Moberg, with his years of experience and intuition, used a paper clip with a wire diameter of about 0.9 mm for testing sensibility with precision and meaning, a paper clip is not recommended for the unskilled examiner. The manufacturing process results in a sharp barb on one end of the clip, and this will elicit the perception of pain not touch.

Instead, the Disk-Criminator (Figure 4.97a), a Boley gauge or other caliper with blunt ends is recommended. The Boley gauge measures the exact distance between the points in millimeters and can be adjusted in increments of 1 mm. The tester must be careful to avoid applying too much pressure, as the Boley gauge is rather heavy (Figure 4.97b). Although the Boley gauge is not a threshold test, the pressure applied should be light—about 5 g. The higher the pressure, the wider is the area of skin that is deformed and stimulated (Brand, 1985).

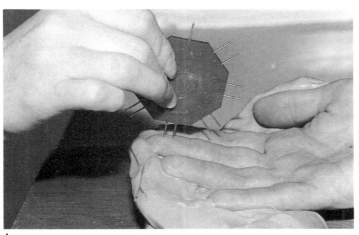

A

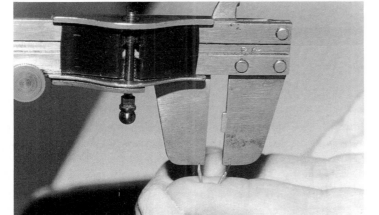

B

Figure 4.97. Recommended instruments for testing two-point discrimination include (A), the Disk-Criminator and (B), the Boley gauge. Increased pressure on the skin applied by the examiner in testing two point discrimination with the Boley gauge depresses a larger area of skin and the test will become unreliable. With light pressure, the two point discrimination will be 5 mm, but if the pressure is increased, at 3 mm distance will be appreciated as if it were a 12 mm distance.

Although using the weight of the instrument as a control is an improvement over a random force application, the hand-held force application of any two-point discrimination instrument (applying one or two points) that does not bend can vary across a wide range of several grams when the instrument is held against the skin. The variation in force is further increased by the vibration of the examiner's hand. Blanching of the skin is used as a control, but it has been shown that blanching can occur at different forces in various fingers.

Current instruments for testing two-point discrimination have been found to produce a heavier force when one point is applied than when two are applied. This means that the responses by the patient are based on his recognition of heavier or lighter pressure, and may have nothing to do with the recognition of two versus one-point (Bell-Krotoski and Buford, 1988; LaMotte, 1979; Bell-Krotoski et al, 1993). It is as important to consider this variable in testing as it is to consider its changes in overall application force from one examiner to another. Automated controlled instruments could help rule out hand-held variables in the test (Horch et al, 1992a and b).

One or two points are touched in random sequence along a longitudinal axis in the center of the finger tip. Investigators have differed in regard to the proper threshold value for this test (Moberg, 1962 and Onne, 1962). The American Society for Surgery of the Hand recommends seven correct answers out of 10 for two-point discrimination. The value of this test has been variously assessed. Moberg (1960, 1962) stated that there is no better test for evaluating tactile gnosis, although he conceded that the test is not ideal because it requires the patient's co-operation.

Two-point discrimination is most useful in the fingertips and has been used as a quick test of normal versus abnormal sensibility. It has, however, been found to lack the necessary sensitivity for detection of entrapment syndromes in clinical testing. Bell-Krotoski and Buford (1988) reported that, when using currently recommended protocols with current hand held tests, it was common to find that some patients had a two-point discrimination "within normal limits" although abnormality could be demonstrated by filament testing. She also noted that filament testing is only rarely found to be normal when two-point is abnormal.

Moving two-point discrimination
Dellon's (1981) moving two-point discrimination test provides an earlier means of assessing the return of discrimination than the constant two-point test. Moving two-point discrimination depends on quickly adapting fibers, which return sooner and in greater density than slowly adapting fibers, on which constant touch depends.

As with constant two-point discrimination, a Boley gauge is used. Testing is begun with the instrument set at 8 mm distance between the two points. One or two points are moved proximally to distally on the finger tip, parallel to the long axis of the finger, with the testing ends side by side. The patient is required to respond to seven out of 10 stimuli before the distance is narrowed. Testing is stopped at 2 mm as this represents normal moving two-point discrimination.

Dellon reported that moving two-point discrimination returns earlier and is usually 8–10 mm better than constant two-point discrimination during nerve regeneration. Moving two-point discrimination gives a measure of the hand's ability to feel objects, provided hand motion is possible. Constant two-point discrimination indicates the capacity of the hand to be aware of held still objects; this usually returns when constant two-point discrimination is less than 15 mm. This means that a patient whose hand has 10 mm of moving two-point discrimination can detect and identify objects unseen, but once the object is lifted and held immobile, the patient cannot identify it (Lister, 1984). The classic two-point discrimination test is still recommended, therefore, to provide this information.

Localization

Point localization is a useful test in demonstrating referred touch. Werner and Omer (1970) used the Semmes–Weinstein monofilaments to classify the patient's response according to point localization instead of area localization, as in the von Prince study (1967). They defined area localization as the ability to recognize the stimulus but not at the exact point. Point localization was considered a reflection of higher level integration than that perceived by light touch perception.

Bell-Krotoski et al (1993) reported that, although point localization is most useful for demonstrating referred touch and re-education, it is hard to quantify. It requires cortical interpretation and spatial reasoning. Since the more a patient uses a hand with referred touch, the more he is doing self training, the use of this test for measurement of return of nerve function could be misleading. Interpretations of test results should be made with this in mind—improvement does not necessarily mean physiologic improvement (Bell-Krotoski et al, 1993).

With vision blocked, the examiner touches the skin with a given filament. If the patient perceives the stimulation, he opens his eyes and localizes the touch point. If the patient correctly localizes the stimulus, a dot is marked in the corresponding zone on a worksheet (Figure 4.98). If the stimulus is incorrectly localized, an arrow is drawn on the worksheet from the point of stimulation to the point where the touch is referred (Figure 4.99). This mapping of responses gives a picture of the patient's level of localization. Serial testing in conjunction with re-education should show fewer and shorter arrows (Callahan, 1984).

Moberg pick-up test

Tactile gnosis is the fine sensibility of the finger pulps that permits recognition of what is being touched without the aid of sight. The Moberg pick-up test assesses general sensibility and tactile gnosis. The advantage of the pick-up test is that it combines sensibility with motion, requiring active manipulation and recognition of an object. The patient must pick up nine objects of different shapes and sizes, one at a time, as quickly as possible, and place them in a container. He does this first with eyes open and then with eyes closed. The examiner times the patient with a stopwatch and observes the manner of prehension.

339

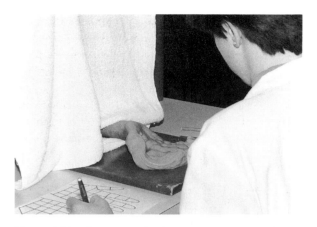

Figure 4.98. Documentation is more accurate with the use of a worksheet that has a grid superimposed on an outline of the hand. The grid is divided into seven palmar zones. The transverse lines correspond to the flexion creases, and the longitudinal lines correspond to the rays of the hand.

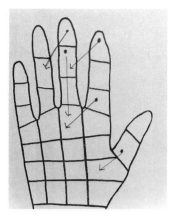

Figure 4.99. Arrows drawn from the point of stimulation to the point where the touch is referred give the examiner and the patient a picture of the patient's level of localization.

Objective tests

Objective tests require only the passive co-operation of the patient, not subjective interpretation of a stimulus. These tests include the ninhydrin sweat test (Moberg, 1958), the wrinkle test (O'Riain, 1973) and nerve conduction studies.

Although these tests do not correlate with functional sensation after nerve repair, the ninhydrin sweat test and the wrinkle test are useful in evaluating nerve function in children and in malingerers, and nerve conduction tests provide useful information about fiber regeneration (Almquist and Eeg-Olofsson, 1970).

Ninhydrin test

The ninhydrin sweat test developed by Aschan and Moberg (1962) is a test of sudomotor activity in the finger. Sweating in an area supplied by a peripheral nerve is generally indicative of peripheral nerve regeneration and the absence of sweating is a sign of peripheral nerve lesion.

The essentials of the test have been described by Perry et al (1974) and Phelps and Walker (1977). The patient's hand is cleansed thoroughly with soap and warm water, rinsed thoroughly, and then wiped with ether, alcohol or acetone. Perry recommends a five-minute waiting period to allow the normal sweating process to ensue, whereas Phelps requires a 20- to 30-minute period to elapse before proceeding with the test. During the waiting period, the patient's fingertips must not come into contact with any surface.

At the end of the waiting period, the fingers are pressed against a good quality of bond paper that has not been previously touched. The fingertips are traced with a pencil and held in place for 15 seconds. The paper is then sprayed with ninhydren spray reagent (N-0507) and allowed to dry for 24 hours or heated in an oven for five to 10 minutes at 93° C. The amino acids and lower peptide components of sweat that have penetrated the paper are stained purple by the ninhydren. After development, the prints are sprayed with ninhydrin fixer reagent (N-0757) for a permanent record of the results (Callahan, 1984).

Normative and reliability data are either limited or not available for this test. It can be useful within limits for the unco-operative patient and for young children unable to respond to other tests (Bell-Krotoski, 1991).

Wrinkle test

The wrinkle test was described by O'Riain in 1973. He observed that a denervated hand placed in warm water (40° C) for 30 minutes does not wrinkle in the denervated area as normal skin does. He associated this phenomenon with an absence of sensory function and the return of wrinkling with a return of sensory function.

Normative and reliability data are limited or not available for this test, but it can be useful within limits for young children unable to respond to other tests (Bell-Krotoski, 1991).

Nerve conduction studies

Nerve conduction studies are valuable for the anatomic localization of a lesion in a peripheral nerve trunk; however, they are dependent upon such variables as temperature, time of day, instrument calibration, and examiner technique (Kimura, 1984)

Sensibility test battery

Sensation is the perception through the senses, or the subjective appreciation of a physical stimulus. Sensibility is the capacity for sensation, that is, the ability to perceive a physical stimulus.

Sensibility testing begins by gathering background information, including:

- an accurate history of the injury;
- a subject description of his symptoms by the patient;
- assessment of trophic changes;
- joint range-of-motion measurements;
- muscle evaluation; and
- quantitative tests of motor function, including grasp and pinch.

After this information has been gathered, the sensibility tests are administered. A detailed evaluation is mandatory if accurate data are to be available for comparison studies. Without such careful evaluation it is impossible to determine whether a patient's recovery after a nerve injury is progressing on schedule or is slower than anticipated.

Testing should be done in a sound-resistant or quiet room with only the therapist and patient present. A quiet, distraction-free environment is of the utmost importance, since nothing (a child crying, people talking, typing) should interfere with the patient's or examiner's concentration. The room temperature should be comfortable and free of excess humidity.

Brand (1985) emphasized that measurement must be precise and repeatable. Precision requires the therapist's time, but time can be saved by selecting one or two tests to evaluate recovery on a quantitative anatomical basis and one or two tests to evaluate recovery on a functional basis. The time that is saved is spent ensuring the precision and repeatability of measurements and in measuring the patient's progress more frequently.

Callahan (1984) recommends a battery of tests to answer three questions:

1 Is protective sensibility present, as measured by the ability to perceive a sharp object, deep pressure, and (optionally) hot and cold?
2 Is light touch present?
3 If light touch is present, is it present on a gross level only or on a fine discriminative level?

With these questions in mind, we begin our sensibility testing with a patient history.

Background information

History

The patient's age, sex, occupation, and hand dominance, the date of the injury, location of the injury, mechanism of injury, diagnosis, date and type of surgical procedure, and other pertinent information is recorded. The date of the injury and the type of surgical procedure are essential data because each defines a predictable time course for recovery. Each characteristically influences recommendations for treatment, sensibility re-education, and return to work. Notation of the mechanism of injury aids the examiner in understanding differences in individual recovery. If, for example, the patient sustained a severe crushing injury with massive tissue damage, scarring and pain may affect grip strength and loss of muscle power. In contrast, nerve lacerations with little other tissue damage present a better prognosis (Wilgus, 1982).

Subjective description of symptoms by the patient

One should include the patient's description of his symptoms and ability to use his hand (numbness, pins and needles, tingling, pain, burning, improvement noted with rest, and ability to use it in activities of daily living). The activities and hand positions that make his condition worse give clues to the etiology of nerve problems. Patients with carpal tunnel syndrome (CTS) may report "numbness" in their hand when they awake in the morning; however, not all patients are good historians. A patient who states that his hand "feels fine" may show a measurable loss of sensibility. Another patient who states that he "feels nothing" in the median nerve distribution may be amazed at how much he does "feel" after the surgeon uses a local anesthetic to block the ulnar nerve.

Assessment of trophic changes

One includes observation of atrophy and nail changes. Burns, blisters, cuts, or bruises on the fingers are indicative of the insensitive hand. The skin condition must be noted (dry, scaly, moist, mottled, pale, shiny). The presence of edema or infection may affect the true validity of the evaluation. Does the patient complain of cold intolerance? Sweating in an area supplied by a peripheral nerve is indicative of peripheral nerve regeneration, and the absence of sweating indicates a peripheral nerve lesion. A patient with a laceration in the peripheral nerve area will not sweat, and therefore his skin will have a very dry appearance. Although sweating is an indication of sudomotor activity in the finger, there is no relationship between the return of sweat production and the quality of sensibility recovery.

Joint range-of-motion

Active and passive range-of-motion measurements are evaluated with a goniometer. The goniometer should barely touch the digit during measurement of active motion, otherwise it may give assistance.

Muscle evaluation

A voluntary muscle test will establish the level of function and provide an estimate of the strength of the active muscles. Manual grading of weak muscles and the identification of normal muscles must be accurately recorded. Trick movements must be detected. If there is questionable motor activity, a local anesthetic may be indicated to block competing innervation. Muscle bulk in the involved forearm is measured and compared with that of the uninvolved extremity. The examiner should describe the patient's co-ordination and the presence of pain as related to muscle function.

Grasp and prehension

Prehension and grasp measurements are checked and compared with those of the uninvolved extremity. The grip of the non-dominant hand is generally slightly less than that of the dominant hand. Grip strength is measured on the adjustable Jamar dynamometer (Figure 4.100). The combined efforts of the intrinsic and extrinsic muscles are evaluated on levels 1, 2, and 3. Primarily extrinsic muscle function is evaluated on levels 4 and 5. The patient's co-operation will be demonstrated during the Jamar dynamometer test.

Normal adult grip measurements for the five consecutive handle positions create a bell curve. The first position is the least favorable for strong grip, followed by the fourth and fifth positions. The strongest grip measurement occurs at the second and third handles (Bechtol 1954, Aulicino and Dupuy, 1990).

Pinch can be quantitated on the pinch meter. Pulp pinch as well as key pinch should be evaluated and recorded (Figure 4.101). The pinch meter should be held lightly by the therapist and never fixed in any way while the patient is testing his strength. If the therapist holds the pinch meter firmly, the patient is able to use the stability to produce a higher reading.

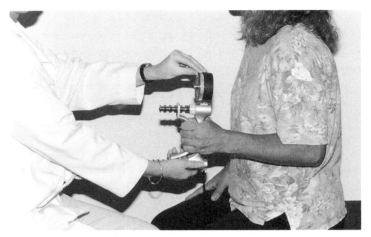

Figure 4.100. Grip strength is measured on the five levels of the adjustable Jamar dynamometer.

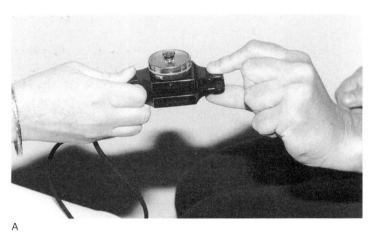

Figure 4.101. Finger pinch is measured on the pinch meter. (A) Pulp pinch. (B) Key pinch.

A

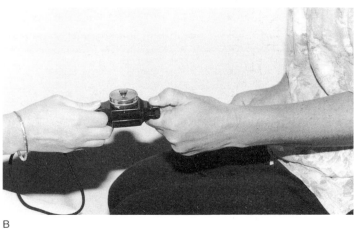

B

Proprioception

With normal sensation, the patient can, with vision blocked, identify the positional and directional change in a finger when performing passive movements of the interphalangeal joints (Omer, 1981). To test proprioception, the examiner supports the patient's finger laterally and moves it 0.5–1.0 cm in any direction. The patient must identify the angle through which the joint is moved.

Threshold test (Semmes–Weinstein monofilaments)

Attention to detail by the examiner will affect the test results. Testing takes place in a quiet room where the patient will not be disturbed.

Brand (1985) reported that a source of error in testing is that the patient can be given cues other than the intended stimuli. He reported that a fiber weighing 1 g can move a finger that is passive and free to move. Movement is perceived proximally in the forearm by tendon–muscle movement even when the finger is insensitive; the patient then points to the totally insensitive finger and says that it has been touched. For this reason, the patient's hand must be fully supported during testing. Brand suggests supporting the hand in putty (see Figure 4.93).

Visual clues are also helpful to the patient. The tester may observe carefully when touching the digit, but pay less attention when not touching it. Patients can respond to facial expressions with a "yes" or "no". To prevent such visual clues, the patient is blindfolded or a screen is used. The patient must also be in a position that does not cause discomfort in the arm (Figure 4.102).

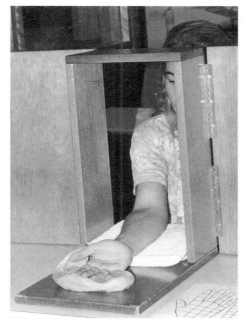

Figure 4.102. Patient must be in a position that does not cause discomfort in the arm.

345

Evaluation of sensibility is done more quickly and is more precise when the therapist maps out the area of dysfunction before testing begins. The examiner draws a probe lightly across the patient's hand, beginning with an area of normal sensibility and progressing slowly to an area of suspected abnormal sensibility (Figure 4.103a). The blunt end of a pen or any instrument that is not sharp or too wide may be used. The patient, whose vision is occluded, is asked to indicate immediately whether and when he perceives a change in feeling. The examiner marks the skin with a felt tip pen where the sensory change occurs (Figure 4.103b). The process is repeated until the proximal, distal, and lateral borders of sensory dysfunction have been determined. The examiner then tests for light touch within this area.

Mapping makes the testing quicker and more effective, because follow-up evaluations require only that the area of dysfunction in the initial examination be re-evaluated. The process may be repeated during successive evaluations. It gives the patient and the examiner the opportunity to note whether the area mapped out diminishes in size or remains the same over a period of time. An alternative method is to have the patient himself outline the area of dysfunction in his hand. The results of the mapping can be recorded on an outline of a hand for serial comparison (Callahan, 1984).

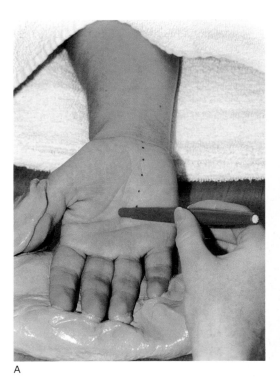 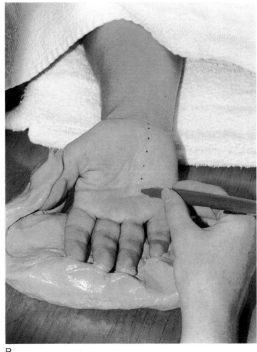

A   B

Figure 4.103. (A) The examiner draws a probe across the skin to determine the proximal, distal and lateral borders of sensory dysfunction. Vision is blocked by having the patient close his eyes or by the use of a wooden screen. (B) The examiner marks the skin with a felt tip pen where the sensory change occurs.

When monitoring nerve recovery, testing becomes more systematic and documentation more accurate if a grid superimposed on an outline of the hand is used (Figure 4.104). The grid, devised by von Prince and Butler (1967), is divided into squares or zones. Transverse lines correspond to the flexion creases of the digits and palm. Longitudinal lines are parallel with the rays of the hand. The examiner visualizes the grid on the patient's hand, applies the filament to the center of a given zone in random sequence, and asks the patient to respond. Correct or incorrect responses can be recorded in the corresponding zone on the worksheet (Callahan, 1984).

Clinical testing techniques using the Semmes–Weinstein monofilaments have been developed by von Prince and Butler (1967), Werner and Omer (1970), and Bell (1984). Testing should begin with the uninvolved extremity. This allows the patient to become familiar with the testing procedure, and the examiner can establish the patient's normal level of sensibility. Higher values may be considered normal when the measurements of the uninvolved extremity are higher than established normal values. However, one cannot always rely on using the contralateral hand as a normal control, as the contralateral hand may not be normal.

The initial test following a nerve laceration or crush includes both surfaces of the involved hand, with special emphasis on the area of dysfunction as determined by mapping. The examiner envisions the "grid" on the patient's hand and applies the monofilament at the center of any given zone. Should a more detailed evaluation be needed (e.g. following digital nerve repair), the zones can be subdivided. Some examiners may prefer to mark the responses with a felt pen directly on the patient's hand for easier reference.

The direction in which the monofilament is applied can affect the accuracy of threshold testing. When it is applied at an angle, the applied force is lessened. The monofilaments are most accurate and repeatable when applied to the skin surface perpendicular to the length of the filament (Bell-Krotoski and Buford, 1988; Bell-Krotoski et al, 1993) (See

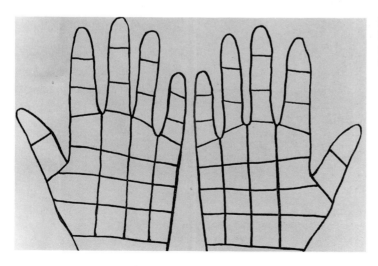

Figure 4.104. Testing becomes more systematic and documentation more accurate if a grid is used.

Figure 4.93). To attain a repeatable touch threshold measurement, the time of filament application is standardized and the test area varied (Brand, 1985). Testing is begun with filament 2.83, which is considered normal light-touch sensibility. With patients who have severe dysfunction, the examiner may choose to begin testing with a higher numbered filament. Skin that is calloused will have a higher sensory threshold than uncalloused skin. These areas should be noted and considered in the interpretation of the results.

The detection threshold of the 2.83 monofilament that is considered normal does not mean that a person with normal sensibility will feel the filament 100 per cent of the time. Usually, a person with normal sensibility can feel the stimulus of 2.83, if given a few attempts. Bell-Krotoski et al (1993) report that in order to differentiate a false-positive response from a true detection, the examiner may stimulate with the 2.83 filament up to (about) five times to ensure that it is not felt.

It is suggested that, in the application of the filaments, the patient should have the opportunity to have a high probability of responding to the normal stimulus level (2.83). A series of a minimum of three applications in a chosen zone ensures that one of the three is the intended threshold, and improves the reliability of the test (Bell and Buford, 1988). Weinstein (1993) states that up to five applications are desirable.

Filaments should be applied and removed in a uniform manner. The examiner should begin moving the monofilament slowly toward the skin from a height of about 2.5 cm (Weinstein, 1993). It should touch the skin in about 1.5 seconds, be held in place for about 1.5 seconds and then lifted to the starting position (less than 2.5 cm above the skin) over a period of 1.5 seconds and then applied two more times in the same manner. The monofilament should not touch the skin before pressing to produce the bend, or else a different force–time shape of stimulus is produced, and the test may be compromised. Bouncing the filaments against the skin will cause an overshoot of the applied force, and removing the filaments too quickly is also contraindicated (Bell-Krotoski and Tomancik, 1987; Weinstein, 1993). The filament must not slip on the skin when it is being applied, for this will give an additional stimulus clue to the patient.

With the patient's hand supported in putty and his vision blocked, the examiner touches a spot with a filament. As soon as the patient perceives the pressure of the stimulus, he responds by saying the word "touch". As discussed previously, in order to allow the patient to have a high probability of responding to the normal stimulus (2.83) if he does not respond to the first application, a minimum of two more may be given. This assures that one of the applications is the intended threshold. When the responses are inaccurate with a given filament in a particular zone, the examiner returns to that zone at varying intervals with successively thicker filaments until a correct response is elicited. When filaments in the range 4.17 to 6.65 are used, only one stimulation is applied in a chosen zone. Successive testing is always scattered randomly to prevent the patient anticipating the next stimulus. If a response is not obtained with the thickest filament (marked 6.65) in a particular zone, the pin-prick test is used as a final test of sensibility in that zone.

Bell-Krotoski et al (1993) report that there are situations in which the application of forces lower than the 2.83 filament are important. They cite a situation in which a patient with CTS can detect 2.83 overall, but can additionally detect 2.44 only in the ulnar nerve distribution. Thus the examiner may surmise that there is a loss of function in the median nerve distribution. When the tester is looking for the earliest possible change in a patient, the full set of monofilaments, including the lower force filaments, are sometimes useful; however, for the majority of patients, they state that it is not necessary to determine that the patient feels better than average, only whether he is worse than average.

Callahan (1984) emphasizes the importance of accurate recording of responses, because it is easy to forget where the stimulus has been applied previously and how the patient responded. Careful recording makes the test shorter, more accurate, and more valid in serial comparison tests. It also documents inconsistencies in the responses of a suspected malingerer. Examples of a suggested code for the worksheet include:

- +2.83: positive response to 2.83 monofilament, testing complete in that zone
- −2.83: negative response to 2.83, test at random intervals with thicker filaments until accurate responses are obtained
- +3.22: positive response to 3.22.

Detailed documentation requires a worksheet with a life-sized outline of the hand to provide space for notations. The examiner may prefer to devise his own code.

The scale of interpretation shown in Table 4.2 enables the examiner to make a meaningful interpretation of the sensibility test results. The norms in the scale, although not standardized, are based on clinical testing of hundreds of nerve-injured hands (Werner and Omer, 1970; Bell, 1984). The numerical values of the filaments recorded on the worksheet are transferred to a color-coded outline of a hand for easy reference and serial comparison (Bell, 1984). The colors correspond to the sensibility levels in the scale of interpretation. For example, the color green indicates normal light touch (2.83) perceived, blue indicates diminished light touch (3.22–3.61) perceived, purple indicates diminished protective sensation (3.84–4.31) perceived, and red (4.56–6.65) indicates loss of protective sensation. A red lined area indicates that no filament was perceived.

		Filament markings	Calculated force (gm)
Green	Normal	1.65–2.83	0.0045–0.068
Blue	Diminished light touch	3.22–3.61	0.166–0.408
Purple	Diminished protective sensation	3.84–4.31	0.697–2.06
Red	Loss of protective sensation	4.56–6.65	3.63–447
Red-lined	Untestable	>6.65	>447

Table 4.2. Scale of interpretation of monofilaments (data from Semmes et al, 1960)

According to a study conducted by Levin et al (1978), an advantage of the Semmes–Weinstein filaments in measuring threshold sensitivity is their ease of application. However, correct interpretation of the results requires an understanding of the factors that can affect those results.

Their engineering analysis found that the principal factors that can lead to variations in the stress required to buckle or bend a filament are the method of application by the examiner, variations in the elastic modules due to elevated temperatures of high humidity, differences on the ends of the filaments, and variations in the attachment of the filaments to the handles. Extreme humidity affects the strength of the lighter Semmes–Weinstein monofilaments and therefore changes the pressure that they exert on the skin. The filaments should be stored where they will not be affected by humidity. With continued use or mistreatment, the filaments become bent. Filaments are no longer in calibration when permanently bent (Bell-Krotoski and Tomancik, 1987).

Functional tests

Constant two-point discrimination

The Weber two-point discrimination test is used to qualify further the level of sensibility that has returned; it therefore assesses the digit's ability to function as a sensory organ (Bell, 1984). The test determines the minimal distance at which a patient can discriminate between being touched with one or two points.

The test procedure should be explained and demonstrated first while the patient observes. His hand should be fully supported in putty. During testing, the patient's vision is blocked with the use of a screen (Callahan, 1984), or he is blindfolded or asked to close his eyes or look in another direction when the stimulus is applied. The gauge is set with a distance of 5 mm between the two points. One point or two points are touched in random sequence along a longitudinal axis in the center of the finger tip. In applying two points, both points should contact the skin simultaneously. The instrument is applied lightly to the point of blanching of the skin (Omer and Spinner, 1975). The patient must respond each time he feels the stimulus. If he cannot recognize whether he has been touched with one or two points, he should guess. Ten separate stimuli are given. Seven out of 10 responses must be correctly identified. If the patient cannot distinguish seven out of the 10 stimulations correctly, the distance between the two points is increased and the stimulation is repeated until the patient gives the required accurate responses. Testing is stopped at 15 mm if the response is non-discriminatory.

The interpretation of scores is based on the American Society for Surgery of the Hand Clinical Assessment Recommendations:

Normal: less than 6 mm.
Fair: 6 to 10 mm.
Poor: 11 to 15 mm.
Protective: one point perceived
Anesthetic: no point perceived.

Moberg (1958) observed that 6 mm of two-point discrimination is necessary on both sides of the pinch to wind a watch or to put a 5 mm nut on a screw; 6–8 mm for sewing with an ordinary needle or buttoning a small button; and 12–15 mm for handling small precision tools. Above 15 mm two-point discrimination, gross tool handling may be possible but only with decreased speed and skill. The test values are recorded on a serial test form.

Moving two-point discrimination
As with constant two-point discrimination, a Boley gauge is used. Testing is begun with the instrument set at an 8 mm distance between the two points. The gauge is moved proximally to distally on the fingertip, parallel to the long axis of the finger, with the testing ends side by side. The patient is required to respond to seven out of 10 stimuli before the distance is narrowed. Testing is stopped at 2 mm, which represents normal moving two-point discrimination (Callahan, 1984).

Point localization
Point localization using the Semmes–Weinstein monofilaments is treated as a separate functional test at The Philadelphia Hand Foundation. It is considered to reflect a higher level of integration than that provided by light touch perception.

With the patient's hand fully supported in putty and his vision blocked, the examiner applies a filament to the center of a particular zone (Figure 4.105a). The examiner begins with the lowest numbered filament that resulted in a positive response during light-touch testing. As soon as the patient perceives the stimulus, he opens his eyes and localizes the touch point by pointing to it (Figure 4.105b). The filament is applied only once to each zone. If the patient correctly localizes the stimulus, a dot is marked in the corresponding zone on a worksheet. A worksheet with the grid superimposed on the outline of a hand is again more useful for documentation of the testing results. If the stimulus is incorrectly localized, an arrow is drawn on the worksheet from the point of the stimulation to the point, area, or finger where the touch is referred (see Figure 4.99). This mapping of the patient's responses gives the patient and the examiner a picture of the patient's level of localization. Serial testing in conjunction with sensory reeducation should show fewer and shorter arrows (Callahan, 1984).

Moberg pick-up test
Tactile gnosis is the fine sensibility of the finger pulps that permits recognition of what is being touched without the aid of sight. Moberg (1978b) stated that a hand without tactile gnosis is "blind" and is useless without the aid of vision.

The pick-up test introduced by Moberg (1958) assesses general sensibility and tactile gnosis. The advantage of the pick-up test is that it combines sensibility with motion, and so requires active manipulation and recognition of an object. The patient is required to pick up nine objects of different shapes and sizes, one at a time, as quickly as he can and place them in a container. The objects can include such items as a safety pin, a paper clip, a screw, a key, a marble, coins, and a nut and bolt. The test is first done

351

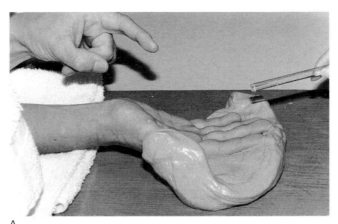

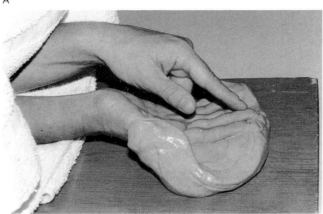

Figure 4.105. (A) The examiner applies a filament to the center of a particular zone. (B) The patient localizes the touch point by pointing to it.

A

B

with the involved hand and then with the uninvolved hand. The patient is then asked to close his eyes and the test is repeated. The patient is timed with a stopwatch each time he performs the test.

The rapidity and the manner of prehension are recorded, and a comparison is made between the involved and uninvolved hands. When picking up objects with his vision blocked, the patient will not use regions of poor sensibility. If sensibility in the median nerve is impaired, the patient will pick up the object with his thumb and ring and little fingers instead of using the thumb and index finger as he normally would.

The test can be made more difficult by asking the patient to name or describe the objects as he picks them up with his eyes closed (Moberg, 1958). Omer (1981) suggests that on occasion a piece of chalk be used as an object so that the chalk residue remains to show the functional surfaces of the hand.

Periodic tests will indicate the changing status of coordination. Omer (1981) found that the normal time for picking up nine objects is less than 10 seconds. However, the importance of this test is that the examiner can observe the patient's functional aptitude for picking up the objects. Dellon (1979) modified the test by standardizing test items and by requiring correct object identification.

Nerve conduction studies
Nerve conduction studies help to provide a complete clinical evaluation, with data on the nature, location, degree of nerve involvement and viability of the involved muscle.

Stress testing in nerve compression

The most common nerve entrapment is CTS. Some cases of suspected CTS have been found in which all the testing of neural status described is within normal limits, and a patient history is the only indicative finding. It is suspected that in these cases the patient is not always being tested at the time of his symptoms. For instance, he may come in for testing after he has slept late and had a more quietly paced and lighter duty morning than his normal routine.

Sunderland (1978), Gelberman et al (1981), and Rydevik et al (1981) suggested that the position of the wrist affects distal sensory and motor conduction parameters of the median nerve based on intra-compartmental pressure changes and resultant epineural ischemia. Most patients with suspected CTS have an aggravation of symptoms after strenuous use of their hands or after sleeping with their wrist in flexion. For many of these patients, however, conventional resting sensibility evaluation and nerve conduction studies carried out the following day can be within normal limits.

Marin et al (1983) suggest that these patients have an increased intracarpal tunnel pressure, with the resultant changes in nerve conduction ability, while performing their work activities. This is based on the premise that higher muscular tension places more stress on tendons, synovial membranes and the median nerve. They suggest that the cause of these patients' symptoms is vascular ischemic impairment from increased pressure. However, at the time of their sensibility evaluation or nerve conduction studies, these patients have not been performing heavy or repetitive motion activities or sleeping with their wrist flexed and the increased tunnel pressure has therefore diminished to the point where the transient ischemia of the nerve may not be present. Hence the resting test may be normal.

Most patients who present with CTS at The Philadelphia Hand Foundation and whose resting tests are normal are stress tested to simulate their working and/or sleeping wrist positions. The findings in their sensibility and electrodiagnostic evaluations can then be compared with resting baseline tests. This allows for documentation of marginal or early developing or intermittent compartment syndromes based on working position or activity.

Sensibility is tested with the Semmes–Weinstein monofilaments. The same testing protocol is followed in nerve conduction testing:

1 Test at rest or neutral position.
2 Test in end-range dorsal and volar flexion;

3 Retest in end-range position following 5–8 minutes of therapy (putty squeezing).

4 Compare testing of responses in the respective positions before and after dynamic activity and against resting baseline responses.

Summary

No single method of sensibility evaluation may be appropriate for every patient or the choice of every examiner. Different clinicians use different tests. However, the complexity of sensibility is such that no single test or category of tests in clinical use today can provide the full picture of sensibility.

Therefore, the most complete picture will result from a carefully chosen battery of tests selected to answer three questions:

1 Is protective sensation present?

2 Is light touch present?

3 If light touch is present, what is the level of discriminative sensation?

With this in mind, the battery of tests used at The Philadelphia Hand Foundation includes:

- the threshold tests (Semmes–Weinstein pressure aesthesiometer, vibration);
- two point discrimination (constant and moving);
- point localization tests;
- the Moberg pick-up test; and
- nerve conduction studies.

We have found that this battery of tests provides the desired information in the majority of patients referred for sensibility evaluation.

Isolated tests of nerve loss and recovery are of little value. Postoperative results must be compared with the preoperative status to indicate whether and how much improvement has been obtained. An appropriate battery of tests should be repeated at intervals of approximately 12 weeks to chart the changing status of the injured nerve. Since they are quantitative tests, they have meaning for other examiners and for the patient.

Cutaneous sensibility has been studied since the time of Aristotle (350 BC). Von Frey's classic study in 1899 merits special praise. New techniques and ideas have emerged through the clinical studies of Bell-Krotoski, Callahan, Dellon, Gelberman, Lundborg, and Sunderland. Much is yet to be learned, as indicated by the differing opinions that exist and by the strengths and weaknesses of our current testing techniques. Critical scientific investigations by these examiners and others have provided us with the basis from which to draw upon and further develop our methods of assessing the quality of sensibility remaining in the hand following a nerve injury.

4.4 SIGNS OF NEURAL REGENERATION

The clinical signs of neural regeneration

Two general principles must be kept in mind when considering neural regeneration:

- recovery occurs from proximal to distal, and
- the signs of sensory recovery precede those of voluntary motor activity.

Tinel's sign

The first detectable clinical sign of recovery is Tinel's sign. Percutaneous percussion of the nerve trunk distal to the lesion (as far as the level of axonal regeneration) produces a "pins and needles" sensation distally in the territory of distribution of the cutaneous nerve. This sign was described in the same year (1915) by Hoffmann and by Tinel.

In an article that has become a classic, Tinel distinguished between peripheral paresthesia, a sign of axonal regeneration, and local pain, which indicates irritation of the nerve. He emphasized the significance of this test in monitoring regeneration of the nerve, but stressed that the sign is neither constant nor easy to interpret.

Technique

Percussion must be gentle, done with the tip of the finger or, more accurately, with the blunt tip of a felt pen or a rubber eraser. One should avoid inaccurate mechanical stimulation with a large object and restrict percussion to the course of the nerve. Most clinicians percuss from a distal point upward along the course of the nerve trunk until they reach the site at which percussion triggers paresthesia. Others work in reverse from the site of the lesion downward until the induced paresthesia disappears.

The reaction can be compared to that produced by a weak electric current, unpleasant but not painful. It is important to remember that the sensation is felt peripherally, in the area of the cutaneous distribution of the nerve, and differs from the sometimes painful sensation felt at the point of direct pressure on the nerve caused by neuroma formation or by irritation of pain fibers. A similar peripheral reaction can be obtained by electric stimulation using a cathode 1 cm in diameter applied to a point over the course of a nerve, and a broader anode at some other point on the body (Moldaver, 1978). Even when a continuous stimulus is applied, the sensation is felt as an intermittent vibration.

Clinical significance of Tinel's sign

The "pins and needles" sensation resulting from percussion is caused by regeneration of the sensory axons, which are very sensitive to pressure. The sign thus signifies a favorable prognosis and enables one to follow the progress of the regenerating nerve. Only percussion of the tactile fibers (not those transmitting pain, heat, and cold) triggers the pins and needles sensation.

Changes in the results of Tinel's test reflect the progress of axonal regrowth, which varies from person to person and is faster in the proximal part of the limb than at the extremities. It is faster after spontaneous healing than after nerve suturing. In the latter situation axonal regrowth usually occurs at a rate of 1–2 mm per day (Jung, 1941; Sunderland and Bradley, 1952). A positive response over a long segment of nerve suggests unequal rates of growth of various tactile fibers.

Tinel's sign has occasionally fallen into disrepute, because it sometimes has been absent when a nerve was in fact regenerating and at other times has been positive when exploration showed an absence of continuity between the nerve ends (Woodhall and Beebe, 1956). Some authors, however, have attached great significance to the test (Henderson, 1948).

Tinel himself pointed out that the sign is absent in certain circumstances:

1 It is absent in the early stages following injury or nerve suturing. According to Tinel, the sign appears only four to six weeks after the injury. In fact, this is very variable because axonal growth depends on a number of factors, but it can be said that the time is roughly proportional to the severity of the lesion.
2 The sign may be difficult to elicit if the nerve lies deep to a large mass of muscle.
3 Tinel's sign cannot be demonstrated when the lesion is proximal to the posterior root ganglion.

The prognostic value of this sign is not absolute, because not all the regenerating tactile fibers necessarily recover. Some lose their way; others just stop growing. Even if they continue growing within the nerve sheath, they may follow the wrong route. Thus, a false positive result is elicited when sensory fibers grow into motor sheaths.

Finally the test has no quantitative value; it can be positive with only a few fibers regenerating—hence its limited functional significance.

In spite of all these limitations, the sign is clinically useful when, within a few weeks after the injury or suturing, light percussion distal to the lesion triggers the pins and needles sensation peripherally, and when, in the course of the following weeks, percussion at the same level produces a weak response, which increases in strength if tapping is done more distally. This appears to confirm axonal growth. Interrupted progress must be regarded as alarming, and when this persists, and the absence of other signs of regeneration (to be discussed) confirms it, surgical exploration is indicated. Steady distal progression of the sign, unless contradicted by other factors, suggests a good prognosis, even though the sign gives little information concerning the functional quality of reinnervation.

Too much should not be expected of Tinel's sign, which must be interpreted only in conjunction with other clinical findings.

Sensory recovery

Sensory recovery progresses in time and space according to the following successive stages:

1 Perception of pain and temperature (small caliber pain fibers regenerate more rapidly). Protective sensation is thus established.

2 Perception of low frequency vibratory stimuli (30 Hz) as well as moving tact sense.

3 Per static tact sense, at the same time as perception of high frequency vibratory stimuli (256 Hz).

4 Two point discrimination (Weber test) is the last form of sensation to develop.

This recovery pattern is used by Dellon (1981) as a guide in his sensory rehabilitation program.

Motor recovery

Motor recovery is always slower than sensory recovery. The first sign of motor recovery is regression of the atrophy in the territory normally supplied by the injured nerve. Later, a weak contraction can be detected in the first muscle supplied by the nerve distal to the lesion. The contraction, however, is not powerful enough to produce movement or to overcome gravity.

It should be pointed out that these early signs of neural regeneration are of limited prognostic value: they suggest a favourable outcome but offer no guarantee of functional recovery.

Although it is necessary to detect the early signs of neural regeneration, it is equally essential to follow its progress. Regeneration can be halted at any stage, and there is frequently a marked difference between motor recovery and sensory recovery.

As far as sensory recovery is concerned, pain usually appears before tactile sensation returns. Sensation returns first to the proximal margin of the anesthetic zone. It is important to record the interval between the reappearance of contraction in the first muscle supplied distal to the nerve suture and that in the next. Regeneration can slow down or even cease before reaching the extremity of the limb.

All these variations make difficult the decision to undertake and the timing of surgical repairs.

Early electrodiagnosis is of limited value after a peripheral nerve lesion. The process of wallerian degeneration can be recorded only from four to five weeks after the nerve division. Apart from helping in the detection of denervation, these tests can record spontaneous changes or changes after a nerve repair.

Electrodiagnosis
by P Seror

Electrodiagnosis is made of two different parts: needle examination and stimulodetection. Electrodiagnosis medicine is a specific area of medical practice in which the physician uses not only the technique of electrodiagnosis but also the information from the clinical history and from the physical examination to diagnose and treat neuromuscular diseases.

The motor unit study is the basis of needle examination. One motor unit is the functional group made up of one motor neuron and its dependent muscle fibers. The size of the motor units varies a great deal from one muscle to another. On the whole the more precise the movement must be, the fewer number of muscle fibers are driven by a single motor neuron: in the intrinsic muscles of the hand, one motor neuron supplies 10 to 20 muscle fibers whereas in the gastrosoleus complex, one motor neuron supplies about 1,000 muscle fibers.

These differences between motor unit sizes are electrically translated by amplitudes and durations of potential differences. Thus, small motor units (face and hand) have low or moderate amplitudes and bi- or triphasic potentials. Large motor units (deltoid, triceps surae) have a large amplitude and tri- or polyphasic potentials.

Normal needle examination
Normal needle examination is done with very fine needle electrodes that allow precise study of motor unit potentials. The needle is inserted into the muscle. At rest, no spontaneous activity is recorded in a normal subject. During voluntary movement the recruitment increases progressively (Figure 4.106).

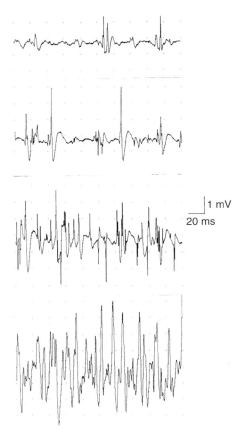

Figure 4.106. Needle examination: normal pattern. The recruitment of motor unit increases with the intensity of muscle contraction: from minimal contraction = single motor unit interference pattern (top) to maximal voluntary contraction: full interference pattern (bottom).

1 mV
20 ms

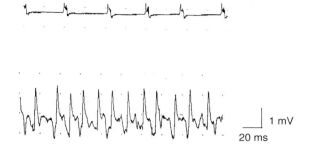

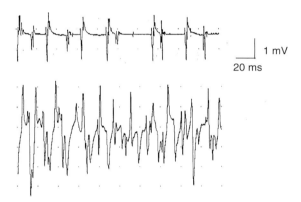

Figure 4.107. Needle examination: different stages of neurogenic pattern. From very severe nerve damage: single unit with high firing rate pattern (top) to moderate lesion: moderate reduced interference pattern (bottom).

In neurogenic lesions, the needle examination shows at rest spontaneous activity (fibrillations and sharp waves), and at voluntary movement a reduced number of motor unit potentials with high firing rate and an increment of polyphasic potential (Figure 4.107).

Stimulodetection

Normal stimulodetection is done with surface electrodes. It permits study of nerve-impulse conduction function along peripheral motor and sensory fibers: motor conduction velocity (MCV) and sensory conduction velocity (SCV) determinations. It is also possible to study conduction of sensory and motor fibers in the central nervous system: somatosensory evoked potential (SEP) and motor evoked potential (MEP).

Motor conduction velocity

The stimulation of a nerve trunk at two different levels allows the recording of two motor action potentials (MAP) of different latencies (Figure 4.108). The distal motor latency (DML) is obtained after stimulation of the most distal point; e.g. the wrist for

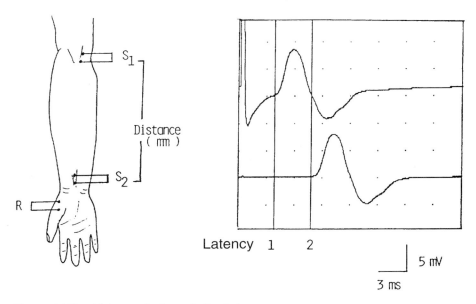

Figure 4.108. Motor conduction velocity study

$$MCV = \frac{\text{distance (mm)}}{\text{conduction delay (ms)}} \quad \text{(in metres per second – m/s)}$$

conduction delay = latency$_2$ − latency$_1$

latency$_1$: distal motor latency

R: recording

S: stimulation

median and ulnar nerves and the ERB point for suprascapular nerve. The relationship between the distance of the two stimulation points (mm) and the latency difference (ms) give the MCV of the segment of a nerve trunk. The normal MCV varies from 50 to 70 metres per second for upper limbs, and from 40 to 55 metres per second for lower limbs. The normal MCV decreases slightly in the elderly.

Stimulation of the sensory fibers

With the sensory fibers, a single stimulation point and a single point of recording are sufficient to calculate sensory conduction velocity (SCV) of a given nerve (Figure 4.109). The sensory action potentials are 1,000 times less ample than the motor action potentials.

The EMG in lesions of peripheral nerves

The EMG is necessary to determine the extent and gravity of peripheral nerve lesions in continuity and to evaluate neural regeneration.

Until wallerian degeneration is completely established, the EMG data remains incomplete. After complete division of a nerve the distal nerve conduction may remain quite normal for five to 15 days, and elective denervation signs (fibrillation, sharp nerve) are

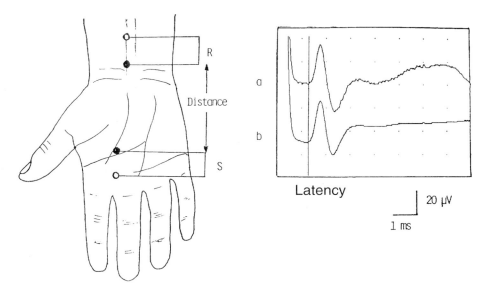

Figure 4.109. Sensory conduction velocity study.

$$SCV = \frac{distance\ (mm)}{conduction\ delay\ =\ latency\ (ms)} = m/s$$

R: recording
S: stimulation
a: direct trace
b: averaged trace

absent. It can cause misdiagnosis or an erroneous prognosis evaluation. The first EMG must therefore not be done before 15 days for the upper extremity and 21 days for the lower extremity. If the EMG is performed before this date, a second one 15 days later must be performed as a control for the first results.

Results of the first EMG
Two different cases can be found:

Complete section. Needle examination tests the extent of the lesion, shows much spontaneous activity and the absence of voluntary activity in denervated territories. Stimulodetection shows the total sensory and motor inexcitability of the nerve below the section.

Incomplete conduction block. Needle examination shows the extent of the lesion. Stimulodetection shows significant motor and sensory conduction changes with slowing and low amplitude of MAP and SAP.

Between these two typical EMG presentations, which are easy to interpret and very well correlated with clinical features, there are many different EMG pictures which do not afford precise diagnosis and prognosis. In all these cases, clinical and EMG examinations should be repeated after *two months*.

In cases of conduction block, there is evidence of abundant direct reinnervation with polyphasic complex potentials of long duration and small amplitude of good conduction improvement.

In the other cases, recovery is late, of poor quality and needs axonal regeneration. The reinnervation is poor, and spontaneous activity remains abundant. Nerve conduction shows little improvement and varies according to the percentage of fibers having a neuropraxic injury as opposed to a more serious lesion.

Next follow-up

For conduction block further EMG examination is usually unnecessary. In other cases with slower recovery, new electrical studies at six and 18 months are useful to follow the recovery.

Electrodiagnosis in carpal tunnel syndrome

Carpal tunnel syndrome (CTS) is the most frequently seen entrapment syndrome. There exists an electrical correlation between compression of the median nerve and localized slowing of nerve conduction velocity (Simpson, 1956). The median nerve conduction velocity is normal at the level of the arm and hand when it is reduced at the wrist. The ulnar nerve conduction is normal at the wrist and at the elbow.

The SCV gives more precise information, usually well correlated with the DML. However, in benign cases, SCV is more often abnormal than DML and sometimes even

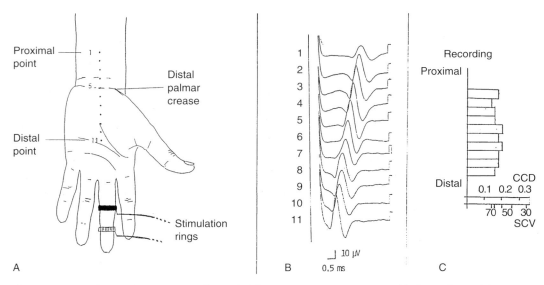

Figure 4.110. The centimetric test of Seror. (A) The eleven recording points. (B) Recordings of the 11 sensitivity potentials in a normal subject. The stimulation artefact has been suppressed. (C) Graph of the values obtained in a normal subject after calculating the 11 centimetric conduction delays (CCD) or the equivalent sensory conduction velocity (SCV).

SCV remains within normal limits. In these cases, a test devised by Kimura (1979) and Seror (1990) provides a functional anatomic study of the median nerve which allows an assessment of the CTS diagnosis (Figure 4.110). The needle examination must always test abductor pollicis brevis and a sample of muscle innervated by the C6 to T1 spinal roots which is essential to evaluate the differential diagnosis or associated cervical radiculopathy, plexopathy or myelopathy.

Factors affecting prognosis after traumatic lesions of peripheral nerves

The prognosis after a traumatic lesion of a peripheral nerve depends on a large number of factors which cannot be enumerated here. Countless neurophysiological studies have been devoted to axonal regeneration and to the reinnervation of muscle fibers and sensory receptors in the skin, yet many questions remain unanswered. However, the surgeon should evaluate the available facts, including results of the clinical examination and electrophysiological studies, and the operative findings.

We distinguish here between local factors, general factors, and factors related to treatment.

Local factors

The nature and severity of the nerve injury, its site, and the associated lesions are important determinants of prognosis.

Nature of the lesion

Traumatic lesions of the peripheral nerves can be classified into two categories—open lacerations and compressions.

From the prognostic point of view, it is probably fair to say that open injuries are more ominous than closed injuries because of the risk of infection and of cicatricial tissue formation. This, however, is a very rough distinction. Partial sectioning may be less damaging than compression caused by a plaster cast or a displaced fracture.

As a general rule, a slowly progressive lesion carries a better prognosis than one that produces sudden paralysis, and a partial lesion carries a better prognosis than a total lesion.

Other more accurate methods of classification take into account the histological lesions of the nerve trunk. Thus, Seddon (1943) recognized three groups of lesions:

1 Neuropraxia
2 Axonotmesis
3 Neurotmesis.

Neuropraxia

Neuropraxia implies interruption of nerve conduction with preservation of anatomical continuity of all neural structures. Its main clinical feature is a dissociated and transitory paralysis that affects primarily large-diameter fibers. It is thus predominantly motor, but also gives rise to sensory changes: the proprioceptive fibers are affected more than the touch fibers, and the latter more than the pain fibers. Recovery occurs in the reverse order.

These transitory paralyses were described as long ago as 1864 by Mitchell, who observed them following bullet injuries in which the bullet passed close to the nerve without hitting it. This type of paralysis can also be triggered by momentary traction or by compression, such as that resulting from the use of crutches.

Electrical tests show no sign of degeneration, conduction is preserved, and fibrillations may be present. This type of paralysis is typically transitory.

Studies have been designed to elucidate these transitory paralyses, which were thought at first to be due to ischemia resulting from transitory compression (Denny-Brown and Brenner, 1944). More recently Lundborg (1970) postulated anoxia in the fascicular microcirculation caused by venous obstruction in the epineurium. Kuczynski (1974) suggested an electrolytic imbalance at the nodes of Ranvier. In the same year, Gilliat et al and Ochoa demonstrated microscopic mechanical lesions resulting in demyelination at the nodes. The latter lesions are the slowest to recover; the process of remyelination takes about 60 days.

In cases of incomplete paralysis caused by compression with no axonal degeneration, the prognosis must be good. However, because such neuropraxic lesions are due to a variety of causes, some may take months to recover. If after three months there is no sign of recovery, neurolysis to relieve the compression must be considered (Spinner, 1978). Recovery then occurs in a few days unless demyelination has occurred, in which case reinnervation of the muscles takes two to three months.

Axonotmesis

Axonotmesis is a term coined by Seddon (1943) to describe loss of continuity of axons and of their myelin sheath, while the rest of the nerve trunk is intact: Schwann cells, endoneurium, perineurium, and epineurium. The motor, sensory, and sympathetic paralysis is total, and electrical tests show signs of neural degeneration. Reinnervation can occur spontaneously; its duration depends on the site of the lesion.

Neurotmesis

Finally, there is neurotmesis, which implies either a physical division of the nerve trunk or complete destruction of the intraneural architecture when spontaneous recovery is impossible, despite apparent continuity. Such lesions occur after traction injuries, toxic injections, and prolonged ischemia. Clinically it is impossible to differentiate between axonotmesis and neurotmesis without allowing the lesion to follow its course. Waiting too long for spontaneous recovery, however, is not without danger. Exploration may be necessary to establish the prognosis and attempt surgical repair.

Sunderland's classification

Sunderland's classification (1978) distinguishes five degrees of lesions (Table 4.3):

- the first degree corresponds to neurapraxia;
- the second degree is not unlike axonotmesis;

Seddon	Sunderland
Neurapraxia	First degree
Axonotmesis	{ Second degree { Third degree
Neurotmesis	{ Fourth degree { Fifth degree

Table 4.3. Correlation between Seddon's and Sunderland's classifications

- the third degree implies, in addition to axonal destruction and wallerian degeneration, destruction of the internal fascicular structure by edema, stasis, ischemia, segmental hemorrhage, or other factors. This gives rise to intrafascicular fibrosis, which in turn impedes regeneration. The period of denervation of the peripheral tissues is more prolonged than that occurring after a second degree lesion; in the course of regeneration there may be an exchange of fibers, and the quality of functional recovery suffers;

- the fourth degree is characterized by complete disruption of the fascicular organization. The perineurium is destroyed, and although the continuity of the nerve trunk is preserved, it is reduced to a cord of connective tissue. This type of lesion necessitates partial resection of the cicatricial tissues;

- the fifth degree lesion implies a break in continuity of the nerve.

When the nerve has been severed, the prognosis depends to some extent on the amount of nerve tissue lost. Other local factors are also relevant—the type of nerve and whether it is sensory, motor, or mixed. The extent of contusion and subsequent fibrosis also has a considerable influence on the nerve repair.

Site of the lesion
The site of the lesion can influence the prognosis in a number of ways. The more proximal the lesion, the farther the axons have to travel to reinnervate the extremity of the limb. In addition to the distance, there are the dangers inherent in the delay in reinnervation. The obstacles include exhaustion of the nerve cell, interstitial fibrosis, progressive atrophy, and degeneration of the muscle fibers.

Recovery of the intrinsic muscles of the hand following a high nerve lesion is exceptional in adults.

Another factor that worsens the prognosis in proximal lesions is the extent of retrograde axonal degeneration, which is always greater in lesions close to the cell body. This phenomenon can lead to the death of nerve cells, or at best reduces the regenerating capacity of the axon, which may be unable to reach the extremity of the limb. Retrograde degeneration is also influenced by the severity of the trauma, the site of nerve division, and the nature of the injury. It is more marked after avulsions and after injuries by high velocity missiles.

The nerve involved

From a prognostic standpoint, risks of directional errors concerning the axons seem greater when the nerve is "mixed." All motor nerves contain sensory fibers. Repair of predominantly motor nerves (e.g. the radial nerve) carries a better prognosis than that of "mixed" nerves containing a high percentage of sensory fibers (e.g. the ulnar and above all the median nerve).

Associated lesions

Associated traumatic lesions of muscle, bone, and blood vessels increase the scarring around and ischemia of the damaged nerve. The state of the "nerve bed" also influences the quality of the repair.

Emergency repair of the vessels, as is increasingly widely practiced, probably has a beneficial effect on the state of the muscle fibers, avoiding or delaying their degeneration and thus permitting late reinnervation.

General factors

The age of the patient is of such importance that any analysis of results must be made by age groups if it is to be valid. Every series published so far confirms that the best results are obtained in young subjects (Hallin et al, 1981). After the age of 30 the chances of success are reduced. It has been suggested that in children the axons have a shorter distance to travel because the limbs are shorter, the capacity for regeneration is greater, and there is probably the possibility of participation by a still adaptable nervous system.

The effect of age on conduction velocity has been studied by several investigators. Thomas and Lambert (1960) reported that in children five years old or less, conduction velocity is slower than that in the adult. This is readily explained by the fact that the rate of conduction is directly proportional to the diameter of the fibers, and this changes little after the age of five. At the other end of the scale, conduction velocity decreases with age, by about 10 per cent at the age of 60, owing to local ischemia and reduced permeability of the cell membrane (Wagman and Lesse, 1952).

The effect of delay on the prognosis

This problem is far from simple, and one must differentiate between delays in spontaneous regeneration compatible with functional recovery and delays between the injury and the repair compatible with functional recovery.

Delays prior to spontaneous recovery

These include:

1 the initial latent period (Sunderland, 1968), which corresponds to the time needed by the axon to cover the distance of the retrograde degeneration in addition to that needed for it to cross the injured zone of the nerve;

2 the period taken by the axons to cover the distance between the site of injury and the peripheral connections; and

3 the time required for the regrown axons and their reinnervated terminal corpuscles to be converted into functional units.

These delays are inevitably longer after proximal lesions, because retrograde degeneration is more marked, the axons have farther to travel, and the peripheral tissues remain denervated longer.

It appears that, in practice, the latent period is proportional to the severity of the lesion. In the majority of cases the first signs suggesting regeneration appear after six months, although in some proximal lesions the latent period may be even longer.

Delays prior to nerve repair

It has now been virtually established that the limiting factor is not so much the regeneration capacity of the nerve cell as the degeneration of the denervated muscles (Sunderland, 1950). Some nerve cells probably retain for years the capacity to grow new axons. By contrast, the period during which a denervated muscle can recover useful function is shorter. This delay in muscle recovery depends on the number of useful axons reaching the muscle and the number of surviving muscle fibers capable of reinnervation. Each of these must be considered in more detail.

The number of functional axons reaching the denervated muscles is necessarily smaller than normal by an amount that varies with the number of neurons surviving retrograde degeneration, the number of axons whose growth is stopped by fibrosis at the level of the injury, the number of axons misdirected outside the fascicles, and the number of axons misdirected within the fascicles.

The number of muscle fibers capable of reinnervation depends on the degree of destruction at the time of injury, the secondary degenerative changes in the muscles (leading to atrophy and sclerosis), the capacity for connection between the extremities of the nerve fibers reaching the motor end plates, and the restoration of sufficient neuromuscular units to achieve useful motor function.

Gutmann and Young (1944) believed that the longer the delay in reinnervation, the less the chances of return of motor function, because the proportion of reinnervated motor end plates is rapidly reduced when atrophy sets in. Also, the formation of new end plates slows because they are probably less efficient than the old. The number of fibers destined not to be reinnervated increases with time. It follows, therefore, that the earlier reinnervation occurs, the better are the chances for functional recovery.

It has been shown that the delay prior to a nerve repair affects the quality of the results. Figures published by the US Army Medical Services concerning nerve suturing performed during World War II showed that every delay of six days before the repair reduced the quality of the result by 1 per cent (Woodhall and Beebe, 1956). Analyzing their results in microsurgical repair of nerve injuries. Zilch and Buck-Gramcko (1975) found that 85 per cent of their failures occurred when the repair was performed more than four months after the injury. Delay between injury and nerve repair seems to have much stronger effects on the functional scores than on the electrophysiological measures.

Delays compatible with reinnervation after nerve repair

The delay usually noted as being compatible with good recovery of muscle function ranges from 12 to 18 months. It seems unlikely that muscles that have been denervated for 18 months will regain useful function (Zachary and Roaf, 1954). However, Bowden and Gutmann (1944) have shown in muscle biopsy studies that reinnervation remains possible for up to three years. Now that repairs after brachial plexus lesions are more frequent, reinnervation has been seen to occur after more than two years.

It should be pointed out, however, that the late reinnervations occurred in young patients and in muscles relatively free of atrophy and sclerosis as a result of regular physiotherapy. It is important to point out that function continues to improve for at least four years (Nicholson and Seddon, 1957; Önne, 1962). This notion is perhaps not widely appreciated by surgeons. Assessments of final results of nerve repair therefore require follow-up times in excess of four years.

From a practical viewpoint, it is worth stressing that:

1 Nerve repair should be carried out as soon as local conditions are favorable.
2 As soon as paralysis has been diagnosed, a course of physiotherapy should be prescribed to keep the joints supple and to prevent muscle fibrosis.
3 The more proximal a lesion, the earlier the repair should be performed.
4 When assessing the theoretical chances for recovery, the surgeon should add the preoperative delay to the time needed for the growing axon to reach the paralyzed muscle (on the basis of an average of 1 mm a day). If the total is greater than 18 months, it is often wiser, especially if the patient is not young, to combine a nerve repair with palliative surgery to correct the motor deficit resulting from lack of function of the paralyzed muscles, provided this does not produce a further deficit.
5 By contrast, sensation (or at least protective sensation) can return after much longer delays—seven years or more in some of our cases. Protective sensation, however, should not be confused with the return of "stereognosis," which is difficult to obtain even with early repair.

Prognostic factors pertaining to treatment

The prognostic factors pertaining to treatment are extremely important. It is now agreed that the surgical procedure should be delicate and non-traumatic, that the "nerve bed" (at the site of the repair) should be cleared of scar tissue, and that excessive dissection and suturing under tension should be avoided. The use of operating microscopes, bipolar coagulation, microinstruments, and microsutures has now become commonplace. Accurate realignment of the nerve ends is always desirable but difficult to achieve. Median or ulnar nerve lesions are often accompanied by interruption of the radial or ulnar artery. The beneficial influence of arterial repair on the ultimate functional result has often been demonstrated (Merle et al, 1988).

Emphasis should be placed on the influence on prognosis of the experience and careful technique of the surgeon.

Prognostic factors relating to other aspects of treatment and the patient

The functional prognosis is in great part dependent upon the state of the paralyzed limb, e.g. the remaining muscles and the suppleness of the joints. Hence, the fundamental importance of physiotherapy, which as soon as paralysis is present must be undertaken to overcome abnormal positions and stiffness, maintain the strength of the remaining muscles, and enforce maximal use of the limb by the patient. This treatment is continued throughout the course of nerve regeneration.

A will to recover on the part of the patient and his ability to play a role was long unrecognized. This explains why certain individuals are capable of discriminative use of the hands in spite of severely disturbed sensitivity test results. Rehabilitation of sensitivity is also based upon the possibility of improving use of the regenerated nerve potential. After motor paralysis, the efforts of the patient to use his limb and obtain best use of the reinnervated muscles help considerably in his adaptation to the new circumstances.

REFERENCES

Adson AW, Coffey JR (1927) Cervical rib: a method of anterior approach for relief of symptoms by division of the scalemus anticus. *Ann Surg*, **85**:839–57.

Albinus BS (1724) *Historia musculorum hominis* (Leiden).

Almquist EE, Eeg-Olofsson O (1970) Sensory nerve conduction velocity and two-point discrimination in sutured nerves, *J Bone Joint Surg*, **52A**:791.

American Society for Surgery of the Hand (1976) *Clinical Assessment Committee Report* (ASSH).

Arkless R (1966) Cineradiography in normal and abnormal wrists, *Am J Roentgenol*, **96**:837–44.

Aschan W, Moberg E (1962) The Ninhydrin finger print test used to map out partial lesions to hand nerves, *Acta Chir Scand*, **123**.

Aubriot JH (1981) The metacarpophalangeal joint of the thumb. In: Tubiana R, ed, *The Hand*, volume 1 (WB Saunders: Philadelphia).

Aulicino PL, Dupuy TE (1990) Clinical examination of the hand. In: Hunter JM, Schneider LH, Mackin EJ et al, eds, *Rehabilitation of the Hand: Surgery and Therapy*, 3rd edn (CF Mosby: St Louis).

Backhouse KM (1968) Functional anatomy of the hand. *Physiotherapy*, **54**:114–17.

Barreiro FJJ, Valdecasas Huelin JM (1981) Radiological studies on the vascular anatomy of the forearm and hand. In: Tubiana R, ed, *The Hand*, volume I (WB Saunders: Philadelphia).

Baumann JA, Patry G (1943) Observations microscopiques sur la texture fibreuse et la vascularisation de l'ensemble tendineux extenseur du doigt et de la main, chez l'homme (considérations fonctionnelles), *Rev Méd Suisse Romande*, **36**:900–12.

Bechtol CD (1954) Grip test: use of a dynamometer with adjustable handle spacing, *J Bone Joint Surg*, **36A**:820.

Bell C (1833) *The Hand. Its Mechanism and Vital Endowments as Evincing Design* (William Pickering: London).

Bell J (1978) Sensibility evaluation. In: Hunter JM, Schneider LH, Mackin EJ et al, eds, *Rehabilitation of the Hand*, 1st edn (CV Mosby: St Louis).

Bell J (1984) Light touch–deep pressure testing using Semmes–Weinstein monofilaments. In: Hunter JM, Schneider LH, Mackin EJ et al, eds, *Rehabilitation of the Hand*, 2nd edn (CV Mosby: St Louis).

Bell-Krotoski JA (1990a) Light touch–deep pressure testing using the Semmes–Weinstein monofilaments. In: Hunter JM, Schneider LH, Mackin EJ, eds, *Rehabilitation of the Hand: Surgery and Therapy*, 3rd edn (CV Mosby: St Louis) 585–93.

Bell-Krotoski JA (1990b) Pocket filaments and specifications for the Semmes–Weinstein monofilaments, *J Hand Therapy*, **3**:26.

Bell-Krotoski JA (1991) Advances in sensibility evaluation, *Hand Clin*, 7: 4.

Bell-Krotoski JA (1992) Pocket filaments and specifications for the Semmes–Weinstein monofilaments. In: Amadio PC, Hentz VR, eds, *Year Book of Hand Surgery* (CV Mosby: Chicago) 293–4.

Bell-Krotoski JA, Buford WL (1988) The force time relationship of clinically used sensory testing instruments, *J Hand Therapy*, **1**:76.

Bell-Krotoski JA, Tomancik E (1987) The repeatability of testing with Semmes–Weinstein monofilaments, *J Hand Surg*, **12A**:155–61.

Bell-Krotoski JA, Weinstein S, Weinstein C (1993) Testing sensibility, including touch-pressure, two-point discrimination, point localization and vibration. *J Hand Therapy*, **6**:114–23.

Belsole J, Hibelin D (1986) Scaphoid orientation and location from computed three dimensional carpal models, *Orthop Clin North Am*, **17**:505–10.

Bichat X (1855) *Recherches physiologiques sur la vie et la mort*, 3rd edn (A Delahays: Paris).

Biesalski K, Mayer L (1916) *Die physiologische Sehnerverpflanzung* (Springer: Berlin) 330.

Biondetti PR, Vannier MW, Gilula LA et al (1987) Wrist coronal and transaxial CT scanning, *Radiology*, **163**:149–51.

Björkensten G (1946) Position of fingers and function deficiency in ulnar paralysis. *Acta Chir Scand*, **93**:99.

Blix M (1894) Due Länge und die Spannung des Muskels, *Skand Arch Physiol*, **5**:149.

Blonstein A, Doyon D, Harry G (1977) L'arteriographie de la main traumatique. Indications, methode, resultats à propos de 150 observations, *J Radiol*, **58**:93–102.

Bonnel F (1985) Histologic structure of the ulnar nerve in the hand, *J Hand Surg*, **10A** (2):264–9.

Bonnel F (1994) The distal radio-ulnar joint (personal communication).

Bonnel F, Allieu Y (1984) Les articulations radio cubito carpienne et medio carpienne: organisation anatomique et bases bioméchaniques, *Ann Chir Main*, **3**: 287–96.

Bonnel F, Durand J, Blotman F et al (1978) Anatomie et systématisation fasciculaire du nerf médian. In: Simon L, ed, *Actualités rééducationelles, fonctionelles et réadaptives*, 4th series. (Masson: Paris) 113–19.

Bonnel F, Mailhe P, Allieu Y et al (1980) Bases anatomiques de la chirurgie fasciculaire du nerf médian au poignet, *Ann Chir*, **34**:707–10.

Botte MJ, Cohen MS, Lavergna CJ et al (1990) The dorsal branch of the ulnar nerve: an anatomic study, *J Hand Surg*, **15A**:603–7.

Boussy J Cited by Rabischong, 1971.

Bouvier (1851) Note sur un cas de paralysie de la main, *Bull Acad Med*, **27**:125.

Bowden REM, Gutmann E (1944) Denervation and re-innervation of human voluntary muscle, *Brain*, **67**:273.

Bowers WH (1988) The distal radioulnar joint. In: Green DP, ed, *Operative Hand Surgery*, 2nd edn volume 2 (Churchill Livingstone: New York) 939.

Boyes JH (1962) Selection for a donor muscle for tendon transfer, *J Hosp Joint Dis*, **23**:1.

Boyes JH (1964, 1970) *Bunnell's Surgery of the Hand* (JB Lippincott: Philadelphia).

Brand PW (1974) Biomechanics of tendon transfer, *Orthop Clin North Am*, **5**:205.

Brand PW (1980) Functional manifestations of sensory loss. Presented at Symposium on Assessment of Levels of Cutaneous Sensibility, USPHS Hospital: Carville, Louisiana.

Brand PW (1985) *Clinical Mechanics of the Hand* (CV Mosby: St Louis).

Brand PW, Beach RB, Thomsen DE (1981) Relative tension and potential excursion of muscles in the forearm and hand, *J Hand Surg*, **6**:201–9.

Brand PW, Cramer KC, Ellis JC (1975) Tendon and pulleys at the metacarpophalangeal joint of a finger, *J Bone Joint Surg*, **57A**:779.

Braunstein EM, Louis DS, Greene TL et al (1985) Fluoroscopic and arthrographic evaluation of carpal instability, *Am J Roentgenol*, **144**:1259–62.

Braunstein EM, Vydareny KH, Louis DS et al (1986) Cost effectiveness of wrist fluoroscopy and arthrography in evaluation of obscure wrist pain, *Orthopedics*, **9**:1504–6.

Bridgman CF (1949) Radiography of the carpal navicular bone, *Med Radiogr Photogr*, **25**:104–5.

Brooks HSJ (1886) Variations in the nerve supply of the flexor pollicis brevis muscle, *J Anat*, **20**:641.

Brun J (1963) *La Main et l'esprit* (Presses Universitaires de France: Paris).

Brunelli F (1993) Le lambeau dorso cubital du ponce, *Ann Chir Main*, **12**:105–14.

Brunelli F, Mathoulin C (1991) Presentation d'un nouveau lambeau en clot homodigital sensible à contre–courant, *Ann Chir Main*, **10**:48–53.

Brunelli F, Brunelli G, Nanfito F (1991) An anatomical study of the vascularization of the first dorsal interosseous space in the hand and a description of a bony pedicle graft arising from bone, *Surg Rad Anat*, **13**:73–5.

Brunelli F, Peguin Z, Cabral J (1991) Dorsal arterial supply to the thumb, *Surg Radiol Anat*, **13**:240–2.

Brunelli F, Brunelli G (1991) Vascular anatomy of the distal phalanx. In: Foucher G, ed, *Fingertip and Nailbed Injuries* (Churchill Livingstone: Edinburgh).

Buck–Gramcko D, Dietrich FE, Gogge S (1976) Bewertungs Kriterien bei Nachuntersuchungen von beugeschnenwieder Herstellungen. *Handchirurgie* **8**:65–9.

Bunnell S (1938) Opposition of the thumb, *J Bone Joint Surg*, **20**:269–84.

Bunnell S (1956) *Surgery of the Hand*, 5th edn (revised by Boyes J) (JB Lippincott: Philadelphia).

Burton AC (1939) The range and variation of the blood flow in the human fingers, *Am J Physiol*, **127**:437.

Bush CH, Gillespy III T, Dell PC (1987) High-resolution CT of the wrist: initial experience, *Am J Roentgenol*, **149**:757–60.

Caffinière JY de la (1970) L'Articulation trapéziometacarpienne, approche bioméchanique et appareil ligamentaire, *Arch Anat Pathol*, **18**:277–84.

Caffinière JY de la (1971) Anatomie fonctionelle de la poulie proximale des doigts, *Arch Anat Pathol*, **19**:35.

Caffinière JY de la (1981) Topographic anatomy of the hand. In: Tubiana R, ed, *The Hand*, volume 1 (WB Saunders: Philadelphia).

Callahan A (1984) Sensibility testing: clinical methods. In: Hunter JM, Schneider LH, Mackin EJ et al, eds, *Rehabilitation of the Hand*, 2nd edn (CV Mosby: St Louis).

Callahan AD (1990) Sensibility testing: clinical methods. In: Hunter JM, Schneider LH, Mackin EJ et al, eds, *Rehabilitation of the Hand: Surgery and Therapy*, 3rd edn (CV Mosby: St Louis) 432–42.

Cannieu JMA (1897) Recherches sur une anastomose entre la branche profonde du cubital et le médian, *Bull Soc Anat Physiol Bordeaux*, **18**:339–40.

Capener N (1956) The hand in surgery, *J Bone Joint Surg*, **38B**:128.

Cauna N (1954) Nature and functions of the papillary ridges of the digital skin, *Anat Rec*, **119**:449.

Cauna N, Ross LL (1960) The fine structure of Meissner's touch corpuscles of human fingers, *J Biophys Biochem,* **8**:476.

Chow SP (1980) Digital nerves in the terminl phalangeal region of the thumb, *The Hand*, **12**:1993–6.

Cleland J (1878) The cutaneous ligaments of the phalanges, *J Anat Physiol*, **12**:526.

Coene LN (1985) Axillary nerve lesions and associated injuries. Thesis, Leiden Kempenaer, Oegstgeest, Netherlands.

Coleman HM (1956) Tears of the fibrocartilagineous disc at the wrist, *J Bone Joint Surg*, **38B**:782.

Coleman HM (1960) Injuries of the articular wrist, *J Bone Joint Surg*, **42B**:522.

Cone RO, Szabo R, Resnick D et al (1983) Computed tomography of the normal soft tissues of the wrist, *Invest Radiol*, **18**:546–51.

Cooney WP, Chao EYS (1977) Biomechanical analysis of static forces in the thumb during hand function, *J Bone Joint Surg*, **59A**:27.

Cruveilhier J (1843) *Traité d'anatomie descriptive* (Labe: Paris).

Dalinka MK, Turner ML, Osterman AL et al (1981) Wrist arthrography, *Radiol Clin North Am*, **19**:217–26.

Daniels L, Williams M, Worthingham C (1956) *Muscle Testing* (WB Saunders: Philadelphia).

Dautel G, Merle M (1993) Tests dynamiques arthroscopiques pour le diagnostic des instabilités scapho-lunaires. *Ann Chir Main,* **12**:206–9.

DeFrenne HA (1977) Les structures aponevnotiques au niveau de la première commissure, *Ann Chir,* **31**:1017–19.

Delay J (1935) *Les Astéreognosies. Pathologie du toucher* (Masson: Paris).

Delay J (1952) *Les Dissolutions de la mémoire* (Presses Universitaires de France: Paris).

Dellon AL (1979) The paper clip: light hardware to evaluate sensibility in the hand, *Contemp Orthop,* **1**:39.

Dellon AL (1981) *Evaluation of sensibility and reeducation of sensation in the hand* (Williams and Wilkins: Baltimore).

Denny-Brown D, Brenner C (1944) Paralysis of nerve induced by direct pressure and by tourniquet, *Arch Neurol Psychiat,* **51**:1–26.

Destot E (1923) *Traumatismes du poignet et rayons* (Masson: Paris).

Dobyns JH, Linscheid RL, Chao EYS et al (1975) Traumatic instability of the wrist, *American Academy of Orthopaedic Surgeons Instructional Course Lectures,* **24**:182.

Doyle JR, Blythe W (1975) The finger flexor tendon sheath and pulleys: anatomy in reconstruction. In: American Academy of Orthopedic Surgeons, *Symposium on Tendon Surgery in the Hand* (CV Mosby: St Louis).

Dubousset J (1971) Anatomie fonctionnelle de l'appareil capsulo-ligamentaire des articulations des doigts. In: Vilain R, ed, *Traumatismes ostéo-articulaires de la main.* Monographie du GEM (Expansion Scientifique Française: Paris).

Duchenne GB (1867) *Physiologie des mouvements* (JB Baillière: Paris).

Duchenne GB (1949) *Physiology of Motion* (translated and edited by Kaplan EB) (JB Lippincott: Philadelphia).

Duparc J, Caffinière JY de la, Pineau H (1971) Approche bioméchanique et rotation des mouvements du première métacarpien, *Rev Chir Orth Rep Appl Moteur,* **57**:3–12.

Dupré E (1903) Psychopathies organiques. Agnosies et apraxies. In: Ballet G, ed, *Traité de pathologie mentale:* 1092.

Eaton RG (1971) *Joint Injuries of the Hand* (Charles C Thomas: Springfield, Illinois).

Ebskov B (1970) *De motibus motoribusque pollicis humani.* Thesis, Copenhagen.

Ekenstam FW (1985) The distal radioulnar joint. Doctoral Thesis, Acta Universitatis Upsaliensis 505: 1–55.

Ekenstam F, Hagert C (1985) Anatomical studies on the geometry and stability of the distal radioulnar joint, *Scand J Plast Reconstr Surg,* **19**: 17–25.

Elftman H (1966) Biomechanics of muscle, *J Bone Joint Surg,* **48A**:363.

Engber WD, Gmeiner JG (1980) Palmar cutaneous branch of the ulnar nerve, *J Hand Surg,* **5**:21–4.

Eyler DL, Markee JE (1954) The anatomy and function of the intrinsic musculature of the fingers, *J Bone Joint Surg,* **36A**:1.

Fahrer M (1969) The range of movements of the fourth metacarpal joint. A problem for pianists and anatomists, *J Anat,* **104**:410.

Fahrer M (1971) Considérations sur l'anatomie fonctionelle du muscle fléchisseur commun profond des doigts, *Ann Chir,* **25**:945–50.

Fahrer M (1973) The role of the palmaris longus muscle in the abduction of the thumb, *J Anat (Lond),* **116**:476.

Fahrer M (1975) Considérations sur les insertions d'origine des muscles lombricaux: les systèmes digastriques de la main, *Ann Chir,* **29**:979–82.

Fahrer M (1977) Anatomy of the karate chop, *J Anat (London),* **124**:521.

Fahrer M (1981a) The hypothenar eminence. In: Tubiana R ed, *The Hand,* volume 1 (WB Saunders: Philadelphia).

Fahrer M (1981b) The thenar eminence. In: Tubiana R, ed, *The Hand,* volume 1 (WB Saunders: Philadelphia).

Fahrer M, Pineau H (1976) La force musculaire des longs fléchisseurs de la main, *Ann Chir*, **30**:947–52.

Fahrer M, Tubiana R (1976) Palmaris longus, anteductor of the thumb; an experimental study, *Hand*, **8**:287–9.

Fess E (1986) The need for reliability and validity in hand assessment instruments, *J Hand Surg*, **11A**:621–3.

Fick R (1901) Ergebnisse einer Untersuchung der Handbewegungen mit X-Strahlen, *Verh Anat Ges*, **15**:175.

Fick R (1911) *Handbuch der Anatomie und Mechanik der Gelenke*—3 Teil (G Fischer: Iena).

Finkelstein H (1930) Stenosing tenovaginitis of the radial styloid process. *J Bone Joint Surg*, **12**:509.

Fisk GR (1970) Carpal instability and the fractured scaphoid, *Ann R Coll Surg Engl*, **46**:63.

Flatt AE (1971) The pathomechanics of ulnar drift. Final report. Social and Rehabilitation Services Grant RD 2226 M (Department of Health, Education, and Welfare: Washington DC).

Flatt AE, Fischer GW (1969) Stability during flexion and extension at the metacarpo-phalangeal joints. In: Tubiana R, ed, *La Main Rhumatoïde*, 2nd edn. Monographie du GEM (Expansion Scientifique Française: Paris).

Focillon H (1947) Eloge de la main. In: *Vie des formes* (Presses Universitaires de France: Paris).

Forster O (1934) The motor cortex in man in the light of Hughlings Jackson's doctrines. *Brain*, **59**:135–59.

Foucher G (1985) The kite flaps. In: Tubiana R, ed, *The Hand*, volume 2 (WB Saunders: Philadelphia).

Fowler SB (1949) Extensor apparatus of the digits, *J Bone Joint Surg*, **31B**:447.

Fowler SB (1959) The management of tendon injuries, *J Bone Joint Surg*, **41A**:579–80.

Freehafer A, Peckham PH, Keith MW (1979) Determination of muscle-tendon unit properties during tendon transfer, *J Hand Surg*, **4**:331–9.

Freehafer AA, Peckham PH, Keith MW et al (1988) The brachioradialis: anatomy, properties and value for tendon transfer in the tetraplegic, *J Hand Surg*, **13A**:99.

von Frey M (1924) Physiologische Sensibilitätsprüfungen Verhand d 37°. Kongress für innere Medizin.

von Frey M, Kiesow F (1899) Über die Funktion der Tastorperchen, *Ztschr Psychol Physiol Sinnesorg*, **20**:126–63.

Frohse F, Frankel M (1908) Die Muskeln des menschlichen Armes. *Bardelebens Handbuch der Anatomie des Menschlichen* (Fisher: Iena).

Froment J (1920) Paralysie des muscles de la main et troubles de la préhension, *J Med Lyon*.

Galien (Galen) (1854) *Œuvres anatomiques, physiologiques et médicales* (translated by Daremberg C) (Baillière: Paris).

Ganel A, Engel J, Ditzian R et al (1984) Arthrography as a method of diagnosing soft-tissue injuries of the wrist, *J Trauma*, **19**:376–80.

Gaul J St (1971) The ratio of motion of the interphalangeal joints. Unpublished report.

Gelberman R, Hergenroeder P, Hargens A et al (1981) The carpal tunnel syndrome. A study of carpal tunnel pressures. *J Bone Joint Surg*, **63A**:380.

Gelberman RH, Menon J (1980) The vascularity of the scaphoid bone, *J Hand Surg*, **5**:508.

Gelberman RH, Panagis JS, Taleisnik J et al (1983) The arterial anatomy of the human carpus. Part I: The extraosseous vascularity, *J Hand Surg*, **8**:367.

Gelberman RH, Salamon PB, Jurist JM et al (1975) Ulnar variance in Kienböck's disease, *J Bone Joint Surg*, **57A**:674–6.

Gilbert A et al (1985) Lesions of the volar plates. In: Tubiana R, ed, *The Hand*, Volume 2 (WB Saunders: Philadelphia).

Gilliatt RW, Ochoa J, Rudge P et al (1974) The cause of nerve damage in acute compression, *Trans Am Neurol Assn*, **99**:71–4.

Gilula LA, Destout JM, Weeks PM et al (1987) Roentgenographic diagnosis of the painful wrist, *Clin Orthop*, **187**:52–64.

Gilula LA, Totty WG, Weeks PM (1983) Wrist arteriography – The value of fluoroscopic spot viewing, *Radiology*, **146**:555–6.

Glicenstein J, Dardour JC (1981) Pulp: anatomy and physiology. In: Tubiana R, ed, *The Hand*, Volume I (WB Saunders: Philadelphia).

Gosset J (1972) Anatomie des aponévroses palmo-digitales. In: Tubiana R, Heuston JT, eds, *Maladie de Dupuytren*, 2nd edn. Monographie du GEM (Expansion Scientifique Française: Paris).

Grapow M (1887) Die Anatomie and physiologische Beteudung der palmar aponeurose, *Archiv Anatomie und Physiologie, Anat Abt*, **2–3**:143.

Grayson J (1941) The cutaneous ligaments of the digits, *J Anat*, **75**:164.

Gruber W (1870) Uber die Verbindung des Nervus medianus mit dem Nervus ulnaris am Unterarme des Menschen und der Sängethiere, *Arch Anat Physiol*, **37**:501–22.

Gupta A, Kleinert JM, Layman CD et al (1998) Vascular disease of the upper extremity. In: Tubiana R, ed, *The Hand*, volume 5 (WB Saunders: Philadelphia).

Gutmann E, Young JZ (1944) The re-innervation of muscle after various periods of atrophy, *J Anat*, **78**:15.

Guyon F (1861) Note sur une disposition anatomique propre à la face antérieure de la région du poignet et non encore décrite, *Bull Soc Anat Paris*, 2nd series, **6**:184–6.

Hagert CG (1992) The distal radioulnar joint in relation to the whole forearm, *Clin Orthopaedics*, **275**:56–64.

Haines RW (1944) Mechanism of rotation at first carpo metacarpal joint, *J Anatomy (London)*, **78**:44.

Hakstian RW, Tubiana R (1967) Ulnar deviation of the fingers. The role of joint structure and function, *J Bone Joint Surg*, **49A**:299.

Hallin RG, Wiesenfeld I, Lungnegard H (1981) Neurophysiological studies of peripheral nerve function after neural regeneration following nerve suture in man. *Int Rehab Med*, **3**:187–92.

Harness D, Sekeles E (1971) The double anastomotic innervation of thenar muscles, *J Anat*, **109**:461–6.

Harris C, Rutledge GL (1972) The functional anatomy of the extensor mechanism of the finger, *J Bone Joint Surg*, **54A**: 713–26.

Hart VL, Gaynor V (1941) Roentgenographic study of the canal. *J Bone Joint Surg*, **23A**:382–3.

Hauck G (1923) Die Ruptur der Dorsalaponeurose am ersten Interphalangealgelenk; zugleich ein Beitrag zur Anatomie und Physiologie der Dorsalaponeurose, *Arch Klin Chirurgie*, **123**:197–232.

Hazelton FT, Smidt GL, Flatt AE et al (1975) The influence of wrist position on the force produced by the finger flexors, *J Biomechanics*, **8**:301–6.

Head H (1920) *Studies in Neurology* (Oxford Medical Press: Oxford).

Henderson WR (1948) Clinical assessment of peripheral nerve injuries. Tinel's test, *Lancet*, **2**:801.

Henke W (1859) Die Bewegungen der Handwurzel, *Z Rationelle Med*, **7**:27.

Henle J (1868) *Handbuch der systematischen Anatomie des Menschen* (Friedrich Vieweg und Sohn, Braunschweig).

Highet WB (1942) Procaine nerve block in investigation of peripheral nerve injuries, *J Neurol Psychiatr Lond*, **5**:101.

Highet WB (1943) Innervation and function of the thenar muscles, *Lancet*:227–30.

Hoffmann H (1884) Stereognostische Versuche angestellt zur Ermittelung der Elemente des Gefühlssinnes aus denen die Vorstellungen der Körper im Raume gebildet werden. First Inaugural Dissertation, Strassburg.

Hoffmann P (1915) Uber eine Methode den Erflog einer Nervennaht zu beurteilen, *Med Klin*, **11**:359–60.

Holstein A, Lewis GB (1963) Fractures of the humerus with radial nerve paralysis, *J Bone Joint Surg*, **45A**:1382.

Horch K, Hardy M, Jimenez S et al (1992a) An automated tactile tester for evaluation of cutaneous sensibility, *J Hand Surg*, **17A**:829–37.

Horch K, Hardy M, Jimenez S et al (1992b) Evaluation of nerve compression with the automated tactile tester, *J Hand Surg*, **17A**:838–42.

Hovelacque A (1927) *Anatomie des nerfs craniens et rachidiens et du système grand sympathique chez l'homme* (Gaston Doin: Paris).

Hueston JT (1973) Surgical anatomy of the hand. In: Rank BK, Wakefield AR, Hueston JT, eds, *Surgery of the Hand as Applied to Hand Injuries*, 4th edn (Churchill Livingstone: Edinburgh).

Hunter JM, Ochiai JF, Konikoff J et al (1980) The pulley system, *J Hand Surg*, **5**:283.

Hunter JM, Singer DI, Mackin EJ (1990) Staged flexor tendon reconstruction using passive and active tendon implants. In: Hunter JM, Schneider LH, Mackin EJ et al, eds, *Rehabilitation of the Hand*, 3rd edn (CV Mosby: St Louis).

Imamura K (1987) Cineradiography, *Nippon Seik Gokkai Zashi*, **61**:499–510.

Jabaley ME (1981) Recovery of sensation in flaps and skin grafts. In: Tubiana R, ed, *The Hand*. (WB Saunders: Philadelpha) volume 1, 583–601.

Jabaley ME, Wallace W, Keckler FR (1980) Internal topography of major nerves of the forearm and hand, *J Hand Surg*, **5A**:1.

Jarvilehto T (1977) Neural basis of cutaneous sensations analyzed by microelectrode measurements from human peripheral nerves, *Scand J Psychol*, **18**:348–59.

Jeanne (1915) La déformation du pouce dans la paralysie du cubital, *Bulletin et Mémoires de la Société Chirurgicale de Paris*: 702.

Jones FW (1919) Voluntary muscular movements in cases of nerve lesions, *J Anat*, **54**:41.

Jung R (1941) Die allgemeine Symptomatologie der Nervenverletzungen und ihre physiologischen Grundlagen, *Nervenarzt*, **11**:494.

Jupiter JE, Kleinert HE (1988) Vascular injuries in the upper extremity. In: Tubiana R, ed, *The Hand*, volume 3 (WB Saunders: Philadelphia).

Kapandji AI (1963) *Physiologie articulaire*, volume 1 (Librairie Maloine: Paris).

Kapandji AI (1972) Les mouvements du pouce, *Rev Chir Orth*, **58**:273.

Kapandji AI (1981) Biomechanics of the thumb. In: Tubiana R, ed, *The Hand*, volume 1 (WB Saunders: Philadelphia).

Kapandji AI (1981) The inferior radioulnar joint and pronosupination. In: Tubiana R, ed, *The Hand*, volume 1 (WB Saunders: Philadelphia).

Kapandji AI (1986) Cotation clinique de l'opposition et de la contreopposition du pouce, *Ann Chir Main Memb Super*, **5**:67–73.

Kapandji AI (1992) Clinical evaluation of the thumb's opposition, *J Hand Therapy*, **5**:102–6.

Kapandji A, Moatti E, Raab C (1980) La radiographic spécifique de l'articulation trapézo-métacarpienne, *Ann Chir Main*, **34**:719–26.

Kaplan EB (1954) Anatomical problems of opposition of the thumb, *Bull Hosp Joint Dis*, **15**:56.

Kaplan EB (1965) *Functional and Surgical Anatomy of the Hand*, 2nd edn (JB Lippincott: Philadelphia).

Kaplan EB (1975) Anatomy and kinesiology of the hand. In: Flynn JE, ed, *Hand Surgery*, 2nd edn (Williams and Wilkins: Baltimore).

Kaplan EB, Spinner M (1980) *Normal and Anomalus Innervation of Peripheral Nerve Problems* (WB Saunders: Philadelphia).

Kauer JMG (1964) Een analyse van de carpale flexie. Thesis, Leyden.

Kelleher JC, Robinson JH, Yanik MA (1985) The pattern abdominal pedicle flap. In: Tubiana R, ed, *The Hand*, Volume 2 (WB Saunders: Philadelphia).

Ketchum LD, Thompson D, Pocock G et al (1978) Forces generated by intrinsic muscles of index, *J Hand Surg*, **2**:571.

Ketchum LD, Thompson DE (1985) An experimental investigation into the forces internal to the human hand. In: Brand P, ed, *Clinical Mechanics of the Hand* (CV Mosby: St Louis).

Kilgore ES Jr, Graham WP et al (1975) The extensor plus finger, *Hand* 7:159–65.

Kiloh LG, Nevin S (1952) Isolated neuritis of the anterior interosseous nerve, *Br Med J*, **i**:850–1.

Kimura J (1978) A method for determining median nerve conduction velocity across the carpal tunnel, *J Neurol Sci*, **38**:1.

Kimura J (1979) The carpal tunnel syndrome. Localization of conduction abnormales within the distal segment of median nerve, *Brain*, **102**:619–35.

Kimura J (1984) Principles and pitfalls of nerve conduction studies. *Ann Neurol*, **16**:415–27.

Kleinert HE, Kutz JE et al (1973) Primary repair of flexor tendons, *Orthop Clin North Am*, **4**:865–76.

Kristensen SS, Thomassen E, Christensen F (1986) Ulnar variance determination, *J Hand Surg*, **11**:255–7.

Krukenberg H (1922) Über Ersatz des M Opponens pollicis, *Zeitschrift für Orthopädische Chirurgie*, **42**:178–9.

Kuczynski K (1968) The upper limb. In: Passmore R, Robson JS, eds, *A Companion to Medical Studies*, volume 1 (Blackwell Scientific: Oxford).

Kuczynski K (1974) Functional micro-anatomy of the peripheral nerve trunks, *Hand*, **6**:1–10.

Kuczynski K (1975) Less-known aspects of the proximal interphalangeal joints of the human hand, *Hand*, 7:31–3.

Kuenz (1923) Les géodes du semi-lunaire. Thesis, Lyon.

Kuhlmann JN, Fahrer M, Kapandji AI et al (1985) Stability of the normal wrist. In: Tubiana R, ed, *The Hand* (WB Saunders: Philadelphia) volume 2, 934–44.

Kuhlmann N (1977) Anatomia descriptiva y funcional del carpo en relacion con la pathologia traumatica del mismo, *Rev Esp Cirug Mano*, **5**:13–104.

Kuhlmann N, Gallaire M, Pineau H (1978a) Déplacements du scaphoïde et du semi-lunaire au cours des movements du poignet, *Ann Chir*, **32**:543–53.

Kuhlmann N, Tubiana R, Lisfranc R (1978b) Apport de l'anatomie dans la compréhension du canal carpien et des séquelles des interventions décompressives, *Rev Chir Orthop*, **64**:59–70.

LaMotte RH (1979) Presented in discussions at Symposium on Assessment of Cutaneous Sensibility, Gillis W Long Hansen's Disease Center: Carville, Louisiana.

Landsmeer JMF (1949) Les insertions des muscles interosseux de la main chez l'homme, *C R Assn Anat*, **36**:404–10.

Landsmeer JMF (1955) Anatomical and functional investigations on the articulations of the human fingers, *Acta Anat* (suppl 24), **25**:1.

Landsmeer JMF (1956) Les aponévroses dorsales de la main, *C R Assn Anat*, **43**:443.

Landsmeer JMF (1962) Power grip and precision handling, *Ann Rheum Dis*, **21**:164–70.

Landsmeer JMF (1963) The coordination of finger joint motions, *J Bone Joint Surg*, **45A**:1654–62.

Landsmeer JMF (1968) Les cohérences spatiales et l'équilibre spatial dans la région carpienne, *Acta Anat* (suppl 54), **70**:1–84.

Landsmeer JMF (1976) *Atlas of Anatomy of the Hand* (Churchill Livingstone: Edinburgh).

Landsmeer JMF, Long C (1965) The mechanism of finger control based on electro-myograms and location analysis, *Acta Anat*, **60**:330–47.

von Lanz T, Wachsmuth W (1959) *Praktische Anatomie Arm*, 2nd edn (Springer: Berlin).

Leddy JP, Packer JW (1977) Avulsion of the profundus tendon insertion in athletes, *J Hand Surg* **2**: 66–9.

Lee MLH (1963) The intraosseous arterial pattern of the carpal lunate bone and its relation to avascular necrosis, *Acta Orthop Scand*, **33**:43.

Legré R, Courtes S, Huguet F, Bureau H (1993) Valeur diagnostique de l'arthrographie du poignet dans le bilan des traumatismes ligamentaires du carpe, *Ann Chir Main*, **12**:326–34.

Legueu M, Juvara E (1892) Des aponévroses de la paume de la main, *Bull Soc Anat Paris*.393.

Leroi-Gourhan A (1964) *Le Geste et la parole* (Albin Michel: Paris).

Levame GM, Otero C, Berdugo G (1967) Vascularisation artérielle des téguments de la main et des doigts, *Ann Chir Plast Esthet*, **12**:316–24.

Levin S, Pearsall G, Ruderman R (1978) Von Frey's method of measuring pressure sensibility in the hand: an engineering analysis of the Weinstein–Semmes pressure aesthesiometer, *J Hand Surg*, **3**:211–16.

Levinsohn EM, Palmer AK, Coren AB et al (1987) Wrist arthrography: the value of the three compartment injection technique, *Skeletal Radiol*, **16**:539–44.

Lichtman DM (1988) *The Wrist and its Disorders* (WB Saunders: Philadelphia).

Linburg RM, Comstock RE (1979) Anomalous tendon slips from the flexor pollicis longus to the flexor digitorum profundus. *J Hand Surg* **4**: 79–83.

Linscheid RL (1992) Biomechanics of the distal radioulnar joint, *Clin Orthop Rel Res*, **275**: 46–55.

Linscheid RL, Dobyns JH (1971) Rheumatoid arthritis of the wrist, *Orthop Clin North Am*, **2**:649.

Linscheid RL, Dobyns JH, Beabout JW et al (1972) Traumatic instability of the wrist. Diagnosis, classification and pathomechanics, *J Bone Joint Surg*, **54A**:1612–32.

Lister G (1984) Reconstruction. In: *The Hand: Diagnosis and Indications* (Churchill-Livingstone: New York) 107–191.

Littler JW (1956) Neurovascular pedicle transfer of tissue in reconstructive surgery of the hand, *J Bone Joint Surg*, **38A**: 917.

Littler JW (1959) Neurovascular skin island transfer in reconstruction hand surgery. Transactions of the International Society of Plastic Surgeons (E&S Livingstone: Edinburgh).

Littler JW (1960) The physiology and dynamic function of the hand, *Surg Clin North Am*, **40**:259.

Littler JW (1973) On the adaptability of man's hand, *Hand*, **5**:187.

Littler JW (1974) Hand, wrist and forearm incisions. In: Littler JW, Cramer LM, Smith JW, eds, *Symposium on Reconstructive Hand Surgery* (CV Mosby: St Louis).

Littler JW (1977) The hand and upper extremity. In: Converse JM, ed, *Reconstructive Plastic Surgery*, 2nd edn (WB Saunders: Philadelphia).

Littler JW, Cooley SGE (1963) Opposition of the thumb and its restoration by ADQ transfer, *J Bone Joint Surg* **45A**:1389.

Long C (1975) The moving finger writes . . . An electromyographic study. In: Stack G, Bolton H, eds, *The Second Hand Club* (British Society for Surgery of the Hand: London).

Long C, Brown ME (1964) Electromyographic kinesiology of the hand: muscles moving the long finger, *J Bone Joint Surg*, **46A**:1683–1706.

Lundborg G (1970) Ischemic nerve injury. Experimental studies on intraneural microvascular pathophysiology and nerve function in a limb subjected to temporary circulatory arrest, *Scand J Plast Reconstr Surg* (suppl 6):1–113.

Lundborg G, Myrhage R, Rydevik B (1977) The vascularization of human flexor tendons within the digital synovial region—structural and functional aspects, *J Hand Surg*, **2**:417.

Lundborg G, Lie-Stenstrom AK, Sollerman C et al (1986) Digital vibrogram: a new diagnostic tool for sensory testing in compression neuropathy, *J Hand Surg*, **11A**:693–6.

MacConaill MA (1941) The mechanical anatomy of the carpus and its bearings on some surgical problems, *J Anat*, **75**:166.

MacConaill MA (1946) Studies in the mechanics of synovial joints: displacements of articular surfaces and the significance of saddle joints, *Irish J Med Sci*, **247**:223.

Manaster BJ (1986) Digital wrist arthrography: precision in determinating the site of radio-carpalmidcarpal communication, *Am J Roentgenol*, **147**:563–6.

Mannerfelt L (1966) Studies on the hand in ulnar nerve paralysis. A clinical experimental investigation in normal and anomalous innervation, *Acta Orthop Scand* (suppl 87).

Mannerfelt L, Raven M (1978) Die Äthiologie und Bedeutung der Radius Krypte im Rheumatischen Handgelenk, *Verh Dtsch Ges Rheumatol*, **5**:94–6.

Manske PR, Lecker PA (1982) Nutrient pathways of flexor tendons in primates, *J Hand Surg*, **7**:436.

Marie P, Meige H, Patrikios R (1917) Paralysie radiale dissociée simulant une griffe cubitale, *Rev Neurol*, **24**:123–4.

Marin E, Vernick S, Friedmann LW (1983) Carpal tunnel syndrome: median nerve stress test, *Arch Phys Med Rehabil*, **64**:206–11.

Martin R (1987) *Tal om Nervus allmana Egenskaper i Mannsikans Kropp* (Lars Salvius: Stockholm).

Martineaud JP, Seroussi S (1977) *Physiologie de la circulation cutanée* (Masson: Paris).

Martinek H (1977a) Zur arthrographie des Handgelenks und ihrer Unfallchirugischen Bedeutung, *Fortschr Röntgenstr,* **127**:458–62.

Martinek H (1977b) Zur Traumatologie des Discus Articularis des Handgelenks, 2 teile, *Arch Orthop Unfallchir,* **87**:285.

Masquelet AC (1989) L'examen clinique du poignet, *Ann Chir Main,* **8**:159–67.

Masquelet AC, Gilbert A (1995) *An Atlas of Flaps in Limb Reconstruction* (Martin Dunitz and JB Lippincott: London and Philadelphia).

Masquelet AC, Strube F, Nordin JY (1993) The isolated scapho-trapezio-trapezoïd ligament injury: diagnosis and surgical treatment in four cases, *J Hand Surg,* **18B**:730–5.

McFarlane RM (1962) Observations on the functional anatomy of the intrinsic muscles of the thumb, *J Bone Joint Surg,* **44A**:1073–88.

McFarlane RM (1974) Patterns of diseased fascia in the fingers in Dupuytren's contracture, *Plastic Reconstr Surg,* **54**:31.

McMurtry RY, Youm Y, Flatt A, Gillespie TE (1978) Kinematics of the wrist. Clinical application, *J Bone Joint Surg,* **60A**:955–61.

Medical Research Council (1941) Aids to the investigation of peripheral nerve injuries. War Memorandum number 7 (HMSO: London).

Melki JP, Riche MC, Francheschi C et al (1988) Investigation of the circulation. In: Tubiana R, ed, *The Hand* volume 3 (WB Saunders: Philadephia).

Merle M, Dautel G (1992) *La Main traumatique 1. L'urgence* (Masson: Paris).

Merle M, Dautel G (1995) *La Main traumatique 2. Chirurgie secondaire. Le poignet traumatique* (Masson: Paris).

Merle d'Aubigné R, Benassy J, Ramadier JO (1956) Chirurgie Orthopedique des Paralysies (Masson: Paris).

Merle M, Amend P, Michon J (1988) Microsurgical repair in 150 patients with lesions of the median and ulnar nerves. In: Tubiana R, ed, *The Hand* volume 3 (WB Saunders: Philadelphia).

Mestdagh H, Bailleul JP, Chambon JP et al (1979) The dorsal arterial network of the wrist with reference to the blood supply of the carpal bones, *Acta Morphol Neurol Scand,* **17**:73.

Meyrueis JP, Cameli M, Jan P (1978) Instabilité du carpe. Diagnostic et formes cliniques, *Ann Chir Main,* **32**:555–60.

Mikic ZD (1984) Arthrography of the wrist joint. An experimental study, *J Bone Joint Surg,* **66A**:371–8.

Mikic ZD (1989) Detailed anatomy of the articular disc of the distal radioulnar joint. *Clin Orthop,* **245**: 23–36.

Milford LW (1968) *Retaining Ligaments of the Digits of the Hand* (WB Saunders: Philadelphia).

Mitchell SW, Morehouse GR, Keen WW (1864) *Gunshot Wounds and Other Injuries of Nerves* (JP Lippincott Company: Philadelphia)

Moberg E (1955) Discussion of Brooks D. The place of nerve grafting in orthopedics surgery, *J Bone Joint Surg,* **37A**: 305.

Moberg E (1958) Objective methods for determining the functional value of sensibility in the hand, *J Bone Joint Surg,* **40A**:454–76.

Moberg E (1960) Evaluation of sensibility of the hand, *Surg Clin North Am,* **40**:375.

Moberg E (1962) Criticism and study of methods for examining sensibility in the hand, *Neurology,* **12**:8.

Moberg E (1972) Fingers were made before forks, *Hand,* **4**:201.

Moberg E (1975) Surgical treatment for absent single-hand grip and elbow extension in quadriplegia, *J Bone Joint Surg,* **57A**:196.

Moberg E (1976) Reconstructive hand surgery in tetraplegia, stroke and cerebral palsy. Some basic concepts in physiology and neurology, *J Hand Surg,* **1**:29.

Moberg E (1978a) *The Upper Limb in Tetraplegia* (Georg Thieme: Stuttgart).

Moberg E (1978b) Sensibility in reconstructive limb surgery. In: Fredericks S, Brody GS, eds, *Neurophysiology and Sensation. Symposium on the Neurologic Aspects of Plastic Surgery* (CV Mosby: St Louis) Volume 17:30–5.

Moberg E (1983) The role of cutaneous afferents in position sense, kinaesthesia and motor function of the hand, *Brain*, **106**:1–19.

Moldaver J (1978) Tinel's sign. Its characteristics and significance, *J Bone Joint Surg*, **60A**:412–13.

Montagna W, Fellis R (1961) *Advances in the Biology of Skin* (Pergamon Press: New York).

Morel Fatio D (1985) Surgery of the skin. In: Tubiana R, ed, *The Hand*, volume 2 (WB Saunders: Philadelphia), 224–5.

Mountcastel V (1968) *Medical Physiology*, 12th edn volume 2 (CV Mosby: St Louis): 1345–71.

Murray JF, Wayne C, MacKenzie JK (1977) Transmetacarpal amputation of the index finger: a clinical assessment of hand strength and complications, *J Hand Surg*, **2**:471–81.

Napier JR (1955) Prehensile movements of the human hand, *J Anat*, **89**:564.

Napier JR (1966) Functional aspects of the anatomy of the hand. In: Pulvertaft RG, ed, *The Hand* (Butterworth: London).

Navarro A (1937) Anatomia y fisiologie del carpo, *Ann Inst Clin Quir Chir Exp*, **1**: 162–250.

Nicholson OR, Seddon NJ (1957) Nerve repair in civil practice: results of treatment of median and ulnar nerve lesions, *Br Med J*, **ii**:1065.

Nielsen PT, Hedeboe J (1984) Posttraumatic scapholunate dissociation detected by wrist cineradiography, *J Hand Surg*, **9**:135–8.

Nomina Anatomica (1960) (Excerpta Medica: New York).

O'Riain S (1973) New and simple test of nerve function in the hand, *Br Med J*, **22**:615.

Oberlin C, Sarey JJ, Alnot JY (1988) Apporr arterial cutané de la main. Application à la realisation es lambreaux en îlot, *Ann Chir Main*, **7**:122–5.

Ochiai N et al (1979) Vascular anatomy of flexor tendons. I. Vincular system and blood supply of the profundus tendon in the digital sheath, *J Hand Surg*, **2**:417.

Ochoa J (1974) Schwann cell and myelin changes caused by some toxic agents and trauma, *Proc Roy Soc Med*, **67**:3–4.

Omer GE (1973) Sensibility of the hand as opposed to sensation in the hand, *Ann Chir*, **27**:479–485.

Omer G (1981) Physical diagnosis of peripheral nerve injuries, *Orthop Clin North Am*, **12**:207–28.

Omer GE, Spinner M (1975) *Peripheral Nerve Testing and Suture Techniques. A.A.O.S. Instructional Course* (CV Mosby: St Louis) Volume 24, 122–43.

Omer GE, Spinner M (1980) *Management of Peripheral Nerve Problems* (WB Saunders Company: Philadelphia).

Önne L (1962) Recovery of sensibility and sudomotor activity in the hand after nerve suture, *Acta Chir Scand* (suppl), **300**.

Osborne G (1970) Compression neuritis of the ulnar nerve at the elbow, *Hand*, **2**:10–13.

Pahle JA, Raunio P (1969) The influence of wrist position on finger deviation in the rheumatoid hand, *J Bone Joint Surg*, **51B**:664.

Pallardy G, Chevrot A, Galmichie JM, Galmichie B (1981) Radiographical examination of the hand and wrist. In: Tubiana R, ed, *The Hand*, volume 1 (WB Saunders: Philadelphia), 648–82.

Palmer AK (1987) The distal radioulnar joint, *Hand Clin*, **3**: 31.

Palmer AK, Glisson RR, Werner FW (1982) Ulnar variance determination, *J Hand Surg*, **7**:376–9.

Palmer AK, Levinsohn EM, Kuzma GR (1983) Arthrography of the wrist, *J Hand Surg*, **8**:15–23.

Panagis JS, Gelberman RH, Taleisnik J et al (1983) The arterial anatomy of the human carpus. Part II: The intraosseous vascularity, *J Hand Surg*, **8**:375.

Papilion JD, DuPuy TE, Aulicino PL et al (1988) Radiographic evaluation of the hook of the hamate: a new technique, *J Hand Surg*, **13A**:437–9.

Parks BJ, Abelhez J (1978) Medical and surgical importance of the arterial blood supply of the thumb, *J Hand Surg*, 3:383–5.

Peet RM, Hendrickson JD, Anderson TP et al (1956) Thoracic outlet syndrome: evaluation of therapeutic exercise program, *Mayo Clin Proc*, 31:281–7.

Penfield WG, Boldney EV (1937) Somatic motor and sensory representation in the cerebral cortex of man as studied by electrical stimulation, *Brain*, 60:389–443.

Penfield WG, Rasmussen T (1950) *The Cerebral Cortex of Man* (Macmillan: New York).

Perry JF, Hamilton GF, Lachenbruch PA et al (1974) Protective sensation in the hand and its correlation to the Ninhydrin sweat test following nerve laceration, *Am J Phys Med*, 53:133.

Phalen GS (1951) Spontaneous compression of the median nerve at the wrist, *JAMA*, 145:1128.

Phelps P, Walker E (1977) Comparison of the finger wrinkling test results to established sensory tests in peripheral nerve injury, *Am J Occup Ther*, 31:9.

Pieron AP (1973) The mechanism of the first carpometacarpal joint, *Acta Orthop Scand*, (suppl) 48.

Pieron AP (1981) The first carpometacarpal joint. In: Tubiana R, ed, *The Hand*, volume 1 (WB Saunders: Philadelphia).

Pigeau I, Frija G, Semaan I et al (1992) Advantages of MRI in the study of the wrist ligaments. In: Brunelli G, Saffar P, eds, *Wrist Imaging* (Springer: Paris).

Piveteau J (1955) *"La Genèse humaine" en biologie* (Encyclopédie de la Pléiade: Paris).

Poirier P, Charpy A (1926) *Traité d'anatomie humaine* (Masson: Paris).

von Prince K, Butler B (1967) Measuring sensory function of the hand in peripheral nerve injuries, *Am J Occup Ther*, 21:385–96.

Protas JM, Jackson WT (1980) Evaluating carpal instabilities with fluoroscopy, *Am J Roentgenol*, 135:137–40.

Quinn SF, Pittman CC, Belsole R et al (1988) Digital subtraction wrist arthrography: evaluation of the multiple compartement technique.

Rabischong P (1963) Innervation proprioceptive des muscles lombricaux de la main chez l'homme, *Rev Chir Orthop*, 25:927.

Rabischong P (1971) Les problèmes fondamentaux du rétablissement de la préhension, *Ann Chir*, 25:927.

Rabischong P (1981) Physiology of sensation. In: Tubiana R, ed, *The Hand*, volume 1 (WB Saunders: Philadelphia).

Reagan DS, Linscheid RL, Dobyns JH (1984) Lunotrichetral sprains, *J Hand Surg*, 9A:502–14.

Resnick D, André M, Kerr R et al (1984) Digital arthrography of the wrist: a radiographic pathologic investigation, *Am J Roentgenol*, 142:1187–90.

Riche P (1897) Le nerf cubital et les muscles de l'eminence thénar, *Bull Mem Soc Anat Paris*: 251–2.

Rieunau G, Gay R, Martinez C et al (1971) Lésion de l'articulation radio-cubitale inférieure dans les traumatismes de l'avant-bras et du poignet. Intérêt de l'arthrographie, *Rev Chir Orthop* (suppl 1):253.

Ross DB (1987) Thoracic outlet syndromes; update, *Am J Surg*, 154:568.

Ross DB (1992) Thoracic outlet syndromes in musicians, *J Hand Ther*, 5:65–72.

Rowntree T (1959) Anomalous innervation of the hand muscles, *J Bone Joint Surg*, 31B:505–10.

Rydevik B, Lundborg G, Bagge V (1981) Effects of graded compression on intraneural blood flow: an *in vivo* study on rabbit tibial nerves, *J Hand Surg*, 6A:3–11.

Saffar PH (1989) *Les Traumatismes du carpe* (Springer-Verlag: Paris).

Saffar PH, Cooney WP (1995) *Fractures of the Distal Radius* (Martin Dunitz and Lippincott: London and Philadelphia).

Salisbury RC (1936) The interosseous muscles of the hand, *J Anat*, 71:395.

Salmon M (1936) *Artères de la peau* (Masson: Paris).

Santos-Gutierez L (1964) Précisions morpho-fonctionnelles à propos du condyle carpien, *C R Assn Anat*, 2:1565.

Sarrafian SK, Melamed JL, Goshgarian GM (1977) Study of wrist motion in flexion and extension, *Clin Orthop*, **126**:153–9.

Schernberg F, Gerard Y (1983) L'exploration radiologie dynamique du poignet, *Rev Chir Orthop*, **69**:521–31.

Schmitt R, Lanz U (1992) Computerized tomography of the wrist. In: Brunelli G, Saffar P, eds, *Wrist Imaging* (Springer: Paris).

Schnek F (1933) Zur Röntgenologischen Diagnose von Kahnbeinbrüchen der Hand, *Zbl Chir*, **60**:1954–6.

Schwartz AM, Ruby LK (1982) Wrist arthrography revised, *Orthopedics*, **5**:883–8.

Seddon HJ (1943) Three types of nerve injury, *Brain*, **66**:237.

Seddon HJ (1954) *Peripheral Nerve Injuries*. Medical Research Council Special Report Service, Number 282 (HMSO: London).

Seddon HJ (1975) *Surgical Disorders of the Peripheral Nerves*, 2nd edn (Churchill Livingstone: Edinburgh).

Semmes J, Weinstein S, Ghent L et al (1960) *Somatosensory Changes after Penetrating Brain Wounds in Man* (Harvard University Press: Cambridge, Massachusetts).

Seror P (1988) Phalen's test in the diagnosis of carpal tunnel syndrome, *J Hand Surg*, **13B**:383.

Seror P (1990) Le test centimetrique: test diagnostique du syndrome du canal carpien débutant, *Neurophysiol Clin*, **20**:137–44.

Seror P (1991) Electromyography of the upper limb: technique, application and limits. In: Tubiana R, ed, *The Hand* volume 4 (WB Saunders: Philadelphia).

Shapiro JS (1970) A new factor in the etiology of ulnar drift, *Clin Orthop*, **68**:32.

Sherrington CS (1896) On the anatomical constitution of skeletal muscles, with remarks on recurrent fibres in the ventral spine nerve root, *J Physiol Lond*, **17**:211–58.

Simpson JA (1956) Electrical signs in the diagnosis of carpal tunnel and related syndromes, *J Neurol Neurosurg Psychiatry*, **19**:275–80.

Smith EM, Juvinall R, Bender L et al (1964) Role of the finger flexors in rheumatoid deformities of the metacarpophalangeal joints, *Arthritis Rheum*, **7**:467.

Smith RJ, Kaplan EB (1967) Rheumatoid deformities at the metacarpophalangeal joints of the fingers. A correlative study of anatomy and pathology, *J Bone Joint Surg*, **49A**:31.

Soleilhac R (1970) L'arthrographie opaque du poignet, Thesis. Toulouse.

Spinner M (1978) *Injuries to the Major Branches of the Peripheral Nerves of the Forearm*, 2nd edn (WB Saunders: Philadelphia).

Stack GH (1962) Muscle function in the fingers, *J Bone Joint Surg*, **44B**:899–909.

Stack GH (1973) *The Palmar Fascia* (Churchill Livingstone: Edinburgh).

Stack GH, Vaughan-Jackson OJ (1971) The zig-zag deformity in the rheumatoid hand, *Hand*, **3**:62–7.

Stanley J, Saffar P (1994) *Wrist Arthroscopy* (Martin Dunitz and WB Saunders: London and Philadelphia).

Stark HH, Zemev NP, Boyes JH et al (1977) Flexor tendon graft through intact superficialis tendon, *J Hand Surg*, **2**:456.

Stecher WR (1937) Roentgenography of the carpal navicular, *Am J Roentgenol*, **37**:704–5.

Steindler A (1940) *Orthopedic Operations* (Charles C Thomas: Springfield, Illinois).

Steyers CM, Blai WF (1989) Measuring ulnar variance: a comparison of techniques, *J Hand Surg*, **14A**:607–12.

Struthers J (1854) On some points in the abnormal anatomy of the arm, *Br For Med Chir Rev*, **14**:170.

Sunderland S (1946) The innervation of the first dorsal interosseous muscle of the hand, *Anat Rec*, **95**:7.

Sunderland S (1950) Capacity of reinnervated muscles to function efficiently after prolonged denervation, *Arch Neurol Psychiat*, **64**:755.

Sunderland S (1968) *Nerves and Nerve Injuries* (Williams and Wilkins: Baltimore).

Sunderland S (1978) *Nerves and Nerve Injuries*, 2nd edn (Williams and Wilkins: Baltimore).

Sunderland S, Bradley KC (1952) Rate of advance of Hohmann-Tinel sign in regenerating nerves, *Arch Neurol Psychiat*, **67**:650.

Swanson AB (1960) Surgery of the hand in cerebral palsy and the swan-neck deformity, *J Bone Joint Surg*, **42A**:951–64.

Taleisnik J (1976) The ligaments of the wrist, *J Hand Surg*, **1**:110.

Taleisnik J (1985) *The Wrist* (Churchill Livingstone: New York).

Taleisnik J, Kelly PJ (1966) The extraosseous and intraosseous blood supply of the scaphoid bone, *J Bone Joint Surg*, **48A**:1125.

Testut L, Kuenz (1928) In: Testut L, Tatarjet A, eds, *Traité d'anatomie humaine*, volume 1 (Douin: Paris).

Thieffry S (1973) *La Main de l'homme* (Hachette Littérature: Paris).

Thomas JE, Lambert EH (1960) Ulnar nerve conduction velocity and H-reflex in infants and children, *J Appl Physiol*, **15**:1.

Thomine JM (1965) Conjonctif d'enveloppe des doigts et squelette fibreux des commissures interdigitales, *Ann Chir Plast*, **10**:194.

Tinel J (1915) Le signe du "fourmillement" dans les lésions des nerfs périphériques, *Presse Med*, **47**:388–9.

Tirman RM, Weben ER, Snyder LL et al (1985) Midcarpal wrist arthrography for detection of tears of the scapholunate and lunotriquetral ligaments, *Am J Roentgenol*, **144**:107–8.

Tubiana R (1960) Greffe des tendons flechisseurs des doigts et du pouce, *Rev Chir Orthop*, **46**:191–214.

Tubiana R (1981) Architecture and functions of the hand. In: Tubiana R, ed, *The Hand*, volume I (WB Saunders: Philadelphia).

Tubiana R (1981) *The Hand* volume 1 Anatomy, Physiology and Research (WB Saunders: Philadelphia).

Tubiana R (1985) *The Hand* volume 2 Hand injuries, surgery of the skin, bone and joint (WB Saunders: Philadelphia).

Tubiana R (1988) *The Hand* volume 3 Surgery of tendons, nerves, mutilations (WB Saunders: Philadelphia).

Tubiana R (1993) *The Hand* volume 4 Neurologic disorders (WB Saunders: Philadelphia).

Tubiana R (1998a) *The Hand* volume 5 Vascular, rheumatoid, Dupuytren's diseases, congenital malformations, tumours, infections (WB Saunders: Philadelphia).

Tubiana R (1998b) Indications for surgical treatment of the rheumatoid hand. In: Tubiana R, ed, *The Hand* volume 5 (WB Saunders: Philadelphia).

Tubiana R, Brockman R (1991) Tendon transfers: Theoretical and practical considerations. In: Tubiana R, ed, *The Hand* volume 4 (WB Saunders: Philadelphia), 79–92.

Tubiana R, Duparc J (1959) Operation palliative pour paralysie sensitive de la main, *Mem Acad Chir*, **85**:666.

Tubiana R, Hakstian R (1969) Les déviations cubitales normales et pathologiques des doigts. In: Tubiana R, ed, *La Main rhumatoïde* (Expansion Scientifique Française: Paris) 33–4.

Tubiana R, Malek R (1968) Paralysis of the intrinsic muscles of the fingers, *Surg Clin North Am*, **48**:1140.

Tubiana R, Roux JP (1974) Phalangization of the first and fifth metacarpals, *J Bone Joint Surg*, **56A**:447.

Tubiana R, Thomine JM (1990) *La Main: anatomie fonctionnelle et examen clinique* (Masson: Paris).

Tubiana R, Valentin P (1963) L'Extension des doigts, *Rev Chir Orthop*, **49**:543.

Tubiana R, Valentin P (1964) Anatomy of the extensor apparatus and The physiology of the extension of the fingers, *Surg Clin North Am*, **44**:897–906 and 907–18.

Tubiana R, Michon J, Thomine JM (1974) Assessment of deformity in Dupuytren's disease. In: Hueston JT, Tubiana R, eds, *Dupuytren's Disease*, 3rd edn (Churchill Livingstone: Edinburgh).

Tubiana R, McCullough CJ, Masquelet AC (1990) *An Atlas of Surgical Exposures of the Upper Extremity* (Martin Dunitz and JB Lippincott: London and Philadelphia).

Tubiana R, McMeniman P, Gordon S (1979) Evaluation des resultats après reparation des tendons longs plichisseurs des doigts, *Annales Chir*, 33:659–62.

Tubiana R, Miller HW, Reed S (1989) Restoration of wrist extension after paralysis, *Hand Clin*, 5:53.

Tubiana R, Simmons BP, De Frenne H (1982) Location of Dupuytren's Disease on the radial aspect of the hand, *Clin Orthop*, 168:222–9.

Tubiana R, Thomine JM, Mackin EJ (1984) *Examination of the Hand and Upper Limb* (WB Saunders: Philadelphia).

Valentin P (1962) *Contribution à l'Étude anatomique physiologique et clinique de l'appareil extenseur des doigts*. Thesis, Paris.

Valentin P (1985) The interossei and lumbricals. In: Tubiana R, ed, *The Hand*, volume 2 (WB Saunders: Philadelphia) 244–54.

Valery P (1938) Discours d'ouverture au Congrès de Chirurgie (Nouvelle Revue Française: Paris).

Vallbo AB, Johansson RS (1978) The tactile sensory innervation of the glabrous skin of the human hand. In: Gordon G, ed, *Active Touch* (Pergamon Press: Oxford) 29–49.

Vallois H (1926) In: Poirier P, Charpy A, eds, *Traité d'anatomie humaine* (Masson: Paris) 119–55.

Vasilas A, Grieco V, Bartone NF (1960) Roentgen aspects of injuries to the pisiform bone and pisotriquetral joint, *J Bone Joint Surg*, 42A:1317–28.

Vayssairat M, Housset E (1980) Place de la capillaroscopie dans les acrosyndromes, *Rev Practicien*, 30:1923–53.

Verdan C (1954) Le rôle du ligament antérieur radio-carpien dans les fractures du scaphoïde. Déductions thérapeutiques, *Z Unfallmed Berufskr*, 4:299.

Verdan C (1960) Syndrome of the quadriga, *Surg Clin North Am*, 40:425.

Verdan C (1976) *Chirurgie des Tendons de la Main* (Expansion Scientifique Français: Paris).

Vesalius A (1543) *De humani corporis fabrica* (Liber 7: Basel).

Vichard P, Tropet Y, Laudecy G et al (1982) Paralysies radiales contemporaines des fractures de la diaphyse humérale, *Chirurgie*, 108:791–5.

Wagman IH, Lesse H (1952) Maximum conduction velocities of motor fibers of ulnar nerve in human subjects of various ages and sizes, *J Neurophysiol*, 15:235.

Watson HK, Ashmead IVD, Makhlouf MV (1988) Examination of the scaphoid, *J Hand Surg*, 13A:657–60.

Weber EH (1835) Über den Tastinn. *Arch Anat Physiol Wissensch Med*, 152–60.

Weber ER (1985) Concepts governing the rotational shift of the intercalated segment of the carpus. In: Tubiana R, ed, *The Hand* (WB Saunders: Philadelphia) volume 2, 945–58.

Weeks PM, Vannier MW, Stevens G et al (1985) Three dimensional imaging of the wrist, *J Hand Surg*, 10A:32–9.

Weeks PM, Wray RC (1978) *Management of Acute Hand Surgery. A Biologic Approach*, 2nd edn (CV Mosby: St Louis) 314.

Weinstein S (1993) Fifty years of somatosensory research: from the Semmes–Weinstein monofilaments to the Weinstein Enhanced Sensory Test, *J Hand Therapy*, 6:11–22.

Werner JL, Omer GE (1970) Evaluating cutaneous pressure sensitivity of the hand, *Am J Occup Ther*, 24:5.

White SJ, Louis DS, Braunstein EM et al (1984) Capitate–lunate instability: recognition by manipulation under fluoroscopy, *Am J Roentgenol*, 143:361–4.

Wilgus EFS (1982) Techniques for diagnosis of peripheral nerve loss, *Clin Orthop*, 163:8–14.

Winslow JB (1752) *Exposition anatomique de la structure du corps humain*, 2nd edn (Amsterdam).

Woodhall B, Beebe GW (1956) *Peripheral Nerve Regeneration* (United States Government Printing Office: Washington DC).

Wood-Jones F (1942) *The Principles of Anatomy as Seen in the Hand*, 2nd edn (Williams and Wilkins: Baltimore) 305.

Wuttge R, Küfferg HD, Bauer J et al (1988) Die Handgelenksarthrographie zur Bestimmung des Prothesenlagers, *Digit Bilddiagn*, 8:39–44.

Wynn Parry CB (1966) Diagnosis and after care of peripheral nerve lesions in the upper limb, *J Bone Joint Surg*, 48A:607.

Wynn Parry CB (1981a) Recent trends in surgery of peripheral nerves, *Int Rehab Med*, 3:169–73.

Wynn Parry CB (1981b) *Rehabilitation of the Hand*, 4th edn (Butterworth: London).

Youm Y, McMurtry RY, Flatt AE et al (1978) Kinematics of the wrist. I. An experimental study of radial-ulnar deviation and flexion-extension, *J Bone Joint Surg*, 60A:423–31.

Zachary RB (1946) Tendon transplantation for radial paralysis, *Br J Surg*, 33:358.

Zachary RB, Roaf R (1954) Lesions in continuity. In: Seddon HJ, ed, *Peripheral Nerve Injuries*, Medical Research Council Special Report Series Number 282 (HMSO: London) 57.

Zancolli E (1977) *Traitement palliatif des paralysies du membre supérieur* (Réunion d'automne du GEM: Paris).

Zancolli E (1979) *Structural and Dynamic Basis of Hand Surgery*, 3rd edn (JB Lippincott: Philadelphia).

Zancolli EA, Cozzi EP (1992) *Atlas of Surgical Anatomy of the Hand* (Churchill Livingstone: New York).

Zilch H, Buck-Gramcko D (1975) Ergebnisse der Nervenwiederherstellungen an der oberen Extremität durch Mikrochirurgie, *Handchirurgie*, 7:21–31.

Zlatkin MB, Chao PC, Osterman AL et al (1989) Chronic wrist pain: evaluation with high resolution MR imaging, *Radiology*, 173:731–3.

Zook EG (1981) Anatomy, physiology and care of injuries, *Clin Plas Surg*, 8:21–31.

Zweifler AJ, Cushing G, Conway J (1967) The relationship between pulse volume and blood flow in the finger, *J Vasc Dis*, 18: 591–8.

van Zwieten KJ (1980) The extensor assembly of the finger in man and non-human primates. Thesis, Leiden.

INDEX

Note: References in *italics* refer to illustrations or tables.

Abduction, terminology, 195, *196*
Abductor digiti minimi, *123*, 123, 125, *309*, 309
Abductor digiti quinti, *48*, *51*, 305
Abductor indicis (first dorsal interosseous), *48*, *51*, *206*
Abductor pollicis brevis, 119–20, *120*, 121, *122*
   clinical examination, *205*
   innervation, 123
   muscle work, *117*
   relative strength, *48*, *51*
   thumb movement analysis, 310, *314*, 315
Abductor pollicis longus, 118–19
   in carpal canal, *11*
   clinical examination, *205*, 205
   maximal excursion, *53*
   muscular work, *117*
   posterior retinaculum, *37*
   relative strength, *48*, *51*
   strength value, *45*
   thumb movement analysis, 310, *313*, 313, 317
   wrist movement analysis, 301
Activities of daily living, 325
   see also Sensibility, tests
Adductor pollicis, 119, *120*, 121, *122*
   clinical examination, *205*
   Froment's sign, 327
   grip strength, *115*
   innervation, 123
   muscular work, *117*
   relative strength, *48*, *51*
   thumb movement analysis, 310, 315, *316*
Adson test, 262
Age factors, neural regeneration, 366
Allen test, 181–2, *183*
Anastomoses arcades, digital arteries, 139, *140*

Anatomy,
   fibrous skeleton of hand, 16–27
   fibrous skeleton of wrist, 29–38
   hand function, 156–74
   hand and wrist movements, 40–127
   osseous skeleton of hand, 4–16
   osseous skeleton of wrist, 28–9
   skin cover, 128–55
   vascular system, 38–9, 243–57
Anconeus, 296, *297*
Angiography, 258–9, *259*
Anteposition, terminology, 195, *196*, 197, *198*, 310
Anterior interosseous nerve syndrome, *274*, 274
Anteroposterior movements, 59
Aponeuroses, 16–23, 25, 176–81
Arches,
   arterial, 247–9
   of hand, 9–16, *25*
Arms *see* Upper limbs
Arterial system *see* Vascular system
Arthrography, 237–8
Arthroscans, *241*, 241
Articular system, 41–2
Atrophied skin, signs of, 176
Attrition ruptures, flexor tendons, 218
Automatic longitudinal rotation, thumb, 197, *198*
Automatism, 173
Axial pattern flaps, *138*, 138
Axillary artery, *244*, 244
Axillary nerve, 264–5, *265*, *266*
Axis, of a joint, definition, 47
Axonotmesis, 363, 364, *365*

Ballotment (shear) tests, *189*, 189
Basal layer, epidermis, 128
Benediction sign, 274
Biceps, 289, *290*, 296, *297*
Biceps brachii, *298*, 298

387